Surgery for the Painful, Dysfunctional Sacroiliac Joint

Bruce E. Dall • Sonia V. Eden
Michael D. Rahl

Editors

Surgery for the Painful, Dysfunctional Sacroiliac Joint

A Clinical Guide

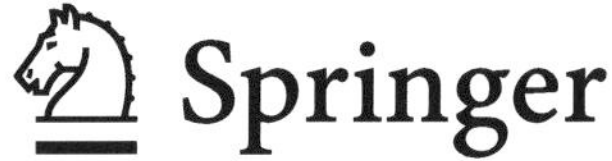

Editors
Bruce E. Dall, MD
Orthopedic Spine Surgeon
Borgess Brain and Spine Institute
Western Michigan University School
 of Medicine
Kalamazoo, MI, USA

Sonia V. Eden, MD
Neurosurgeon
Borgess Brain and Spine Institute
Western Michigan University School
 of Medicine
Kalamazoo, MI, USA

Michael D. Rahl, PT, DPT, OCS, CSCS
Full Potenial Physical Therapy
Holland, MI, USA

ISBN 978-3-319-10725-7   ISBN 978-3-319-10726-4 (eBook)
DOI 10.1007/978-3-319-10726-4
Springer Cham Heidelberg New York Dordrecht London

Library of Congress Control Number: 2014954252

Printed on acid-free paper

Springer is part of Springer Science+Business Media (www.springer.com)

Preface

This textbook is a first of its kind in the medical surgical literature. Despite the fact that surgeries on the painful, relatively stable, sacroiliac joint have been discussed in the literature for almost a century, there has never been a textbook written to bring all this information together for the surgeon or for the clinician dealing with surgical options for intractable sacroiliac joint pain. The authors creating this detailed discussion have very early on understood that the sacroiliac joint does cause pain, that this pain can be extremely disabling, and that in our modern medical society it is still grossly ignored or misunderstood. These practitioners have each spent a considerable portion of their careers working to further understand the painful, dysfunctional sacroiliac joint and creating ways, both conservative and surgical, to help patients with this diagnosis. This book shares with its audience the vast knowledge base that is being amassed concerning sacroiliac joint pain, the severe disability it can cause, associated pathological conditions, ways to navigate through making a definitive diagnosis and creating a valid treatment plan, multiple ways to operate on this joint and avoid the multiple pitfalls that may present themselves, and how to rehabilitate the postoperative patient with this condition. The authors are all very excited to share their years of experience treating patients with disabling pain from a dysfunctional sacroiliac joint and hope, as a result of reading this material, that surgeons and clinicians will develop the necessary learning to proactively be diagnosing and appropriately be treating this condition in their respective practices.

Kalamazoo, MI, USA   Bruce E. Dall, M.D.

Contents

Contributors

Brandon Bucklen, Ph.D Globus Medical Inc., Audubon, PA, USA

Bruce E. Dall, M.D. Neurosurgery of Kalamazoo, Borgess Brain and Spine Institute, Kalamazoo, MI, USA
Orthopedic Spine Division, Western Michigan University Medical School, Kalamazoo, MI, USA

E. Jeffrey Donner, M.D. The Spine Institute, Loveland, CO, USA

Sonia V. Eden, M.D. Department of Neurological Surgery, Borgess Brain and Spine Institute, Kalamazoo, MI, USA
Western Michigan University Medical School, Kalamazoo, MI, USA

Robert W. McNutt, B.S., M.S. Statistical Consulting Center, Western Michigan University, Kalamazoo, MI, USA

Mark Moldavsky, B.S., M.S. Globus Medical Inc., Audubon, PA, USA

Michael R. Moore, M.D. Department of Surgery, University of North Dakota Medical School, Bismarck, ND, USA
The Bone and Joint Center, Bismarck, ND, USA

David W. Polly, Jr., M.D. Department of Orthopaedic Surgery, University of Minnesota, Minneapolis, MN, USA

Michael D. Rahl, PT, DPT, OCS, CSCS Full Potential Physical Therapy, Holland, MI, USA

Arnold Graham Smith, M.D., P.A. Orthopaedic Surgery, Baptist Medical Center – South, Jacksonville, FL, USA

Introduction

1

Bruce E. Dall

Introduction

This chapter defines the diagnosis of "dysfunctional sacroiliac joint" and explains why a book on this subject matter is needed in the literature. It covers high points in the surgical history of treatment for a sacroiliac joint (SIJ) having this diagnosis and the evolution of that treatment during the past century. After discussing what this book intends to cover, the sources for the material covered in this book are explained. The objectives hoping to be accomplished for both the surgeon treating a dysfunctional SIJ and the therapist rehabilitating a patient after surgical intervention are discussed.

Definition of a Dysfunctional Sacroiliac Joint

The definition that will be used in this book for the dysfunctional SIJ is "a SIJ that is chronically painful, essentially stable, and has become disabling to the patient" [1, 2]. It will be understood that there are a myriad of causes for a SIJ to become dysfunctional, each of which will be discussed (Chap. 5); however, acute fracture, infection, and tumor will not be considered in this book as each of those represents entities that have their own well-discussed treatment methods in the literature and surgical treatments discussed here, in general, will not apply.

Current Literature

Currently, there are no surgical textbooks available that discuss surgery for the painful, stable, dysfunctional SIJ despite the fact that surgery has been performed for this diagnosis for almost a century. The first publication discussing surgery was by Smith-Pedersen in 1926 [3]. It was published when most all low back and radiating leg pain was considered to be emanating from the SIJ. In 1934, when Mixter and Barr published their landmark article on the injured herniated lumbar disk, the SIJ as a pain generator slipped into obscurity [4]. This continued until the 1980s when the SIJ once again made its debut in the

B.E. Dall, M.D. (✉)
Neurosurgery of Kalamazoo, Borgess Brain
and Spine Institute, 1541 Gull Road, Kalamazoo,
MI 49048, USA

Orthopedic Spine Division, Western Michigan
University Medical School, Kalamazoo, MI, USA
e-mail: dall.bruce@yahoo.com

B.E. Dall et al. (eds.), *Surgery for the Painful, Dysfunctional Sacroiliac Joint*,
DOI 10.1007/978-3-319-10726-4_1, © Springer International Publishing Switzerland 2015

surgical literature as a cause for chronic pain [5]. Since that time, there has been a steady increase of papers on surgery for the dysfunctional SIJ; however, the majority of these have consisted of series of cases followed retrospectively (Chap. 2).

The FDA and Surgery for the Sacroiliac Joint

In 2008, the Federal Drug Administration (FDA) granted a 510(k) to SI-BONE, Inc. for the iFuse™ minimally invasive SI Joint Fusion System to treat conditions including degenerative sacroiliitis and SIJ disruptions [6]. The 510(k) designation makes it possible for corporations to get a device into the market quickly for far less cost than the other option of "pre-market approval" which typically entails spending tens of millions of dollars and potentially delays getting a device into the market for several years. The SI-BONE surgical method is a lateral approach and is similar to the approach used for decades by trauma surgeons to stabilize an acutely fractured SIJ. Since 2008, there have been several other surgical device companies that have also obtained a 510(k) clearance for their laterally placed fixation/fusion devices. Surgeons now have effective minimally invasive surgical treatment options for elective SIJ fusion. For the first time, because of the availability of these minimally invasive solutions, many surgeons are now interested in and aware of the SIJ as a pain generator. And as a result of the above, many surgeons and other health-care providers now include the evaluation of the SIJ in their diagnostic evaluation of patients with lower back pain.

Current Education and Societal Commitments for This Condition

The SIJ is a subject matter that is thoroughly taught in universities of osteopathy, anesthesiology, physical therapy, physiatry, and chiropractory. The anatomy and physiology are taught as well as a multitude of clinical diagnostic methods and conservative treatment regimens to include a multitude of invasive types of varied injections. It has been and currently remains a very ignored entity in the disciplines of orthopedic surgery, orthopedic spine surgery, and neurosurgery, even though it is the lowest joint in the spine and a key joint in the pelvis. At the time of this writing, no surgical society has laid claim to the dysfunctional SIJ [6]. This will change as the old myths concerning the lack of pain generation from this joint continue to be dispelled, as more and more SIJ injections by pain management doctors are found to be giving temporary relief and as patients continue to be more and more self-educated via the Internet and seeking out surgeons with an interest in treating the painful dysfunctional SIJ.

Sources of Information for This Textbook

The sources for the information covered in this textbook are varied. It should be reiterated that there are no textbooks on the subject and the literature is lacking in prospective and randomized studies from which to ascertain solid information about both conservative treatment and fusion for the dysfunctional SIJ. Thus, we have to rely on individuals and institutions, of which there are several, that have long been involved in the diagnosis and treatment of this dysfunctional joint and have pursued continued research to further their ongoing learning experience. The Borgess Brain and Spine Institute (BBSI, Kalamazoo, MI; Fig. 1.1) has been involved in diagnosing and treating, both conservatively and surgically, the dysfunctional SIJ since 1991. Long before that, it was involved surgically with this joint in terms of trauma and infection.

Since 1991, BBSI has generated several publications in peer review journals [7–10], created an algorithm for the diagnosis and treatment of the dysfunctional SIJ [11], devised new methods of approach to the SIJ, invented new types of SIJ fixation, and worked with engineers in the cadaver lab to further understand the biomechanics of the ligament injured SIJ (Chap. 4). As a result, the BBSI has become an international referral center for patients with the diagnosis of a

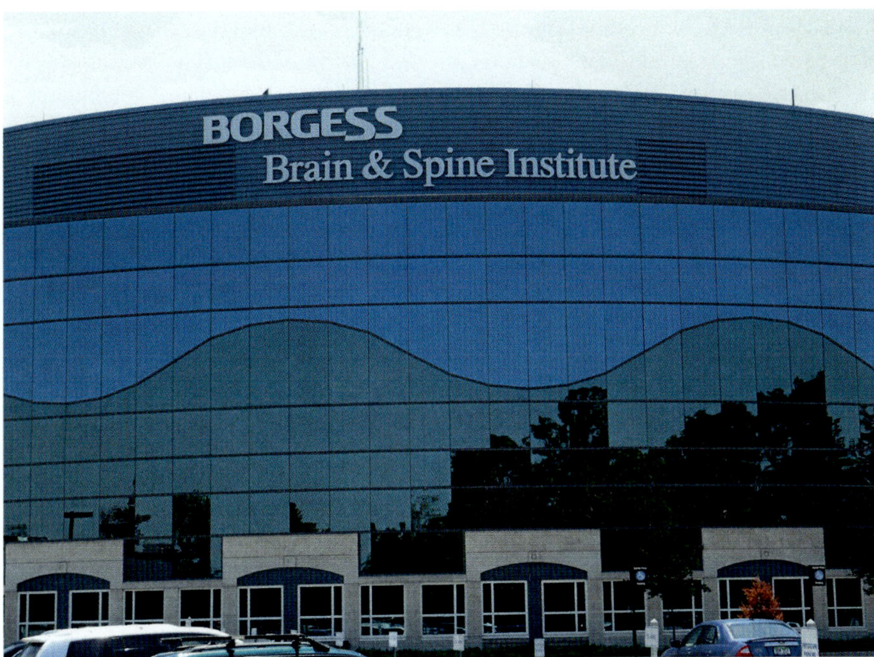

Fig. 1.1 Borgess Brain and Spine Institute (BBSI), Kalamazoo, MI. *Used with permission from Borgess Health*

dysfunctional SIJ. It should be noted that many of the surgeries and illustrations from BBSI in this textbook represent our posterior oriented surgical experience prior to 2008 and the subsequent development of adequate lateral instrumentation to perform straight lateral minimally invasive fusions. The posterior midline approach was used extensively by us for the treatment of the dysfunctional SIJ for many years as the only other option available was the trauma way of placing two screws laterally across the joint with no real fusion as part of the process. Since the advent of very good lateral fixation devices, the current main operation now being used at BBSI is the minimally invasive lateral approach. As a result of having such a varied surgical history with the SIJ, BBSI is in the unique position of being able to choose between multiple techniques to obtain the desired fusion of the SIJ depending on the individual circumstances of the patient. These different circumstances will be discussed throughout this book, as well as the many varied ways to approach, instrument, and fuse the SIJ.

The authors responsible for the creation of this textbook comprise between them over 80 years of performing surgeries on the dysfunctional SIJ and bring their collected experience of thousands of patients from major referral centers covering all parts of the country. Each author will provide their reasons for using a certain approach and define situations where it is best utilized and possibly where it should be avoided.

The current literature (Chap. 2), published in peer review journals since the 1980s, contains unique information that will also be sited throughout this book by multiple chapter authors.

The Philosophical Approach for the Creation of This Textbook

The philosophical approach to the organization of surgical information in this textbook is to discuss the various previously published techniques along with new techniques in groups according to the approach used to perform them. The approaches are defined by their potential to be invasive and their anatomical locations with reference to the SIJ. So, for example, one of the most utilized surgeries today would be found in the chapter entitled "the lateral approach, minimally invasive." The emphasis in this book is to provide information on approaches and not specific types of instrumentation to perform those approach-driven procedures. It should be noted here that the anterior approach will not be discussed in this textbook. All the authors agree that this is a very rarely used approach for the dysfunctional SIJ, and only in an extremely unusual circumstance would a surgeon consider using that approach. These types of rare situations would most likely be associated with some acute event or a trauma. In this book, different authors do favor different types of instrumentation, and their bias will show through in their illustrations and images. It is the editors' expectation that all the writings in this textbook are being provided for general SIJ treatment information and not as a medium for solicitation of devices.

Book Objectives

Through the writing of this book, the authors hope to accomplish several objectives for the surgeon treating a dysfunctional SIJ patient and the physical therapist in charge of rehabilitating such a patient, either in the midst of conservative treatment or postoperatively after a SIJ fusion. The surgeon will be educated about the anatomy and physiology of the SIJ as a pain generator. They will understand how to diagnose a dysfunctional SIJ and learn the conservative and all the available surgical methods to treat a patient with this diagnosis. Surgeons will understand the multiple pitfalls that can exist when operating on the SIJ and the complications most common with each surgical approach. They will learn methods from various authors to choose the most appropriate procedure for a given patient and the best ways to rehabilitate the patient postsurgery. The physical therapist will learn the latest anatomy and physiology of the dysfunctional SIJ and learn the most recent successful techniques in treating a patient with this diagnosis. They will understand what an important role they play in the algorithm for treating the dysfunctional SIJ and the appropriate

measures to take when treating the postoperative SIJ fusion patient. The final chapter in this textbook (Chap. 16) is a "Roundtable Discussion" concerning important timely questions that a surgeon or a physical therapist might have as asked and discussed by the chapter authors. Hopefully, it will serve as a springboard for those on the edge of wanting to learn more about the dysfunctional SIJ to get started doing so.

"Off-Label" Uses of Products

Except for Chap. 8, the lateral approach, minimally invasive, and portions of Chap. 11, the lateral approach, open, all the material discussing instrumentation going through or into the SIJ and the use of bone morphogenic protein (Infuse, Medtronic) is used "off-label." Within each chapter, the individual authors will restate the FDA status of the devices they are discussing as they are presented.

Disclaimer There currently is no established standard for the surgical treatment of the dysfunctional SIJ or for the resulting rehabilitation of the patient after such a surgery. The reader must understand that this textbook represents a collection of techniques to diagnose and treat the dysfunctional SIJ from multiple sources. Not all these techniques have been fully tested or have been published in peer-reviewed journals. Those that have are listed as such throughout the book. The information provided here represents procedures and techniques that have worked well for these authors for the patients they have treated. Any surgeon or therapist deciding to use these procedures and techniques to treat patients does so knowing that the authors claim no responsibility for the related outcomes of such treatments.

References

1. Zelle BA, Gruen GS, Brown S, George S. Sacroiliac joint dysfunction: evaluation and management. Clin J Pain. 2005;21:446–55.
2. Dreyfuss P, Michaelsen M, Pauza K, McLarty J. The value of medical history and physical examination in diagnosing sacroiliac joint pain. Spine. 1996;21:2594–602.
3. Smith-Petersen MN, Rogers WA. End-result study of arthrodesis of the sacroiliac joint for arthritis-traumatic and non-traumatic. J Bone Joint Surg Am. 1926;8:118–36.

4. Mixter WJ, Barr JS. Rupture of the intervertebral disc with involvement of the spinal canal. N Engl J Med. 1934;211:210–5.

5. Waisbrod H, Krainick JU, Gerbershagen HU. Sacroiliac joint arthrodesis for chronic lower back pain. Arch Orthop Trauma Surg. 1987;106:238–40.

6. http://www.accessdata.fda.gov/cdrh_docs/pdf12/K122o74.pdf

7. Dall BE. Someone needs to claim it. Spine J. 2009;2:190–1.

8. Hutchinson MR, Dall BE. Midline fascial splitting approach to the iliac crest for bone graft: a new approach. Spine. 1994;1:62–6.

9. Belanger TA, Dall BE. Sacroiliac arthrodesis using a posterior midline fascial splitting approach and pedicle screw instrumentation: a new technique. J Spinal Disord. 2001;2:118–24.

10. Wise CL, Dall BE. Minimally invasive sacroiliac arthrodesis: outcomes of a new technique. J Spinal Disord Tech. 2008;8:579–84.

11. http://www.borgess.com/files/bbsi/pdf/si_joint_white.pdf

Surgical Treatment for the Painful, Stable Sacroiliac Joint: What Does the Literature Tell Us?

Sonia V. Eden

Introduction

Low back pain (LBP) represents the second most common cause of visits to primary care physicians with the loss of productivity, income, and associated medical expenses resulting in a $60 billion expenditure in the USA on an annual basis [1]. The sacroiliac joint (SIJ) has been identified as one of the causes of LBP 15–30 % of the time at the initial office visit [1]. The SIJ is a true synovial joint that primarily handles forces between the spine and pelvis [2, 3]. In its normal state, the SIJ gains all of its stability from numerous associated ligamentous structures and its undulating oblique structure allows it to withstand significant loads under normal physiologic conditions [3].

The painful, stable SIJ has recently been designated as a dysfunctional SIJ [4]. Although this is a recent definition, procedures to treat this joint have been in existence for nearly a century. The first publication offering evidence in support of this condition with a primary diagnosis of

traumatic arthritis was published in 1926 [5]. Consideration for the SIJ's potential to cause pain temporarily slipped into obscurity when Mixter and Barr published their work on the injured herniated lumbar disc in 1934 [6]. Interest in the SIJ as a treatable pain generator has resurfaced, especially during the last decade. This is partially due to the emergence of pain clinics and the increasing number of diagnostic and potentially therapeutic SIJ injections being performed. In addition, with the increased utilization of instrumented lumbar or lumbosacral fusions to treat various spinal pathologies, the awareness of adjacent level degeneration affecting the SIJ and resulting in the painful, stable SIJ has surfaced [7–9]. Common causes for painful, stable SIJs include inflammatory arthritis, postpartum syndrome, adjacent osteoporosis, Paget's disease, direct or indirect trauma, and adjacent segmental degeneration secondary to a previous lumbosacral fusion [10, 11].

When patients suffering from painful, dysfunctional SIJs have failed conservative treatment measures and their symptoms result in significant inhibition of function, arthrodesis and/or stabilization of the joint may be considered. Again, along with an increase in diagnosis, there has been a resurgence of operations to fuse and/or stabilize the stable, painful SIJ during the past decade. Despite evidence of the existence of the painful, stable SIJ in the general population, the knowledge base for surgically treating the painful, stable SIJ remains limited.

S.V. Eden, M.D. (✉)
Department of Neurological Surgery, Borgess Brain and Spine Institute, Western Michigan University Medical School, Kalamazoo, MI, USA
e-mail: soniaeden@borgess.com

B.E. Dall et al. (eds.), *Surgery for the Painful, Dysfunctional Sacroiliac Joint*,
DOI 10.1007/978-3-319-10726-4_2, © Springer International Publishing Switzerland 2015

This article will systematically review the literature to better understand what our current knowledge base is concerning surgeries for the painful, stable SIJ. We will examine the indications for SIJ surgical procedures as well as the published surgical techniques, outcomes, and complications following these procedures in hopes of gaining a better understanding of the optimal treatment options for patients with painful, stable SIJs.

Methods Used to Review the Literature

In order to generate the initial source articles, we conducted an electronic search in MEDLINE (OVID), EMBASE, CINAHL, and Web of Knowledge databases using the following Medical Subject Heading (MESH) terms: sacroiliac concept, surgery, fusion concept, outcomes concept, and complications concept. The search was restricted to articles related to human subjects and included articles in peer-reviewed journals between January 1, 1966, and April 1, 2013. Similar searches were conducted in each of the databases. Please refer to Appendix A for the complete search document. This search was performed using the established criteria laid out in the Quorum Statement for the conduct and reporting of systematic reviews [12, 13].

Studies of varying design, scale, and duration were included in this review. Studies were deemed eligible for this review if they (1) were published in English in peer-reviewed journals; (2) had relevant surgical treatment of the degenerative, stable sacroiliac joint; (3) were either randomized controlled trials, retrospective series, prospective series, observational or population-based studies, or case series; (4) reported quantitative results; and (5) studied patient populations within the USA. Studies were classified as randomized controlled trials, prospective cohort studies, or retrospective studies [14]. Case reports were excluded from this review. Studies pertaining to surgical treatment of the SIJ for trauma, tumor, or infection were also excluded from this review. Please refer to Appendix A for the full search strategies.

Results of the Literature Review

Of the 281,909 articles indexed in MEDLINE related to the surgical treatment of the SIJ, 18 (0.00006 %) of the articles pertained to the surgical treatment of the painful, stable SIJ. A total of 277 items pertaining to the dysfunctional SIJ were identified in MEDLINE (OVID), EMBASE, CINAHL, and Web of Science. One reviewer (SE) examined abstracts from all of the publications identified by the search and eliminated irrelevant articles and duplicates. Once the duplicates were discarded, the remaining 195 items were reviewed and screened by the reviewer (SE) for the above inclusion criteria. Of these articles, 11 (0.0004 %) met criteria to be included in this review. One additional article that met inclusion criteria was selected from other database searches, yielding a total of 12 articles.

The results of the review are summarized based on the surgical approach used in the included studies. The three approaches utilized are (1) open, dorsal approach (five articles); (2) minimally invasive lateral approach (five articles); and (3) minimally invasive, dorsal approach (two articles). For the purpose of this review, minimally invasive approaches are defined as those performed either via a percutaneous approach or through a skin incision of less than 1 in. [15]. Three of the studies were prospective analyses [16–18]. The remaining nine studies were all retrospective in nature. None of the reviewed studies utilized a randomized control design.

Open, Dorsal Approach

Five of the studies that met our inclusion criteria focused on outcomes following SIJ arthrodesis performed via open, dorsal approaches. A total of 118 patients underwent sacroiliac arthrodesis by this approach, of which 42 patients underwent bilateral SIJ fusions. Four of the studies were retrospective case reviews and one study was a prospective case review. The surgical techniques, treatment indications, and diagnostic and primary outcome measures are summarized in Table 2.1.

Table 2.1 Open, dorsal approach

Article	# joints fused	Study design	Fusion technique	Outcome measures	Outcomes	Complications	Fusion revision rates
Buchowski et. al.	20	Retrospective	Modified Smith-Peterson technique	SF-36 health survey improvements (post–pre)	Physical functioning: (0.0072); bodily pain(0.0009); vitality(0.0047); physical summary (0.0252); mental summary(0.0105)	Two post-op wound infections requiring debridement	15 %
Keating et. al.	26	Retrospective	Joint debridement with allograft bone and compression screws placed across joint	VAS: 1–10 reduction: pre–post	Mean: pre[61.]–post[2.9] ($p<0.01$)	None reported	None reported
Kibsgard et. al.	75	Retrospective	Dorsal trans-iliac fusion or intra-extra-articular fusion	VAS: 1–10 reduction: pre–post	Mean reduction morning: [24](90.029) Mean reduction evening: [28](0.011)	1:icterus 1:pulmonary embolism 1:pin tract infnx. 1:appendicits 1:SBO	None reported
Schutz et. al.	34	Retrospective	Dorsal bilateral interlocking technique	VAS: 1–10 reduction: pre–post		3:excision of scar tissue 10:hardware removal 5:fusion revision	29.4 %
Giannikas et. al.	5	Prospective	Placement of two large bi-cortical bone plugs across the joint	Satisfaction with symptom resolution	4/5 (80 %)	None	0

Table 2.2 Minimally invasive dorsal approach

Article	# Fusions	Study design	Fusion technique	Outcome measures	Outcomes	Complications	Fusion re-vision rates
Wise et. al.	19	Prospective cohort analysis	Posterior MIS approach with threaded cage, BMP	VAS: 1–10 reduction (average)	Lower back pain: 4.9 ($\leq$0.001) Leg pain: 2.9(0.013) Dyspareunia: 2.6(0.0028)	None	5.3 %
Haufe et. al.	38	Retrospective analysis	SIJ debridement without bony fusion	VAS: 1–10 % reduction	23/38: 50–100 % reduction 20/38: >75 % reduction 3/38: 25–50 % reduction Avg. reduction: 4.1	None	0

Two of the five studies showed statistically significant pain reduction scores when comparing the preoperative and postoperative visual analog scores ($p<0.01$ in the Keating study and $p=0.029$ in the Kibsgard study) [10, 19]. Giannikas et al. demonstrated complete resolution of the symptoms in 80 % of the study patients [17]. Buchowski et al. demonstrated a statistically significant improvement in all SF-36 outcomes ($p<0.05$) except for general and mental health ($p<0.4706$ and $p<0.0604$, respectively) [11]. The Schutz study was the outlier of the five studies, reporting an 18 % patient satisfaction rate, a 65 % reoperation rate, and 35 % fusion rate in the patients undergoing SIJ fusions in their series [20]. Moreover, there were minimal improvements in the patients' postoperative pain scores pre- and postsurgery in the study.

Complications were varied and only reported in two of the five studies [10, 11]. The Buchowski study reported a 15 % reoperation rate for nonunion (three patients). Following the revision fusion, two of the three patients developed deep wound infections requiring debridement and delayed pseudoarthrosis requiring additional revision surgery via an anterior approach. A few unusual complications were reported in the Kibsgard study, all of which were self-limiting (Table 2.1). There were no complications in the Giannikas patient cohort and complications were not mentioned in the Keating and Schutz papers.

Minimally Invasive Dorsal Approach

Two studies focused on minimally invasive dorsal techniques to treat the stable, dysfunctional SIJ. A total of 51 patients underwent SIJ surgeries via this approach and six of the patients underwent bilateral SIJ fusions. The Wise study was a prospective study and the Haufe study was retrospective. Wise et al. demonstrated statistically significant reductions in pain as measured on the preoperative and postoperative visual analog scales ($p<0.001$) [16]. They also reported an overall fusion rate of 89 %. A formal statistical hypothesis could not be derived from the Haufe study [15]. However, they reported that 61 % of the fused patients had 50–100 % reductions in their VAS and 53 % of the study patients had greater than 75 % improvement for at least 2 years postoperatively (Table 2.2). The Haufe study utilized a novel technique of debriding the SIJ to treat the pain. There were no reported complications or reoperations in either of these studies.

Minimally Invasive Lateral Approach

The remaining five studies focused on lateral, percutaneous approaches to treat the symptomatic, stable SIJ. One hundred and thirty-nine patients underwent statistical analysis following SIJ arthrodesis via this approach.

The Mason study was a prospective analysis and the four other studies were all retrospective analyses. All studies demonstrated statistically significant improvements in pain levels as measured by various validated outcome scales [1, 18, 21–23]. Significant pre- and postreductions in the visual analog scale were seen in the Al-Khayer, Mason, Rudolf, and Sachs studies ($p < 0.002$, $p < 0.0001$, $p < 0.0001$, and $p < 0.0001$, respectively). The Khurana study showed statistically significant improvements in the SF-36 pain score ($p < 0.031$).

No complications occurred in the Khurana and Sachs studies. The three remaining studies had a 33 % complication rate between them. These complications resulted in a 17 % reoperation rate. It is with this approach that reported complications involved nerve pain, significant post-op hematomas, malpositioning of the hardware, and a fracture of the ilium (Table 2.3).

Discussion

Although the first article describing an SIJ arthrodesis was published in 1926, nearly a century ago, our literature review suggests that data regarding the surgical treatment for the SIJ is remarkably limited [5]. Out of 281,909 articles indexed in MEDLINE related to the surgical treatment of the SIJ, 18 (0.00006 %) of the articles pertained to the surgical treatment of painful, stable SIJ. Only 11 (0.0004 %) of these articles met search criteria for inclusion in our review, with one additional article from the other searched databases.

Waisbrod's 1987 article that was published 60 years after the Smith-Peterson article marks the beginning of the modern era for both the diagnosis and surgical treatment of the painful, stable SIJ [24]. He reported the results of a series of 21 patients who underwent surgery for a painful, stable SIJ. The approach was very similar to the approach described by Smith-Peterson in his sentinel paper. However, this time, in addition to abandoning the drastic gluteal muscular dissection, he inserted ceramic blocks into the posterior ligamentous aspect of the SIJ. His follow-up was

30 months with a 70 % success rate in decreasing patient's original pain by at least 50 %. There were two nonunions, one infection, and no reported revision surgeries. Another hiatus of 14 years occurred before Belanger published the second paper in the modern area on fusing the painful, stable SIJ [2]. In this study he introduces a new approach for reaching the SIJs. This approach is a midline fascial splitting approach, which is the same approach as described by Hutchinson in his paper on a new way to approach the iliac wing and harvest bone graft while avoiding the cluneal nerves, which were cut with the then standard arched incision over the rim of the iliac crest [25]. This was also the first time that pedicle screw instrumentation was used in achieving stabilization for this fusion surgery. This procedure also introduced a new way to fixate a screw to the ilium, allowing for bone graft to be placed directly into the prepared SIJ and allowing for compression across the SIJ by the instrumentation. Patients were braced in a pantaloon brace, and for the first time after such a surgery, they were allowed to be immediately full weight bearing on the surgical side. The four patients in the study were followed for up to 9 years, and all went on to solid fusions. There were no major complications. The long-term success rate was determined to be 80 % with two patients having their hardware removed prior to final follow-up due to one of the pelvic screws being point tender. This pain resolved with hardware removal in each case.

The diagnosis of the painful, stable SIJ up to this time in history had been made by a combination of the surgeon's clinical exam, various imaging studies, and, more recently, extra articular injections of a local anesthetic. The Waisbrod and Belanger studies are significant as they represent attempts to utilize more modern thought and devices to address SIJ dysfunction which translated into more sophisticated methods of diagnosis, treatment, and follow-up methods [2, 24].

It was in 2005 that specific outcome measures (ODI, VAS, and SF-36) were first used to evaluate patients having an SIJ fusion procedure. These studies also used standardized intraarticular injections under image to diagnose SIJ

Table 2.3 Minimally invasive lateral approach

Article	# Fusions	Study design	Fusion technique	Outcome measures	Outcomes	Complications	Fusion revision rates
Khurana et. al.	15	Retrospective	Lateral hollow modular anchorage screw	SF-36 survey and Majeed pain score improvements (pre–post)	SF-36: physical function (0.026); bodily pain (0.0009); vitality (0.0047); physical summary (0.0252); mental summary (0.0105) ($p=0.031$)	None	0
Al-hayer et. al.	12	Retrospective	Placement of one HMA hollow titanium screw filled with autograft bone and bone matrix	VAS (1–10); Oswestry disability index (ODI) reduction	Mean VAS: pre[8.1]–post[4.6] ($p<0.002$)	One deep would infection requiring debridement and intravenous antibiotics	0
Mason et. al.	55	Prospective	Placement of modular anchorage screw	Mean VAS: SF-36; Majeed	Mean VAS: pre[8.05]–post[4.48] ($p=0.00$) SF-36 mean physical function post[42.93]–pre[26.59] ($p=0.00$) Majeed: pre[64.78]–post[36.18] ($p=0.00$)	2: post-op nerve pain requiring re-operation	0 %
Rudolf et. al.	55	Retrospective	Placement of titanium triangular implants	VAS: 1–10; activity difficulty changes	Pain: 3mos. Difference-mean[−3.92] 6 mos. difference mean[−4.36] 12 mos. difference mean[−4.29] ($p\leq0.0001$)	3:superficial cellulitis; 1:deep soft tissue wound infection; 2:large buttock hematomas; 2:implant penetration into neural foraminae req. re-operation; 1:implant malpositioning req. re-operation; 1:non-displaced ileum fracture	0 %
Sachs et. al.	12	Retrospective	Placement of titanium triangular implants	VAS: 1–10 reduction: pre–post	Mean change[−6.2] ($p=0.000$)	None	0 at 1 year

dysfunction. Of these studies, there are 12 publications that met criteria for this systematic review. Only two of these studies were prospective analyses, with the first being published in 2008 [16, 17]. Ten of the reviewed studies documented statistically significant reductions in the pain scores based on reduction in VAS or improvements in the SF-36 scale [1, 10, 11, 16, 18, 19, 21, 22, 26]. Based on a patient satisfaction survey, Giannikas et al. demonstrated an 80 % success rate in the operated patients [17]. Although a statistical hypothesis could not be derived from the Haufe study, 61 % of the patients in the study had 50–100 % reductions in their VAS and 53 % had >75 % improvement for greater than a 2-year follow-up period [15].

Only one of the reviewed articles showed poor outcomes following bilateral posterior SIJ fusions, with an 18 % success rate and a 65 % reoperation rate [20]. These poor results may be attributable to difficulty in patient selection and the surgical technique. The pseudoarthrosis rate was almost 30 % and bony fusion was questionable in 42 % of the patients in this study. Moreover, statistical analyses failed to show any relationship between long-term pain relief and the preoperative test results.

There appears to be a renewed interest in fusing the painful, stable SIJ. Although more studies concerning this topic are being published, this literature review confirms that the data regarding the fusion of the painful, stable SIJ is scarce. Existing literature on this surgical procedure is limited to retrospective and prospective case series. Moreover, there is no uniformity in the surgical approaches to the SIJ, and many of the studies utilize varying outcome measures, making it difficult to directly compare the outcomes and draw meaningful data-driven conclusions.

Despite these limitations, all of the studies reviewed with the exception of the Schutz study showed meaningful or statistically significant pain reduction or improvements in the outcome measures following fusion surgery for the painful, stable SIJ. Moreover, no complications were noted in the minimally invasive posterior approach surgical procedures. Studies focusing on the lateral minimally invasive approach to the SIJ certainly did report higher rates of nerve root injuries than the studies focusing on the other reviewed approaches. This finding suggests that because of the pelvic anatomy, the lateral approach may place the neural elements at more risk of direct injury than the other studied approaches. Nevertheless, the significant reductions in pain noted in 92 % of the reviewed studies certainly suggest that the dysfunctional SIJ does benefit from surgical stabilization and may be amenable to several surgical approaches.

This review is important at this time due to the increasing number of painful, stable SIJs being diagnosed and the current rise in the numbers of fusions being done for this disease. There are various reasons beyond the scope of this chapter as to why there has recently been a dramatic increase in the number of SIJ fusions being performed on the painful, stable SIJ. This is resulting in the immediate need to examine our knowledge base to help us make better educated decisions regarding the best and most appropriate care for patients with painful, stable SIJs.

Conclusion

This is the first review article discussing fusion of the stable, painful SIJ, which looks at almost a century of experience. All papers reviewed consisted of a series of case studies with each varying in indication and technique according to the surgeon performing the surgery. Eleven of the twelve articles demonstrated postoperative patient satisfaction and/or statistically significant improvements in the validated outcome scales. There has been an increase in surgeries to fuse the stable, painful SIJ in recent years. This review helps us understand where we have been historically with this joint when it is in a stable, painful state, but we need good prospective comparison studies to better know how to proceed in the future.

References

1. Sachs D, Capobianco R. One year successful outcomes for novel sacroiliac joint arthrodesis system. Ann Surg Innov Res. 2012;6(1):13.
2. Belanger TA, Dall BE. Sacroiliac arthrodesis using a posterior midline fascial splitting approach and pedicle screw instrumentation: a new technique. J Spinal Disord. 2001;14(2):118–24.
3. Stark JG. The diagnosis and treatment of sacroiliac joint abnormalities. Curr Orthop Pract. 2010;21(4):336–47.
4. Dall BE, Eden SV, Brumbay HG. Sacroiliac joint dysfunction: an algorithm for diagnosis and treatment. 2010. http://www.borgess.com/files/bbsi/pdf/si_joint_white.pdf.
5. Smith-Petersen MN, Rogers WA. End-result study of arthrodesis of the sacro-iliac joint for arthritis: traumatic and non-traumatic. J Bone Joint Surg. 1926;8(1):118–36.
6. Mixter WJ, Barr JS. Rupture of the intervertebral disc with involvement of the spinal canal. N Engl J Med. 1934;211(5):210–5.
7. Ha KY, Lee JS, Kim KW. Degeneration of sacroiliac joint after instrumented lumbar or lumbosacral fusion: a prospective cohort study over five-year follow-up. Spine (Phila Pa 1976). 2008;33(11):1192–8.
8. DePalma MJ, Ketchum JM, Saullo TR. Etiology of chronic low back pain in patients having undergone lumbar fusion. Pain Med. 2011;12(5):732–9.
9. Yoshihara H. Sacroiliac joint pain after lumbar/lumbosacral fusion: current knowledge. Eur Spine J. 2012;21(9):1788–96.
10. Kibsgard TJ, et al. Pelvic joint fusions in patients with chronic pelvic girdle pain: a 23-year follow-up. Eur Spine J. 2013;22(4):871–7.
11. Buchowski JM, et al. Functional and radiographic outcome of sacroiliac arthrodesis for the disorders of the sacroiliac joint. Spine J. 2005;5(5):520–8. Discussion 529.
12. Moher D, Schulz K, Altman D. The CONSORT statement: revised recommendations for improving the quality of reports of parallel group randomized trials. BMC Med Res Methodol. 2001;1(1):2.
13. Ismail K, Winkley K, Rabe-Hesketh S. Systematic review and meta-analysis of randomised controlled trials of psychological interventions to improve glycaemic control in patients with type 2 diabetes. Lancet. 2004;363(9421):1589–97.
14. Egger M, Smith GD, O'Rourke K. Introduction: rationale, potentials, and promise of systematic reviews. In: M. Egger, GD. Smith, D. Altman (Eds.), Systematic reviews in health care. London: BMJ Publishing Group; 2008, p. 1–19
15. Haufe SM, Mork AR. Sacroiliac joint debridement: a novel technique for the treatment of sacroiliac joint pain. Photomed Laser Surg. 2005;23(6):596–8.
16. Wise CL, Dall BE. Minimally invasive sacroiliac arthrodesis: outcomes of a new technique. J Spinal Disord Tech. 2008;21(8):579–84.
17. Giannikas KA, et al. Sacroiliac joint fusion for chronic pain: a simple technique avoiding the use of metalwork. Eur Spine J. 2004;13(3):253–6.
18. Mason LW, Chopra I, Mohanty K. The percutaneous stabilisation of the sacroiliac joint with hollow modular anchorage screws: a prospective outcome study. Eur Spine J. 2013;22(10):2325–31.
19. John G, Keating M. Sacroiliac joint fusion in a chronic low back pain population. In: Vleeming A, editor. The integrated function of the lumbar spine and sacroiliac joints: second interdisciplinary world congress on low back pain. Rotterdam: ECO; 1995. p. 361–5.
20. Schutz U, Grob D. Poor outcome following bilateral sacroiliac joint fusion for degenerative sacroiliac joint syndrome. Acta Orthop Belg. 2006;72(3):296–308.
21. Al-Khayer A, et al. Percutaneous sacroiliac joint arthrodesis: a novel technique. J Spinal Disord Tech. 2008;21(5):359–63.
22. Rudolf L. Sacroiliac joint arthrodesis-MIS technique with titanium implants: report of the first 50 patients and outcomes. Open Orthop J. 2012;6:495–502.
23. Khurana A, et al. Percutaneous fusion of the sacroiliac joint with hollow modular anchorage screws: clinical and radiological outcome. J Bone Joint Surg Br. 2009;91(5):627–31.
24. Waisbrod H, Krainick JU, Gerbershagen HU. Sacroiliac joint arthrodesis for chronic lower back pain. Arch Orthop Trauma Surg. 1987;106(4):238–40.
25. Hutchinson MR, Dall BE. Midline fascial splitting approach to the iliac crest for bone graft: a new approach. Spine. 1994;19(1):62–6.
26. Khurana A, et al. Percutaneous fusion of the sacroiliac joint with hollow modular anchorage screws: clinical and radiological outcome. J Bone Joint Surg. 2009;91(5):627–31.

Michael D. Rahl

Introduction

A detailed anatomic understanding of the sacroiliac joints (SIJ) and surrounding areas is important for all clinicians involved in treating SIJ dysfunction. Prior to any surgical or invasive intervention, it is imperative that the treating clinician has complete knowledge of that particular patient's structural anatomy. Minimizing tissue disruption and sparing major structures in the area of the SIJ can potentially decrease complications, reduce recovery time, and optimize outcomes.

Anatomical variants are common. Although several will be discussed as deemed necessary for this book, it is beyond the scope of this chapter to discuss all possible variations. The locations and distances in relation to other structures noted in this chapter are based on averages.

Osseous Anatomy

Sacroiliac Joint

The lateral surface of the sacrum contains an auricular surface, which articulates with the ilium. This articulation forms the SIJ and is found about

4.5 cm deep to the subcutaneous tissue [32, 43]. The articulating surfaces are chevron shaped and usually extend from the cephalad aspect of S1 to the middle of S3. The caudal limb of the auricular surface is about 5.6 cm long, the cephalad limb is about 4.4 cm long, and they meet to form an angle of about 93° [88] with the apex of the chevron pointing ventrally and inferiorly. The auricular surface has a propeller-like shape (Fig. 3.1).

Relative to the sagittal plane, the angle of the cephalad, middle, and caudal aspects of the joint varies greatly from 0 to 40° and can be oriented anterolateral-posteromedial or anteromedial-posterolateral [16, 19, 43]. The SIJ can be classified as a diarthrodial/synovial joint since it allows for motion and contains a synovial membrane, joint capsule, synovial fluid, cartilage on both articulating surfaces, and ligamentous connections.

The joint space is about 4.5 mm wide [10, 43] and the auricular surfaces are covered with cartilage on both the sacral and iliac sides. The sacral cartilage is from 1.1 to 3.0 mm thick, while the iliac cartilage is from 0.5 to 1.0 mm thick [10, 11, 55, 69] (Fig. 3.2).

Where the cartilage integrates with the underlying bone, the bone end-plate thickness is inversely related to the cartilage thickness with the iliac side being thicker than the sacral side [55]. The thickness of the cartilage on both surfaces decreases with age with more fibrillations and deep fissures forming on the iliac surface [35, 63]. The sacral cartilage is creamy, white, and smooth

M.D. Rahl, PT, DPT, OCS, CSCS (✉)
Full Potential Physical Therapy, 286 Hoover Boulevard,
Holland, MI 49423, USA
e-mail: michael@fullpotentialpt.com

B.E. Dall et al. (eds.), *Surgery for the Painful, Dysfunctional Sacroiliac Joint,*
DOI 10.1007/978-3-319-10726-4_3, © Springer International Publishing Switzerland 2015

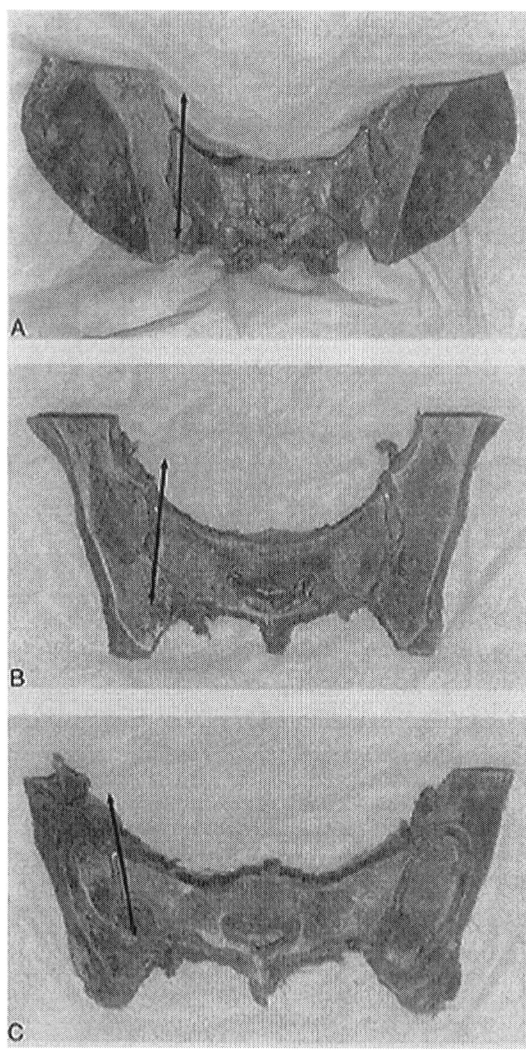

Fig. 3.1 Transverse sections through the (**a**) anterosuperior, (**b**) middle, and (**c**) posteroinferior aspects of the sacroiliac joint. The *arrows* indicate the joint plane orientation of the right sacroiliac joint. Note the different orientations leading to a propeller-like shape of the sacroiliac joint [19]

and appears hyaline in nature, while the iliac cartilage is dull, bluish, and striated and appears more fibrocartilaginous in nature [11, 84]. Substance P and calcitonin gene-related peptide (CGRP) have been identified in the superficial layer of the sacral and iliac cartilage and may contribute to intra-articular nociception [76]. Ridges and corresponding depressions can be found throughout the sacral and iliac cartilage [41, 84]. Increased age is correlated with larger and more numerous ridges and depressions, with females having less pronounced characteristics [84, 90]. These ridges and depression potentially contribute to increased SIJ stability and increase the coefficient of friction at the joint surface.

Sacrum

The most cephalad aspect of the sacrum is the base (Fig. 3.3).

The base is broad and articulates with the fibrocartilaginous intervertebral disc between the fifth lumbar vertebra and the sacrum. The ventral aspect of the sacral base is the sacral promontory. In 18–30 % of the population, structural anomalies known as lumbosacral transitional vertebrae (LSTV) are found [13, 50, 60]. These LSTV can be classified based on whether the fifth lumbar vertebra is sacralized (characteristics of a sacral vertebra) or the first sacral vertebra is lumbarized (characteristics of a lumbar vertebra). Furthermore, these LSTV can be classified as Type I (dysplastic transverse process), Type II (accessory articulation), Type III (bony fusion), or Type IV (mixed) and either "a" (unilateral) or "b" (bilateral) [12]. The size and location of the auricular surfaces may also vary depending on the type of LSTV. A LSTV with a lumbarized S1 segment usually presents with a more cephalad SIJ with the auricular surfaces spanning from cephalad to the S1 vertebral body to the caudal aspect of the S2 vertebral body [51] (Fig. 3.4).

Conversely, a LSTV with a sacralized L5 segment usually presents with a more caudal SIJ with the auricular surfaces spanning from the middle of the S1 vertebral body to the caudal aspect of the S3 vertebral body [51]. Therefore, with a unilateral LSTV, the SIJ on one side may be an entirely different size and be found in a slightly different location than that of the opposite side.

Lateral to the sacral base bilaterally are the pedicles with the most lateral aspect referred to as the sacral ala (Fig. 3.3). The S1 pedicle is about 2.6 cm wide (medial to lateral) and 2.5 cm deep (dorsal to ventral), while the S2 pedicle is about 2.0 cm wide and 1.8 cm deep [18, 22, 56].

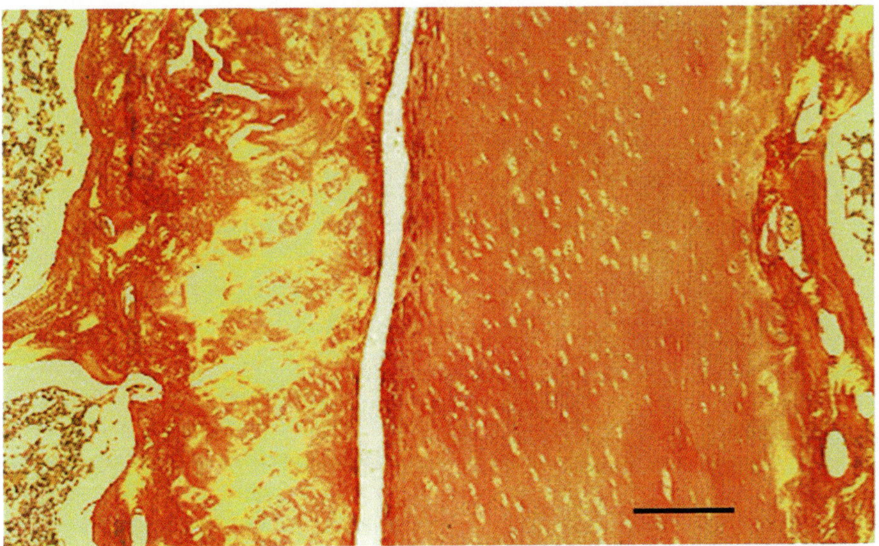

Fig 3.2 Iliac cartilage (*left*) and sacral cartilage (*right*) separated by the sacroiliac joint space. Note the difference in cartilage thickness and collagen arrangement. Scale bar = 0.5 mm [55]

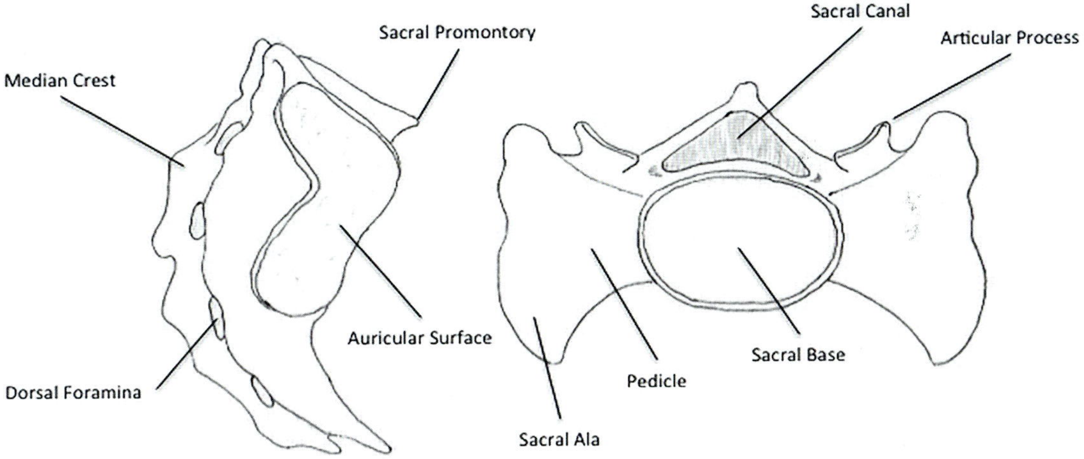

Fig. 3.3 Lateral and cephalad aspects of the sacrum

The sacrum consists primarily of cancellous bone covered by a thin layer of cortical bone. The cancellous bone of the sacrum is denser ventrally [55]. At the S1 level, the sacrum is most dense at the ventral cortex of the sacral pedicle. The ventral cortex of the ala is second densest followed by the ventral cortex of the lateral aspect of the sacral vertebral body [67].

The sacrum is wedge shaped and typically composed of five sacral vertebrae. This wedge shape has evolved to support the body's weight during bipedal gait [1]. Composing most of the sacrum, the sacral vertebral bodies and neural arches have fused to form one continuous bone. The first sacral vertebral body is about 2.8 cm high (cephalad to caudal), 4.3 cm wide

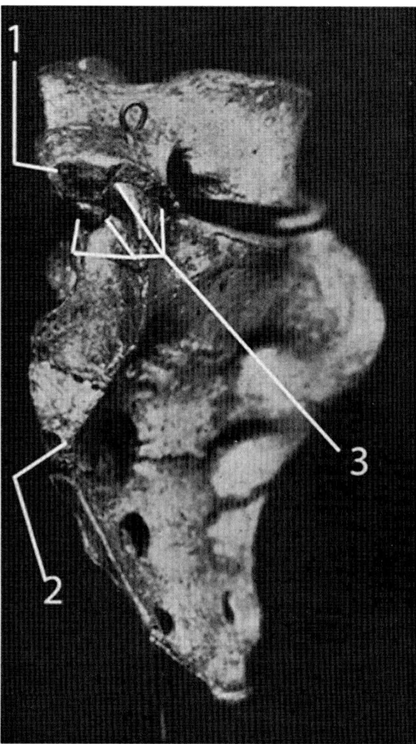

Fig. 3.4 A transitional lumbosacral vertebra and pseudojoint (3) within the auricular surface. Note the variable sacroiliac joint morphology with the superior aspect of the auricular surface (1) cephalad to S1 and the inferior aspect of the auricular surface (2) at the caudal aspect of S2. In a normal sacroiliac joint, the auricular surface spans from S1 to S3 [59]

(medial to lateral), and 2.3 cm deep (dorsal to ventral). The second and third sacral vertebral bodies are about 2.3 cm and 1.9 cm high, 3.0 cm and 2.3 cm wide, and 1.3 cm and 1.0 cm deep, respectively [46].

The sacral canal runs cephalad to caudal through the dorsal aspect of the sacrum and allows the passage of the sacral nerves (Fig. 3.3).

The caudal end of the sacral canal is often deficient and referred to as the sacral hiatus. The coccyx articulates with the caudal end of the sacrum and is composed of 3–5 vertebrae, the most caudal being fused together. This articulation where the sacrum meets the coccyx is a fibrocartilaginous joint and offers minimal movement. The cephalad aspect of the first coccygeal vertebra contains the coccygeal cornua, which articulates to the sacral cornua found on the lateral

aspect of the sacral apex. Sacrococcygeal fusion is common in males and with increasing age and primarily involves the first coccygeal vertebra [77]. It is also correlated with LSTV [77].

The ventral aspect of the sacrum is concave and contains four sacral foramina allowing for the exit of the ventral rami of the first four sacral nerves (Fig. 3.5). The S1 ventral foramen can be found about 2.3 cm below the sacral base and 2.4 cm from the lateral border of the sacrum [26]. Four transverse ridges run horizontally between each foraminal level, indicating the site of osseous fusion of the sacral vertebral bodies.

The dorsal aspect is convex and also contains four sacral foramina allowing for the exit of the dorsal rami of the first four sacral nerves (Fig. 3.5). The S1 dorsal foramen can be found about 2.3 cm below the sacral base and 3.7 cm from the lateral border of the sacrum [26]. Along the midline of the dorsal aspect of the sacrum is the median crest, which is composed of rudimentary spinous processes. The sacral groove is found on each side of the median crest.

Pelvis

The pelvis is made up of three bones bilaterally: the ilium, ischium, and pubis. The ala of the ilium forms the iliac crest. The iliac crest spans from the anterior superior iliac spine (ASIS) ventrally to the posterior superior iliac spine (PSIS) dorsally. The PSIS is approximately level with the second sacral vertebra in the coronal plane and is from 1.7 to 2.2 cm dorsal to the SIJ. The thickness of the ilium overlying the SIJ ranges from 0.8 to 2.2 cm medial to lateral and is generally thicker dorsally [15] (Fig. 3.6).

Just caudal to the PSIS is the posterior inferior iliac spine (PIIS), which forms the dorsal aspect of the greater sciatic notch. Here, the ilium is from 1.5 to 1.7 cm thick in the posterolateral to anteromedial direction [72]. The distance from the PSIS to the greater sciatic notch is about 4.0 cm [72].

The interior aspect of the ilium is smooth and concave and is referred to as the iliac fossa. The medial aspect of the iliac fossa articulates with

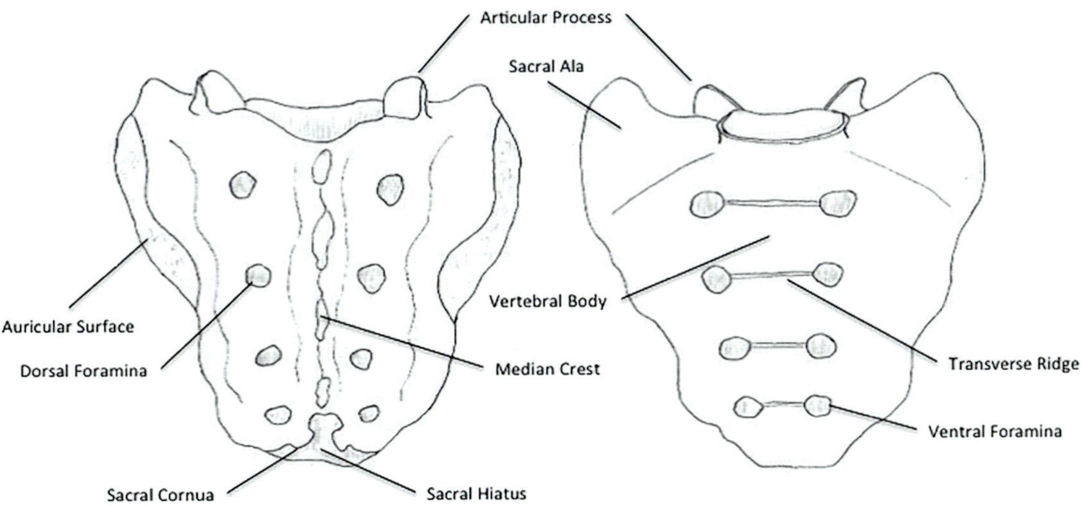

Fig. 3.5 Dorsal and ventral aspects of the sacrum

Fig. 3.6 Relationship of the auricular surface of the sacroiliac joint to the ilium (lateral view)

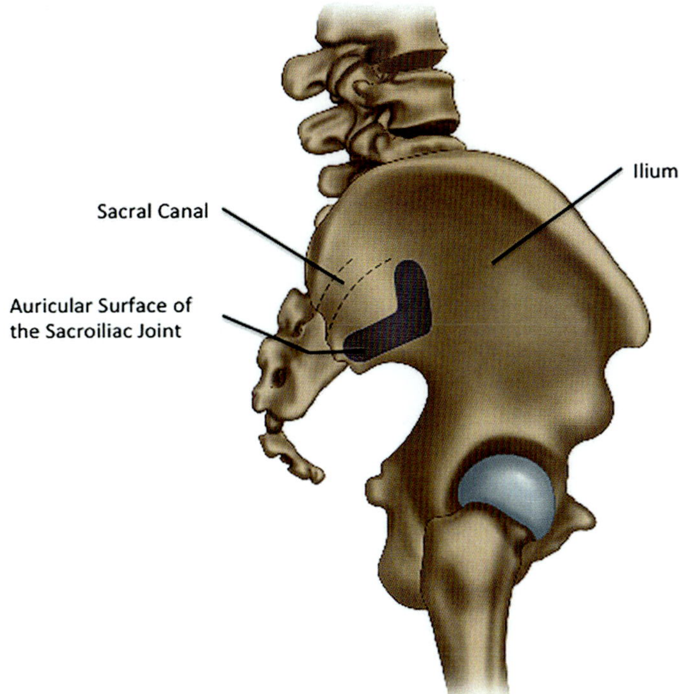

the sacrum to form the SIJ. The arcuate line, or pelvic brim, extends caudal, ventral, and medially over the interior surface of the pelvis. It marks the inferior border of the greater or false pelvis. Below this line is the lesser or true pelvis.

The ischium is dorsal while the pubis is ventral. The most caudal aspect of the ischium is the ischial tuberosity. Located between the ischial spine and ischial tuberosity is the lesser sciatic notch. Both pubic bones meet ventrally and are joined together by fibrocartilage, which collectively is called the pubic symphysis. All three pelvic bones meet laterally to form a deep, cuplike structure called the acetabulum. The head of the femur articulates with the acetabulum to form the hip joint and is the point where the lower extremity transfers the ground reaction force to the pelvis.

Ligaments

Anterior Ligaments

The ventral sacroiliac ligament crosses the SIJ ventrally and caudally at the level of S1–S3 (Fig. 3.7).

It blends with the ventral joint capsule and inserts on the periosteum close to the margins of the auricular surfaces of the sacrum and ilium [34, 63]. Mechanoreceptors and nociceptive fibers, including substance P and CGRP, have

been identified within the ventral sacroiliac ligament and may contribute to the perception of pain from the SIJ [75]. The ventral sacroiliac ligament undergoes the most stress during forward flexion and axial rotation of the sacrum [24].

Posterior Ligaments

The sacrotuberous ligament has its origin at the PSIS, dorsal ligaments, sacral tubercles, sacrum, and superior coccyx [44] (Fig. 3.8).

It has a spiral orientation and runs 6.5–12.2 cm to insert on the ischial tuberosity and, in some, the tendon of the long head of the biceps femoris [44, 80, 83, 85]. The medial fibers originate from the cephalad aspect of sacrum and lateral fibers originate from the caudal aspect of the sacrum [80]. The falciform process runs about 4.6 cm toward the ischioanal fossa and is found in about 87 % of the population [44]. It attaches at various locations including the ischial ramus, obturator fascia,

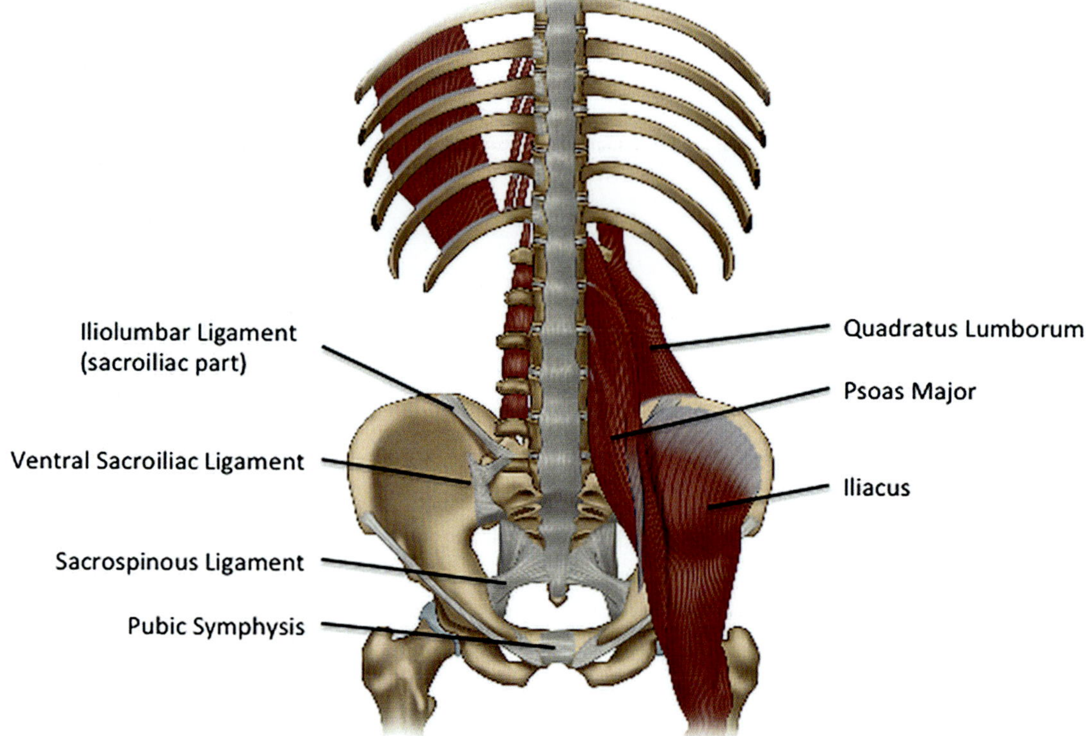

Fig. 3.7 Ventral view of the ligaments and deep musculature

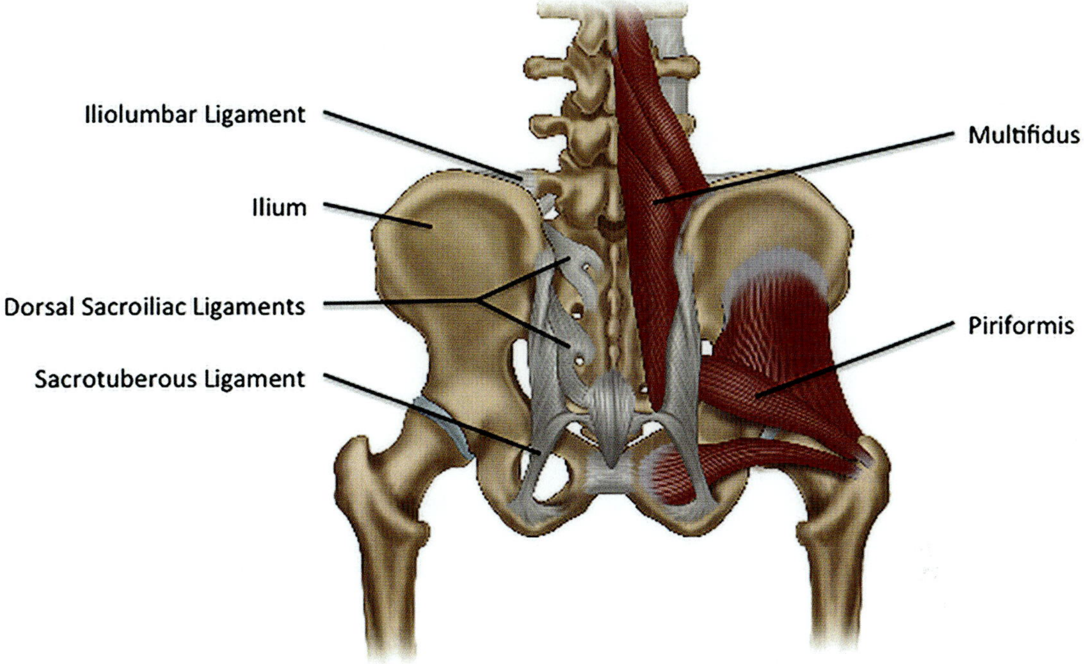

Fig. 3.8 Dorsal view of the ligaments and deep musculature

and anococcygeal ligament [44]. The pudendal nerve and artery pass through Alcock's canal formed by these structures. The fascia from the dorsal aspect of the piriformis is continuous with the sacrotuberous ligament and often has direct muscle fiber attachment to the ventral aspect of the ligament [83]. The gluteus maximus also has attachment to the sacrotuberous ligament. The sacrotuberous ligament resists forward flexion of the sacrum and can impose an extension force on the sacrum via its attachment to the gluteus maximus and long head of the biceps femoris.

Deep to the sacrotuberous ligament is the sacrospinous ligament. It extends from the lateral aspect of the apex of the sacrum and coccyx to the ischial spine. It is the division between the greater and lesser sciatic notches. The sciatic nerve and inferior gluteal artery run dorsal to the sacrospinous ligament, while the pudendal nerve runs ventral to it [40, 78]. The sacrospinous ligament resists forward flexion of the sacrum.

The dorsal sacroiliac ligaments, which are composed of the long and short ligaments, run from the PSIS to the S3–S5 sacral tubercles (Fig. 3.8). The lateral aspect is continuous with the gluteus maximus aponeurosis, while the medial aspect is continuous with the erector spinae aponeurosis and deep lamina of the posterior layer of the thoracolumbar fascia [53, 54, 81]. The lateral branches of the dorsal sacral rami (medial cluneal nerves) penetrate the dorsal ligaments and are surrounded by loose connective tissue within the ligament [53, 54]. Nociceptive fields [68] along with the presence of substance P [27] have been identified in the dorsal ligaments and may contribute to pain in the area of the SIJ. The dorsal ligaments demonstrate the most strain during extension of the sacrum [24].

Deep to the dorsal ligaments and located within the most cephalad aspect between the sacrum and ilium is the interosseous ligament. It consists of several short dense bands and often becomes ossified in people in and beyond their sixth decade of life [64]. The axial interosseous ligament is a component of the interosseous ligament and fills the space between the sacral cavity and iliac prominence just dorsal to the articular surface of the SIJ. It is composed of a mixture of collagen, blood vessels, and adipose tissue in comparison to other ligaments, which are largely composed of collagen [6]. Mechanoreceptors and nociceptive fibers (CGRP) have also been identified within this ligament and may contribute to joint proprioception and pain [75]. The interosseous ligament undergoes the highest strain during forward flexion of the sacrum and axial rotation [24].

Cephalad to the SIJ is the iliolumbar ligament. This ligament is composed of a dorsal band, ventral band, and sacroiliac part. The dorsal band originates at the tip of the L5 transverse process and inserts onto the ventral and cephalad aspect of the iliac tuberosity and crest [62, 65]. It also has direct attachment to the deep layer of the thoracolumbar fascia, erector spinae aponeurosis, and quadratus lumborum [31, 62]. The ventral band originates at the anteroinferior aspect of the L5 transverse process and caudal aspect of the L5 end plate and fans out to insert on the anterosuperior aspect of the iliac tuberosity 2.0–3.0 mm below the dorsal band insertion [62, 65]. The medial iliacus has some connections with the caudal part of the ventral band. The sacroiliac part runs from the cephalad surface of the sacral ala and joins the ventral band at the iliac tuberosity [62] (Fig. 3.7). It also merges with the L5–S1 intertransverse ligament and interosseous ligament [62]. Receptors identified within the iliolumbar ligament include proprioceptive organs and free-nerve endings. The highest concentration of these receptors is found within the ligament at its iliac insertion [39]. The iliolumbar ligament primarily resists forward flexion at L5–S1 (dorsal band) and side bending (ventral band) and becomes more important biomechanically as the intervertebral disc degenerates and loses height [42]. The iliolumbar ligament is protected by activation of the erector spinae muscles [73] (Table 3.1).

Muscles

Anterior Muscles

Several muscles compose the abdominal wall. These muscles include (superficial to deep) the rectus abdominis, external oblique, internal oblique, transversus abdominis, and quadratus lumborum. The rectus abdominis has its origin on the pubic crest and ligaments of the pubic symphysis. It runs cephalad and inserts onto the xiphoid process and fifth to seventh ribs. It is innervated by the lower intercostal nerves and contributes to forward flexion of the trunk.

Table 3.1 Ligaments and associated contributions to the sacroiliac joint

Ligament	Location	Primary restraint	Nerve fibers
Dorsal ligaments *Long ligament* *Short ligament*	PSIS to sacral tubercles	Sacral extension	Nociceptors *Substance P* Penetrated by middle cluneal nerves
Sacrotuberous	PSIS and sacrum to ischial tuberosity	Sacral flexion	–
Sacrospinous	Apex of sacrum to ischial spine	Sacral flexion	–
Ventral ligament	Crosses ventral and caudal aspect of SIJ	Sacral flexion Axial rotation	Mechanoreceptors Nociceptors *CGRP, substance P*
Interosseous	Between sacrum and ilium dorsal to SIJ	Sacral flexion Axial rotation	Mechanoreceptors Nociceptors *CGRP*
Iliolumbar *Ventral band* *Dorsal band* *Sacroiliac part*	Transverse process of L5 to iliac tuberosity and crest	Lateral side bending *Ventral band* Forward flexion *Dorsal band*	Mechanoreceptors Nociceptors

SIJ sacroiliac joint, *CGRP* calcitonin gene-related peptide, *PSIS* posterior superior iliac spine

Deep to the rectus abdominis, the external oblique has its origin on the lower six ribs and inserts inferomedially onto the anterior aspect of the iliac crest, pubis, and aponeurosis of the linea alba. It receives its innervation from many nerves including the lower intercostal, iliohypogastric, and ilioinguinal nerves. It acts to compress the abdominal cavity and assists with forward flexion and rotation of the trunk.

The internal oblique has its origin over the iliopsoas fascia, inguinal ligament, and iliac crest and has variable attachment to the thoracolumbar fascia. Its fibers run superolaterally and insert onto the lower ribs and aponeurosis of the linea alba. Its innervation and primary actions are similar to the external oblique. However, in contrast to the external oblique, rotation will be in the opposite direction. The transversus abdominis has its origin at the middle layer of the thoracolumbar fascia, iliac crest, iliopsoas fascia, and inguinal ligament. It inserts onto the aponeurosis of the linea alba and is innervated by the same nerves as the internal and external oblique muscles. The primary action of the transversus abdominis is compression of the abdominal cavity. It also plays an important role in force closure of the SIJ via its attachment to the thoracolumbar fascia (Fig. 3.9).

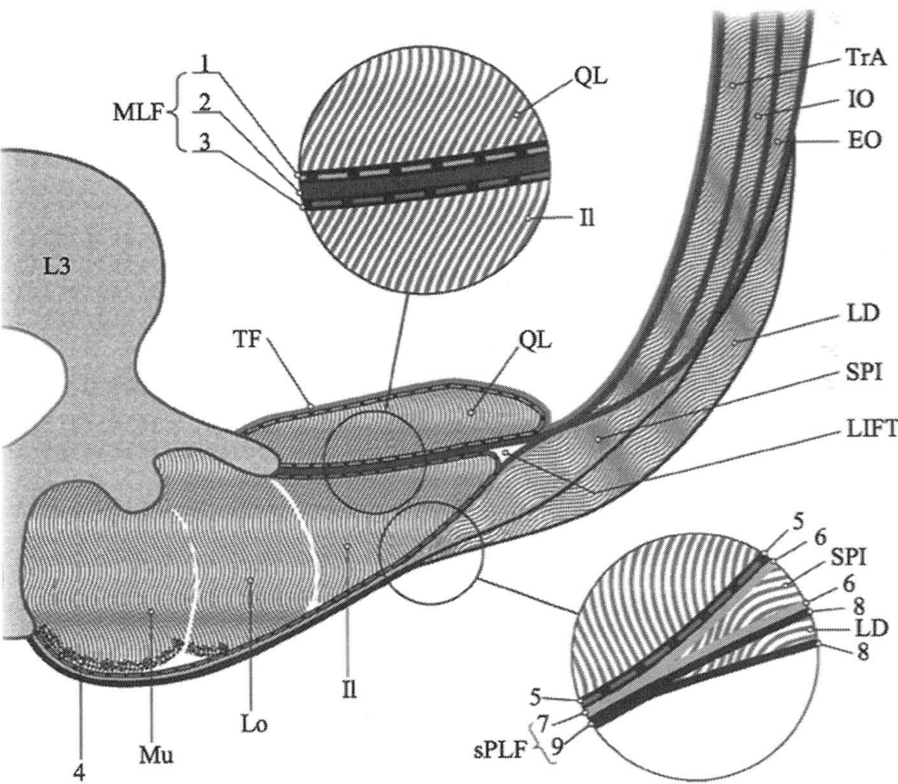

Fig. 3.9 The relationship of the thoracolumbar fascia and surrounding musculature. *EO* external oblique, *Il* iliocostalis lumborum, *IO* internal oblique, *LD* latissimus dorsi, *LIFT* lumbar interfascial triangle, *Lo* longissimus thoracis, *MLF* middle layer of the thoracolumbar fascia, *Mu* multifidus, *QL* quadratus lumborum, *SPI* serratus posterior inferior, *sPLF* superficial lamina of the posterior layer of the thoracolumbar fascia, *TF* transversalis fascia, *TrA* transversus abdominis. 1 = investing fascia of QL, 2 = aponeurosis of the abdominal muscles deriving from TrA, 3 = paraspinal retinacular sheath (PRS), 4 = aponeurosis of the paraspinal muscles, 5 = portion of the PRS composed of the deep lamina of the posterior layer of the thoracolumbar fascia, 6 = investing fascia of SPI, 7 = aponeurosis of SPI, 8 = investing fascia of LD, 9 = aponeurosis of LD [92]

The quadratus lumborum is deep to the transversus abdominis and has its origin over the medial aspect of the iliac crest. It inserts onto the twelfth rib and lower lumbar vertebrae and is innervated by the nerves of T12–L3. The primary action of the quadratus lumborum is lateral flexion of the vertebral column and fixation of the distal ribs to allow for proper contraction of the diaphragm.

The iliopsoas muscle group is composed of two muscles, the psoas major and iliacus. The psoas major has its origin on the bodies and transverse processes of the lumbar vertebrae and runs anteroinferiorly to insert on the lesser trochanter of the femur (Fig. 3.7). It is innervated by the second to fourth lumbar nerves and contributes to hip flexion (open chain) and lumbar flexion (closed chain). The iliacus has its origin over the iliac fossa, ventral sacroiliac ligament, iliolumbar ligament, and base of the sacrum and runs anteroinferiorly to insert on the lesser trochanter of the femur along with the psoas major. The iliacus is innervated by the femoral nerve and aids in hip flexion (open chain) and tilts the pelvis and sacrum ventrally (closed chain). Another muscle in close relation to the iliopsoas group is the psoas minor. The psoas minor is cephalad and ventral to the psoas major and has its origin at the twelfth thoracic and first lumbar vertebrae. It inserts on the superior ramus of the pubis and has the primary action of upward rotation of the pelvis.

The pelvic floor is composed of the levator ani, ischiococcygeus, iliococcygeus, and pubococcygeus. They form a sling through the pelvic ring and make up the floor of the abdominal cavity. The muscles of the pelvic floor activate up to 500 ms prior to any increases in intra-abdominal pressure and help support the pelvic viscera [33, 71]. They are also involved with respiration [33]. Contraction of these muscles can increase the stability of the pelvic ring and stiffness at the SIJ while also causing extension of the sacrum [61].

Posterior Muscles

The gluteus maximus has its origins, arcing from superolateral to inferomedial, at the gluteus medius fascia, ilium, thoracolumbar fascia, erector spinae aponeurosis, dorsal sacroiliac ligaments, sacrum, sacrotuberous ligament, and coccyx. The fascicle orientation runs inferolaterally at 32–45°, and two-thirds inserts onto the iliotibial band at its aponeurotic origin over the greater trochanter and the other one-third inserts onto the gluteal tuberosity [5]. The gluteus maximus attachment to the superficial lamina of the posterior layer of the thoracolumbar fascia is between the lower border of the PSIS and a point 1.0–2.0 cm lateral to the S3 spinous process [5], which then projects across the midline between L3 and S3. These fibers turn into the origin of the transitional component of the latissimus dorsi at L1–L2 and supraspinous ligament. The latissimus dorsi has five other components and origins at the lateral raphe of the thoracolumbar fascia and L3–L5 (raphe component), iliac crest 2.0–5.0 cm lateral to the lateral border of the erector spinae (iliac component), lower three ribs (costal component), lower six thoracic vertebrae and supraspinous ligaments (thoracic component), and inferior angle of scapula (scapular component) [9]. The latissimus dorsi inserts on the intertubercular sulcus of the humerus. In regard to innervation, the gluteus maximus and latissimus dorsi are innervated by the inferior gluteal nerve and thoracolumbar nerve, respectively. These two muscles have a reciprocal relationship during walking and have the ability to add stability to the SIJ, primarily from the action of the gluteus maximus whose fibers are oriented almost perpendicular to the SIJ [5, 9].

The posterior layer of the thoracolumbar fascia also consists of a deep lamina. The fibers of the deep lamina have their origin at the spinous processes of the lumbar vertebrae and run superomedial to inferolateral (30–40°) in contrast to the superficial lamina fibers, which run superolateral to inferomedial [8, 48, 82]. This opposition in fiber orientation gives the posterior layer of the thoracolumbar fascia a crosshatched appearance. The deep lamina has attachments with the sacrotuberous ligament, PSIS, iliac crest, and long dorsal ligament [82]. The deep lamina fuses with the serratus posterior inferior in the thoracic region. These two layers form a retinaculum over the epaxial muscles and are fused at the sacral levels (Fig. 3.9).

The erector spinae, which are a component of the epaxial muscles, consist of both the iliocostalis lumborum and longissimus thoracis. Both muscles have thoracic and lumbar components. The thoracic component of the iliocostalis lumborum runs from the lower ribs to the dorsal PSIS and iliac crest and the lumbar component runs from the tip of the lumbar transverse processes to the ventral iliac crest [47]. The thoracic component of the longissimus thoracis runs from the thoracic transverse processes and ribs to the lumbar and sacral spinous processes, dorsal aspect of the 4th sacral segment, and interspinous region of the posterior ilium. Its lumbar component runs from the lumbar transverse processes and accessory processes to the ventral aspect of the PSIS and iliac crest [47]. The thoracic fibers of the iliocostalis lumborum and longissimus thoracis form the erector spinae aponeurosis, which is freely mobile over the lumbar fibers [47]. The lumbar intermuscular aponeurosis, formed by the caudal tendons of the lumbar component of longissimus thoracis, separates the lumbar components of the iliocostalis lumborum and longissimus thoracis [47]. A cleavage plane separates the erector spinae from the multifidus. This cleavage plane runs from the medial aspect of the PSIS toward the L1 vertebra, curving cranial 2.0 cm lateral to the spinous process [47]. The multifidus originates at the lumbar spinous processes and laminae and inserts at the mammillary processes, inferomedial aspect of the PSIS, erector spinae aponeurosis, dorsal aspect of the sacrum to S4, and dorsal sacroiliac ligaments [49] (Fig. 3.8). It receives its innervation from the medial branch of the dorsal rami of the same segmental number.

The middle layer of the thoracolumbar fascia originates from the tips of the lumbar transverse processes and intertransverse ligaments to the border of the transversus abdominis where it blends with the posterior layer of the thoracolumbar fascia [8] (Fig. 3.9). This attachment lies lateral to the lateral border of the erector spinae and forms a dense lateral raphe. The posterior layer and middle layer of the thoracolumbar fascia form the paraspinal retinacular sheath around the epaxial muscles [71] (Fig. 3.9). Arising from the middle layer of the thoracolumbar fascia between the 12th rib and iliac crest is the transversus abdominis. The internal oblique has variable attachment to the thoracolumbar fascia but primarily arises from the iliac crest. Contraction of the deep abdominal muscles, primarily the transversus abdominis, provides lateral tension on the lateral raphe, which exerts a small extension force on the lumbar spine [48]. Lateral tension on the lateral raphe via the deep abdominal muscles combined with contraction of the epaxial muscles puts tension through the posterior and middle layers of the thoracolumbar fascia which compose the PRS. This tension and pressure can assist with lumbar extension from a flexed position via the hydraulic amplifier mechanism [8, 30, 71].

Ventral to the middle layer of the thoracolumbar fascia is the deep layer of the thoracolumbar fascia and dorsal border of the quadratus lumborum (Fig. 3.9). Ventral to the erector spinae and multifidus are the rotatores. The rotatores muscles have their origin at the sacrum and transverse processes of the vertebrae (lumbar to cervical). They insert on the spinous process of the vertebra one to two segments cephalad.

Lateral and ventral to the gluteus maximus is the gluteus medius. The gluteus medius has its origin over the lateral surface of the ilium between the anterior and posterior gluteal lines (Fig. 3.10).

It inserts onto the greater trochanter of the femur and is innervated by the superior gluteal nerve. Deep to the gluteus medius is the gluteus minimus. The gluteus medius and minimus are the primary hip abductors and play an important role in stabilizing the pelvis in the frontal plane during single-leg stance.

The piriformis muscle has its origin on the ventral surface of the sacrum (Fig. 3.11).

It runs laterally to insert onto the greater trochanter of the femur. It is innervated by the first and second sacral nerves and has the primary action of lateral rotation of the thigh. Other lateral rotators of the hip caudal to the piriformis are the superior gemellus, obturator internus, inferior gemellus, and quadratus femoris (Table 3.2).

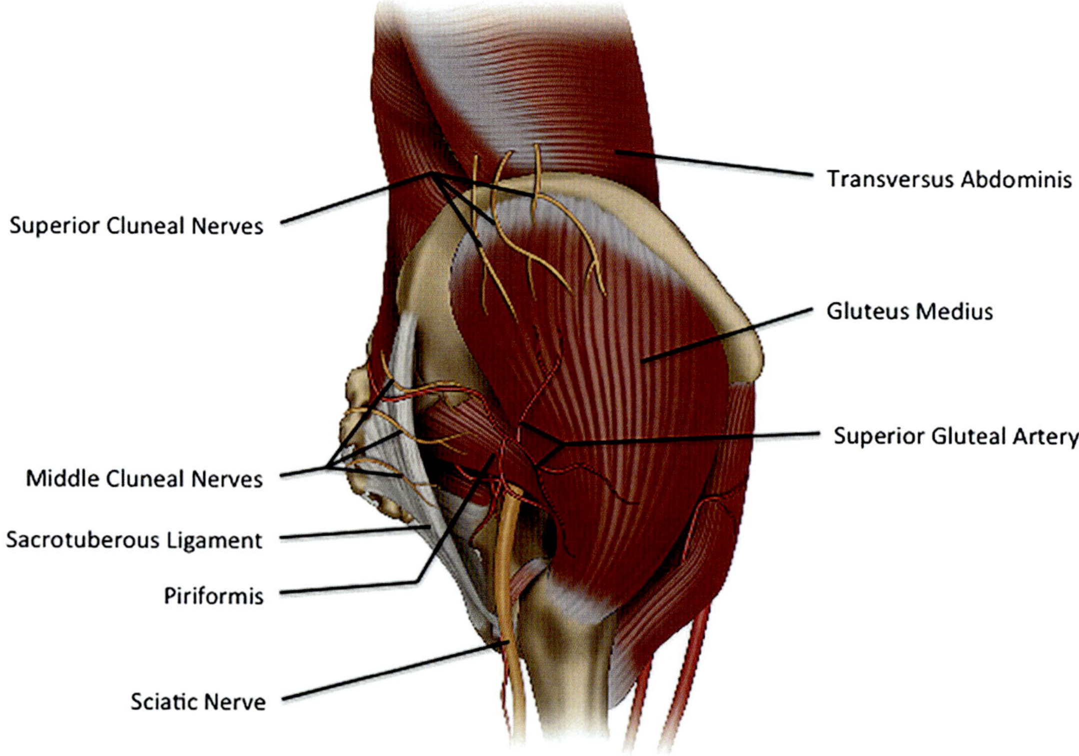

Fig. 3.10 Lateral view of the superficial musculature and neurovascular structures

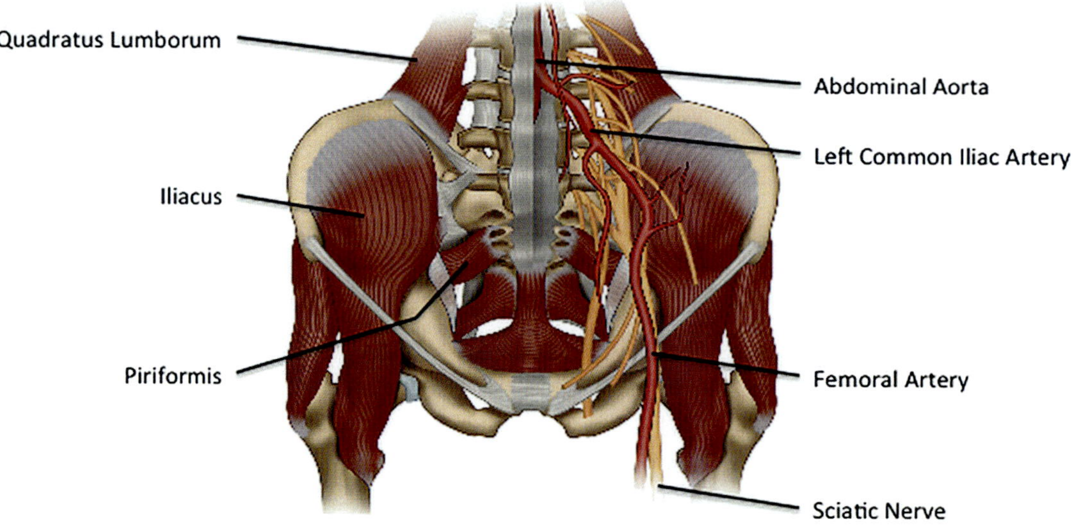

Fig. 3.11 Ventral view of the deep musculature and neurovascular structures

Table 3.2 Muscles and associated effects on the sacroiliac joint

Muscle	Primary action	Effect on SIJ
Erector spinae *Iliocostalis lumborum* *Longissimus thoracis*	Bilateral: back extension Unilateral: side bending	Hydraulic amplifier effect via PRS and TLF
Multifidus	Back extension, side bending, rotation	Imparts sacral flexion, force closure of SIJ with deep abdominals
Gluteus maximus	Hip extension, hip lateral rotation	Stabilizes SIJ due to perpendicular fiber orientation and attachment to TLF
Piriformis	Hip lateral rotation	May alter SIJ motion via direct attachment to ventral aspect of sacrum
Biceps femoris	Hip extension, knee flexion	Long head: Imparts sacral extension via attachment to sacrotuberous ligament
Deep abdominals *Transversus abdominis*	Compression of abdominal cavity	Force closure of SIJ via lateral raphe and TLF
Iliacus	Hip flexion (open chain) and tilts pelvis/sacrum ventrally (closed chain)	Synchronous tilting of the pelvis/sacrum ventrally (closed chain)
Pelvic floor	Support pelvic viscera	Imparts sacral extension

SIJ sacroiliac joint, *PRS* paraspinal retinacular sheath, *TLF* thoracolumbar fascia

Vasculature

Anterior Vasculature

The abdominal aorta descends through the abdomen and bifurcates into the left and right common iliac arteries at about the L4 vertebral body (Fig. 3.11). The common iliac arteries continue to descend, and each bifurcates into the internal and external iliac arteries. The internal iliac artery then divides into a posterior division and anterior division. Its posterior division gives rise to the superior gluteal, iliolumbar, and lateral sacral arteries. The iliolumbar artery begins medial to the SIJ [2] and courses over the cephalad aspect of the joint [26]. It gives off three distinct branches that perforate the medial iliacus and a descending lumbar branch that perforates the psoas major at the level of the greater sciatic notch [66]. The iliac nutrient artery originates off of the iliolumbar artery and courses across the SIJ to the nutrient foramen, located 2.0–2.4 cm cephalad to the pelvic brim and 1.2–1.8 cm lateral to the SIJ [2, 17]. Crossing the SIJ at the level of the first and second sacral foramen, the lateral sacral artery anastomoses with the middle sacral artery which branches off the abdominal aorta proximal to its bifurcation and travels down the midline of the lumbar vertebrae to the coccyx [26]. The anterior division of the internal iliac artery descends and gives off branches to the umbilical, obturator, inferior vesicle, middle rectal, pudendal, and inferior gluteal arteries. The external iliac artery continues caudally and lets off branches to the deep circumflex iliac and inferior epigastric arteries and then becomes the femoral artery as it passes under the inguinal ligament.

The corresponding veins for each artery follow a similar course. Of note, the internal iliac veins lie on the anterolateral surface of the sacral ala at about S1–S2 [58]. Also, the left common iliac vein lies dorsal and medial to the left common iliac artery, while the right common iliac vein lies dorsal and lateral to the right common iliac artery [23] (Table 3.3).

Table 3.3 Anterior vasculature and relationship to the sacroiliac joint

Vessel	Course	Relationship to SIJ
Iliolumbar artery	Medial to lateral	Crosses cephalad aspect of SIJ
Iliac Nutrient artery	Medial to lateral to nutrient foramen	Crosses SIJ
Sacral arteries *Medial* *Lateral*	Caudally over vertebral bodies Lateral to medial	Descends down midline of sacrum Crosses SIJ at S1–S2 level
Internal iliac vein	Superomedially	Lies on anterolateral surface of sacral ala (S1–S2)

SIJ sacroiliac joint

Posterior Vasculature

The superior gluteal artery exits the greater sciatic notch and courses cephalad about 5.4 cm toward the gluteal muscles [52] (Fig. 3.12).

It consists of a superficial branch, deep superior branch, and deep inferior branch. The superficial branch inserts into the gluteus maximus (three perforations), the deep superior branch inserts into the gluteus medius (five perforations) and gluteus minimus (one perforation), and the deep inferior branch inserts into the gluteus medius (four perforations) and gluteus minimus (two perforations) [21]. The distance between the superior gluteal artery, where it exits the greater sciatic notch and the PSIS, is about 6.2 cm [21, 93]. As the superior gluteal artery courses cephalad to the level of the PSIS, it can be found about 3.7 cm lateral to the PSIS and about 10.2 cm caudal to the iliac crest [93]. The deep superior branch is located about 2.9 cm dorsal and lateral to the ASIS at its closest muscular insertion [21].

The inferior gluteal artery originates from the internal iliac artery and passes dorsal to the sciatic nerve and sacrospinous ligament. It exits the pelvis 3.0–5.0 mm dorsal to the cephalad border of the sacrospinous ligament along with the sciatic nerve at the greater sciatic notch [78] (Fig. 3.12) (Table 3.4).

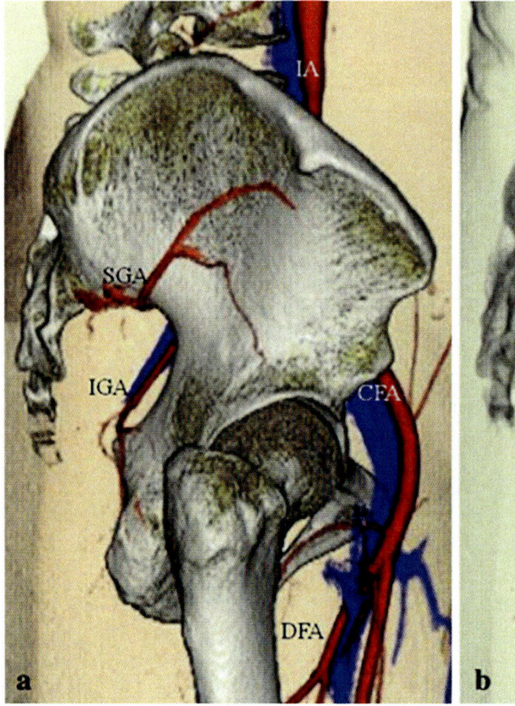

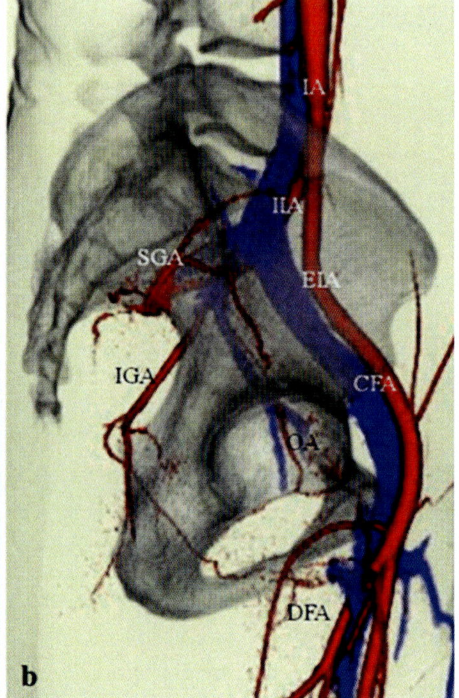

Fig. 3.12 A reconstructed 3D CT image of the right pelvis viewed from the lateral aspect. (**a**) Position of the SGA on the posterior ilium. (**b**) The right femur has been eliminated and the pelvic vasculature is viewed through the pelvis. Note the proximity of the SGA to the auricular surface of the sacroiliac joint. *CFA* common femoral artery, *DFA* deep femoral artery, *EIA* external iliac artery, *IA* iliac artery, *IGA* inferior gluteal artery, *IIA* internal iliac artery, *OA* obturator artery, *SGA* superior gluteal artery [36]

Table 3.4 Posterior vasculature and relationship to the sacroiliac joint

Vessel	Course	Relationship to SIJ
Superior gluteal artery	Exits greater sciatic notch and runs cephalad	From greater sciatic notch to PSIS: 6.2 cm
Inferior gluteal artery	Exits greater sciatic notch and runs caudal	Exits with sciatic nerve: 2.9 cm lateral, 0.7 cm caudal to SIJ

SIJ sacroiliac joint, *PSIS* posterior superior iliac spine

Nerves

Anterior Nerves

The lumbosacral plexus is composed of the distal lumbar nerves (L4 and L5) and sacral nerves (Fig. 3.13).

The L4 and L5 nerves course medial to the SIJ and lateral to the internal iliac vein where they join the S1 nerve root and sacral plexus [58]. The L4 nerve courses from 0.5 to 1.8 cm medial to the SIJ at the level of the sacral ala, while the L5 nerve courses about 1.3 cm medially at the same reference point [4, 87]. The junction where the lumbar nerves join the sacral nerves is found about 1.2 cm medial to the SIJ and is referred to as the lumbosacral trunk [4]. At the pelvic brim, the lumbosacral trunk is at its closest to the SIJ, from 0.1 to 1.0 cm medially [4, 20, 58].

Branches off the lumbar plexus (L1–L4) include the iliohypogastric, ilioinguinal, genitofemoral, lateral femoral cutaneous, femoral, obturator, and accessory obturator nerves. The lateral femoral cutaneous nerve emerges from the lateral border of the psoas major and crosses the iliacus deep to the iliacus fascia to the ASIS. It passes into the thigh medial to the ASIS and dorsal to the inguinal ligament, exiting 1.5–2.0 cm caudally [29]. In some, the lateral femoral cutaneous nerve crosses the iliac crest lateral to the ASIS [29]. The obturator nerve crosses the

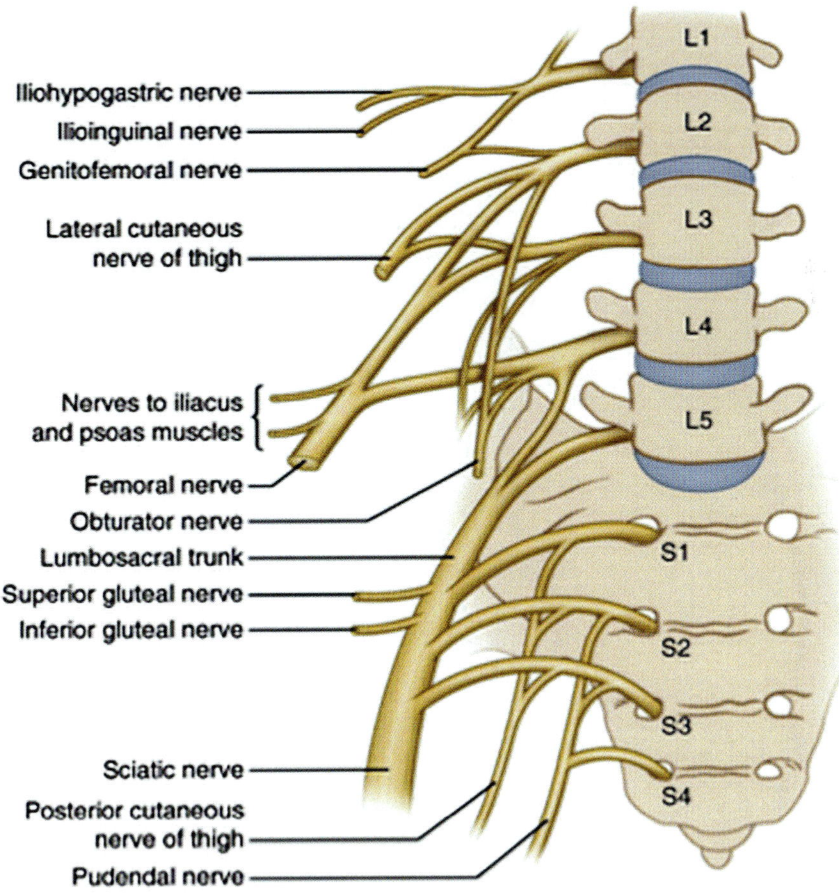

Fig. 3.13 The lumbosacral plexus in relation to the sacroiliac joint [3]

cephalad aspect of the SIJ, but does not contact the sacrum, and can be found about 1.0 cm cephalad from the arcuate line [26, 58]. The obturator and femoral nerves are lateral to the L4 nerve and encased in soft tissue [4].

The sacral nerves are medial to the SIJ and about 0.8 cm from the midline [87]. In relation to the caudal aspect of the SIJ, the S1, S2, and S3 nerves are located about 0.2, 1.7, and 2.4 cm medially in the coronal plane, respectively [87]. Branches off the lumbosacral plexus include the nerve to the quadratus femoris/inferior gemellus, nerve to the obturator internus/superior gemellus, nerve to the piriformis, superior gluteal, inferior gluteal, posterior femoral cutaneous, pudendal, tibial, and common peroneal nerves. The sciatic nerve is composed of the tibial and common peroneal nerves.

Other important neural structures in the area of the sacrum are the sympathetic chains. The sympathetic chains descend bilaterally and are adherent to the anterior sacrum. They course medial to the foramen and join the contralateral chain on the surface of the coccyx to form the ganglion impar [26] (Table 3.5).

Posterior Nerves

The sciatic nerve passes through the greater sciatic notch ventral to the piriformis and exits caudally between the piriformis and superior gemellus (Fig. 3.14).

The sciatic nerve is 0.9–1.5 cm wide and is found 2.9 cm lateral and 0.7 cm caudal to the most caudal aspect of the SIJ [7, 40]. In a small percentage of the population, the peroneal nerve passes through the piriformis muscle, while the tibial nerve passes caudally [7].

The superior cluneal nerves innervate the skin over the gluteus maximus and gluteus medius and are composed of the medial, intermediate, and lateral branches. They run dorsal to the quadratus lumborum and ventral to the deep layer of the thoracolumbar fascia, emerging cephalad to the iliac crest through the thoracolumbar fascia and latissimus dorsi [45, 79] (Figs. 3.10 and 3.14). The medial superior cluneal nerve originates from the L1 nerve root and is located about 8.0 cm lateral to the midline or 5.0–6.8 cm lateral to the PSIS along the iliac crest [45, 79, 93]. The intermediate superior cluneal nerve originates from the L2 nerve root and is located about 7.0 cm lateral to the PSIS along the iliac crest, while the lateral superior cluneal nerve originates from the L3 nerve root and is located about 7.3 cm lateral to the PSIS along the iliac crest [79]. Two to three of the superior cluneal nerves anastomose with each other caudal to the iliac crest.

The dorsal root ganglia of S1 are primarily located intraforaminal, while the dorsal root ganglia of S2, S3, and S4 are located intracanalar [14]. The lateral branch nerves of the dorsal rami exit the foramen lateral to the foraminal midline [94]. These branches take various paths and enter

Table 3.5 Anterior nerves and relationship to the sacroiliac joint

Nerve	Course	Relationship to SIJ
L4	Inferolaterally, medial to SIJ	At pelvic brim (lumbosacral trunk): 0.1–1.0 cm medial to SIJ
L5	Inferolaterally, medial to SIJ	At pelvic brim (lumbosacral trunk): 0.1–1.0 cm medial to SIJ
Sacral *S1* *S2* *S3*	Inferolaterally, medial to SIJ	From caudal aspect of SIJ: 0.2 cm medial 1.7 cm medial 2.4 cm medial
Obturator	Medial to lateral across SIJ	Crosses cephalad SIJ
Sympathetic chain	Caudally over ventral sacrum	Adherent to ventral aspect of sacrum, medial to foramen

SIJ sacroiliac joint

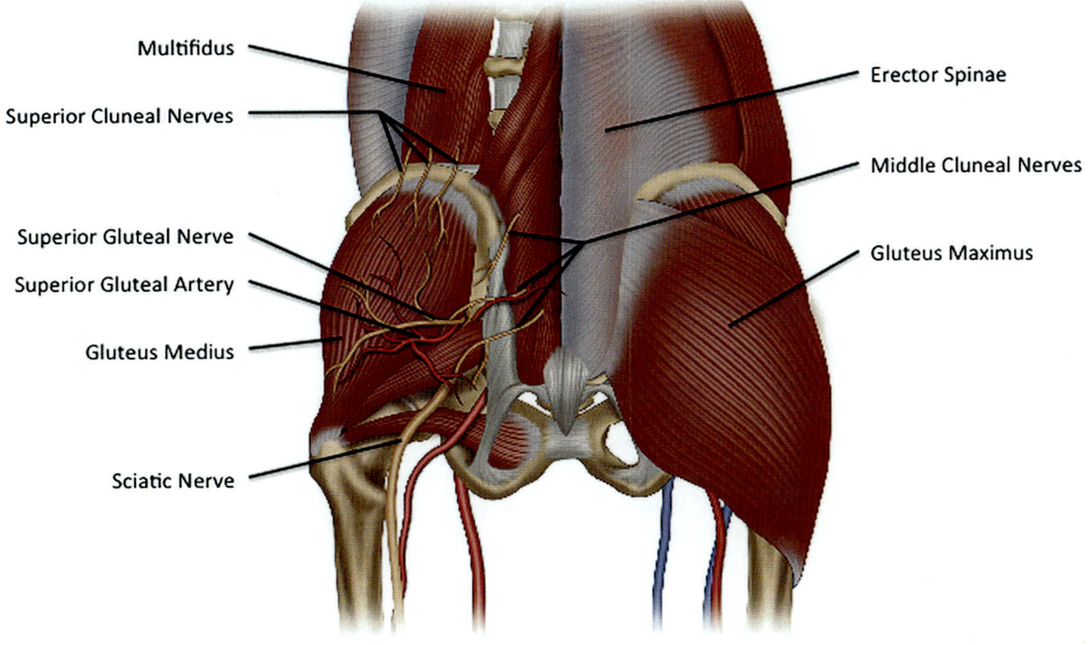

Fig. 3.14 Dorsal view of the superficial musculature and neurovascular structures

Table 3.6 Posterior nerves and relationship to the sacroiliac joint

Nerve	Course	Relationship to SIJ
Sciatic	Exits greater sciatic notch and runs caudal	From caudal aspect of SIJ: 2.9 cm lateral, 0.7 cm caudal
Superior cluneal	Exits cephalad to iliac crest and run caudal	5.0 cm lateral along iliac crest (*medial superior cluneal nerve*)
Middle cluneal	Inferolaterally from dorsal sacral foramina	Penetrate dorsal ligaments

SIJ sacroiliac joint

the dorsal ligaments and interosseous ligament on the way to different areas including the SIJ.

The middle cluneal nerves originate from the dorsal sacral foramina (S1–S3) and exit caudal to the PSIS [79]. They course inferolaterally, entering into the subcutaneous tissue over the gluteus maximus, and anastomose with the medial superior cluneal nerve (Figs. 3.10 and 3.14) (Table 3.6).

Biomechanics of the Sacroiliac Joint

The pelvic ring contains the SIJs dorsally and the pubic symphysis ventrally. Motion at the SIJ consists of a combination of rotation and translation in the sagittal, coronal, and axial planes. Movement of the sacrum in the sagittal plane can be described as sacral flexion or extension. Sacral flexion occurs when the base of the sacrum moves ventrally and the apex of the sacrum moves dorsally. Sacral extension is the opposite, with the sacral base moving dorsally, while the sacral apex moves ventrally. Sacral flexion is also referred to as nutation and sacral extension is referred to as counternutation. Total rotatory motion of the sacrum in the sagittal plane can reach 4°, with nutation and counternutation contributing about 2° each [38, 74, 86]. Translation in the sagittal plane ranges from 0.2 to 1.9 mm and is coupled with rotation [25, 38, 91]. The greatest changes in sagittal plane rotation and translation occur during position changes, especially with going from supine (nearly end-range sacral extension) to standing (nearly end-range sacral flexion).

Motion of the sacrum in the coronal plane is described as lateral side bending and consists of coupled rotation and translation. Rotation of the sacrum in the coronal plane can reach 1.9° with translation of about 1.1 mm during single-leg stance [25, 38]. The sacrum also moves within the axial plane. Motion in the axial plane is described as axial rotation and can reach 0.8° [57].

Force is transferred through the SIJ from the lower extremities to the trunk and from the trunk down to the lower extremities through the SIJs. Force through the SIJ can range from 3.5 to 7.0 MPa and is greatest with forward bending and side bending of the lumbar spine [37]. A leg-length discrepancy can alter biomechanics and lead to asymmetric forces through the SIJ. With a leg-length discrepancy of 2.0–3.0 cm, the force through the SIJ on the side with the longer limb can reach 10–20× that of an individual with relatively equal limb lengths. The force through the SIJ on the side with the shorter limb also increases 5–9× [37].

Motion at the pubic symphysis also consists of translation and rotation in all three planes. Translation in the sagittal, coronal, and axial planes can range from 1.0 to 2.0 mm [28, 89]. Larger translations are found in multiparous females and following traumatic injuries and can range from 3.0 to 10.0 mm [28, 89]. Rotation in the sagittal and coronal planes is about 0.5° [89].

Summary

The anatomy and biomechanics of the SIJs and surrounding areas are complex. The SIJs are relatively stable and allow little motion. Many muscles and ligaments are found in the area of the SIJs and knowledge of their relative influence on the SIJ and each other is important for all clinicians involved in the treatment of SIJ dysfunction. Vital structures, such as nerves and vasculature, are found in close proximity to the SIJs and need to be identified and avoided to prevent injury during invasive procedures. Structural variations are common and great care needs to be taken when operating on the SIJs.

References

1. Abitbol MM. Evolution of the lumbosacral angle. Am J Phys Anthropol. 1987;72:361–72.

2. Alla SR, Roberts CS, Ojike NI. Vascular risk reduction during anterior surgical approach sacroiliac joint plating. Injury. 2013;44(2):175–7.

3. Alpert JN. The neurologic diagnosis: a practical bedside approach. New York: Springer Science + Business Media LLC; 2012.

4. Atlihan D, Tekdemir I, Ates Y, Elhan A. Anatomy of the anterior sacroiliac joint with reference to lumbosacral nerves. Clin Orthop Relat Res. 2000;376:236–41.

5. Barker PJ, Hapuarachchi KS, Ross JA, Sambaiew E, Ranger TA, Briggs CA. Anatomy and biomechanics of gluteus maximus and the thoracolumbar fascia at the sacroiliac joint. Clin Anat. 2014;27(2):234–40. doi:10.1002/ca.22233.

6. Bechtel R. Physical characteristics of the axial interosseous ligament of the human sacroiliac joint. Spine J. 2001;1(4):255–9.

7. Benzon HT, Katz JA, Benzon HA, Iqbal MS. Piriformis syndrome: anatomic considerations, a new injection technique, and a review of the literature. Anesthesiology. 2003;98(6):1442–8.

8. Bogduk N, Macintosh JE. The applied anatomy of the thoracolumbar fascia. Spine. 1984;9:164–70.

9. Bogduk N, Johnson G, Spalding D. The morphology and biomechanics of latissimus dorsi. Clin Biomech (Bristol, Avon). 1998;13(6):377–85.

10. Bollow M, Braun J, Kannenberg J, et al. Normal morphology of sacroiliac joints in children: magnetic resonance studies related to age and sex. Skeletal Radiol. 1997;26(12):697–704.

11. Bowen V, Cassidy JD. Macroscopic and microscopic anatomy of the sacroiliac joint from embryonic life to the eighth decade. Spine (Phila Pa 1976). 1981;6: 620–8.

12. Castellvi AE, Goldstein LA, Chan DP. Lumbosacral transitional vertebrae and their relationship with lumbar extradural defects. Spine. 1984;9:493–5.

13. Delport EG, Cucuzella TR, Kim N, Marley J, Pruitt C, Delport AG. Lumbosacral transitional vertebrae: incidence in a consecutive patient series. Pain Physician. 2006;9:53–6.

14. Ebraheim NA, Lu J. Morphometric evaluation of the sacral dorsal root ganglia: a cadaveric study. Surg Radiol Anat. 1998;20(2):105–8.

15. Ebraheim NA, Lu J, Biyani A, Yeasting RA. Anatomic considerations for posterior approach to the sacroiliac joint. Spine (Phila Pa 1976). 1996; 21(23):2709–12.

16. Ebraheim NA, Lu J, Biyani A, Yeasting RA. Anatomic considerations of an anterior approach to the sacroiliac joint. Am J Orthop (Belle Mead NJ). 1996;25(10): 697–700.

17. Ebraheim NA, Lu J, Biyani A, Yang H. Anatomic considerations of the principle nutrient foramen and artery on internal surface of the ilium. Surg Radiol Anat. 1997;19(4):237–9.

18. Ebraheim NA, Lu J, Yang H, Heck BE, Yeasting RA. Anatomic considerations of the second sacral vertebra and dorsal screw placement. Surg Radiol Anat. 1997;19:353–7.

19. Ebraheim NA, Mekhail AO, Wiley WF, Jackson WT, Yeasting RA. Radiology of the sacroiliac joint. Spine (Phila Pa 1976). 1997;22(8):869–76.

20. Ebraheim NA, Padanilam TG, Waldrop JT, Yeasting RA. Anatomic consideration in the anterior approach to the sacro-iliac joint. Spine (Phila Pa 1976). 1994;19(6):721–5.

21. Ebraheim NA, Olexa TA, Xu R, Georgiadis G, Yeasting RA. The quantitative anatomy of the superior gluteal artery and its location. Am J Orthop (Belle Mead NJ). 1998;27(6):427–31.

22. Ebraheim NA, Xu R, Biyani A, Nadaud MC. Morphologic considerations of the first sacral pedicle for iliosacral screw placement. Spine (Phila Pa 1976). 1997;22(8):841–6.

23. Ebraheim NA, Xu R, Farooq A, Yeasting RA. The quantitative anatomy of the iliac vessels and their relation to anterior lumbosacral approach. J Spinal Disord. 1996;9(5):414–7.

24. Eichenseer PH, Sybert DR, Cotton JR. A finite element analysis of sacroiliac joint ligaments in response to different loading conditions. Spine (Phila Pa 1976). 2011;36:1446–52.

25. Egund N, Ollson TH, Schmid H, Selvik G. Movements in the sacroiliac joints demonstrated with roentgen stereophotogrammetry. Acta Radiol Diagn. 1978;19:833–46.

26. Esses SI, Botsford DJ, Huler RJ, Rauschning W. Surgical anatomy of the sacrum. A guide for rational screw fixation. Spine (Phila Pa 1976). 1991;16(6 Suppl):S283–8.

27. Fortin JD, Vilensky JA, Merkel GJ. Can the sacroiliac joint cause sciatica? Pain Physician. 2003;6:269–71.

28. Garras DN, Carothers JT, Olson SA. Single-leg-stance (flamingo) radiographs to assess pelvic instability: how much motion is normal? J Bone Joint Surg Am. 2008;90:2114–8.

29. Ghent WR. Further studies on meralgia paresthetica. Can Med Assoc J. 1961;85:871–5.

30. Gracovetsky S, Farfan HF, Lamy C. A mathematical model of the lumbar spine using an optimized system to control muscles and ligaments. Orthop Clin North Am. 1977;8:135–53.

31. Hammer N, Steinke H, Bohme J, et al. Description of the iliolumbar ligament for computer-assisted reconstruction. Ann Anat. 2010;192:162–7.

32. Harmon D, O'Sullivan M. Ultrasound-guided sacroiliac joint injection technique. Pain Physician. 2008;11(4):543–7.

33. Hodges PW, Sapsford R, Pengel LH. Postural and respiratory functions of the pelvic floor muscles. Neurourol Urodyn. 2007;26:362–71.

34. Jaovisidha S, Ryu KN, DeMaeseneer M, et al. Ventral sacroiliac ligament: anatomic and pathologic considerations. Invest Radiol. 1996;31(8):532–41.

35. Kampen WU, Tillmann B. Age-related changes in the articular cartilage of human sacroiliac joint. Anat Embryol (Berl). 1998;198(6):505–13.

36. Kawasaki Y, Hiroshi E, Hamada D, Takao S, Nakano S, Yasui N. Location of intrapelvic vessels around the acetabulum assessed by three-dimensional computed tomographic angiography: prevention of vascular related complications in total hip arthroplasty. J Orthop Sci. 2012;17(4):397–406.

37. Kiapour A, Abdelgawad AA, Goel VK, et al. Relationship between limb length discrepancy and load distribution across the sacroiliac joint – a finite element study. J Orthop Res. 2012;30:1577–80.

38. Kissling RO, Jacob HA. The mobility of the sacroiliac joint in healthy subjects. Bull Hosp Jt Dis. 1996;54(3):158–64.

39. Kiter E, Karaboyun T, Tufan AC, et al. Immunohistochemical demonstration of nerve endings in iliolumbar ligament. Spine (Phila Pa 1976). 2010;35:E101–4.

40. Lanzieri CG, Hilal SK. Computed tomography of the sacral plexus and sciatic nerve in the greater sciatic foramen. AJR Am J Roentgenol. 1984;143:165–8.

41. LeBlanche AF, Mabi C, Bigot JM, et al. The sacroiliac joint: anatomical study in the coronal plane and MR correlation. Surg Radiol Anat. 1996;18:215–20.

42. Leong JCY, Luk KDK, Chow DHK, Woo CW. The biomechanical functions of the iliolumbar ligament in maintaining stability of the lumbosacral junction. Spine. 1987;12:669–74.

43. Ling BC, Lee JW, Man HS, Jhangri GS, Grace MG, Lambert RG. Transverse morphology of the sacroiliac joint: effect of angulation and implications for fluoroscopically guided sacroiliac joint injection. Skeletal Radiol. 2006;35(11):838–46.

44. Loukas M, Louis RG, Hallner B, et al. Anatomical and surgical considerations of the sacrotuberous ligament and its relevance in pudendal nerve entrapment syndrome. Surg Radiol Anat. 2006;28(2):163–9.

45. Lu J, Ebraheim NA, Huntoon M, Heck BE, Yeasting RA. Anatomic considerations of superior cluneal nerve at posterior iliac crest region. Clin Orthop Relat Res. 1998;347:224–8.

46. Lu J, Ebraheim NA, Yang H, Heck BE. Anatomic evaluation of the first three sacral vertebrae and dorsal screw placement. Am J Orthop (Belle Mead NJ). 2000;29(5):376–9.

47. Macintosh JE, Bogduk N. The morphology of the lumbar erector spinae. Spine. 1987;12:658–68.

48. Macintosh JE, Bogduk N, Gracovetsky S. The biomechanics of the thoracolumbar fascia. Clin Biomech (Bristol, Avon). 1987;2:78–83.

49. Macintosh JE, Valencia FP, Bogduk N, et al. The morphology of the human lumbar multifidus. Clin Biomech. 1986;1:196–204.

50. Mahato NK. Redefining lumbosacral transitional vertebrae (LSTV) classification: integrating the full spectrum of morphological alterations in a biomechanical

continuum. Med Hypotheses. 2013, http://dx.doi.org/10.1016/j.mehy.2013.02.026

51. Mahato NK. Relationship of sacral articular surfaces and gender with occurrence of lumbosacral transitional vertebrae. Spine J. 2011;11:961–5.

52. Marmor M, Lynch T, Matityahu A. Superior gluteal artery injury during iliosacral screw placement due to aberrant anatomy. Orthopedics. 2010;33(2):117–20.

53. McGrath C, Nicholson H, Hurst P. The long posterior sacroiliac ligament: a histological study of morphological relations in the posterior sacroiliac region. Joint Bone Spine. 2009;76(1):57–62.

54. McGrath MC, Zhang M. Lateral braches of dorsal sacral nerve plexus and the long posterior sacroiliac ligament. Surg Radiol Anat. 2005;27:327–30.

55. McLauchlan GJ, Gardner DL. Sacral and iliac articular cartilage thickness and cellularity: relationship to subchondral bone end-plate thickness and cancellous bone density. Rheumatology. 2002;41:375–80.

56. Miller MD, Cain JE, Lauerman WC, et al. Posterior sacroiliac fixation using a sacral pedicle targeting device: an anatomical study. J Orthop Trauma. 1993;7(6):514–20.

57. Miller JA, Schultz AB, Andersson GB. Load-displacement behavior of sacroiliac joints. J Orthop Res. 1987;5:92–101.

58. Mirkovic S, Abitbol JJ, Steinman J, et al. Anatomic consideration for sacral screw placement. Spine (Phila Pa 1976). 1991;16(6 Suppl):S289–94.

59. Mitchell GAG. The significance of lumbosacral transitional vertebrae. Br J Surg. 1936;24(93):147–58.

60. Nardo L, Alizai H, Virayavanich W, Liu F, Hernandez A, Lynch JA, Nevitt MC, McCulloch CE, Lane NE, Link TM. Lumbosacral transitional vertebrae: association with low back pain. Radiology. 2012;265(2):497–503.

61. Pool-Goudzwaard AL, van Dijke GA H, van Gurp M, Mulder P, Snijders CJ, Stoeckart R. Contribution of pelvic floor muscles to stiffness of the pelvic ring. Clin Biomech. 2004;19:564–71.

62. Pool-Goudzwaard AL, Kleinrensink GJ, Entius C, Snijders CJ, Stoeckart R. The sacroiliac part of the iliolumbar ligament. J Anat. 2001;199:457–63.

63. Puhakka KB, Melsen F, Jurik AG, et al. MR imaging of the normal sacroiliac joint with correlation to histology. Skeletal Radiol. 2004;33(1):15–28.

64. Rosatelli AL, Agur AM, Chhaya S. Anatomy of the interosseous region of the sacroiliac joint. J Orthop Sports Phys Ther. 2006;36:200–8.

65. Rucco V, Basadonna PT, Gasparini D. Anatomy of the iliolumbar ligament. Am J Phys Med Rehab. 1996;75:451–5.

66. Rusu MC, Cergan R, Dermengiu D, et al. The iliolumbar artery-anatomic considerations and details on the common iliac artery trifurcation. Clin Anat. 2010;23(1):93–100.

67. Sabry FF, Xu R, Nadim Y, Ebraheim NA. Bone density of the first sacral vertebra in relation to sacral screw placement: a computer tomography study. Orthopedics. 2001;24(5):475–7.

68. Sakamoto N, Yamashita T, Takabayashi EA. An electrophysiologic study of mechanoreceptors in the sacroiliac joint and adjacent tissues. Spine (Phila Pa 1976). 2001;26:E468–71.

69. Salsabili N, Valojerdy MR, Hogg DA. Variations in thickness of articular cartilage in the human sacroiliac joint. Clin Anat. 1995;8(6):388–90.

70. Sapsford RR, Hodges PW. Contraction of the pelvic floor muscles during abdominal manoeuvres. Arch Phys Med Rehabil. 2001;82:1081–8.

71. Schuenke MD, Vleeming A, Van Hoof T, et al. A description of the lumbar interfascial triangle and its relation with the lateral raphe: anatomical constituents of load transfer through the lateral margin of the thoracolumbar fascia. J Anat. 2012;221:568–76. doi:10.1111/j.1469-7580.2012.01517.x.

72. Smucker JD, Akhavan S, Furey C. Understanding bony safety zones in the posterior iliac crest: an anatomic study from the Hamann-Todd collection. Spine (Phila Pa 1976). 2010;35(7):725–9.

73. Snijders CJ, Hermans PF, Niesing R, et al. Effects of slouching and muscle contraction on the strain of the iliolumbar ligament. Man Ther. 2008;13:325–33.

74. Sturesson B, Uden A, Vleeming A. A radiostereometric analysis of movements of the sacroiliac joints during the standing hip flexion test. Spine. 2000;25(3):364–8.

75. Szadek KM, Hoogland PV, Zuurmond WW, et al. Nociceptive nerve fibers in the sacroiliac joint in humans. Reg Anesth Pain Med. 2008;33:36–43.

76. Szadek KM, Hoogland PV, Zuurmond WW, et al. Possible nociceptive structures in the sacroiliac joint cartilage: an immunohistochemical study. Clin Anat. 2010;23:192–8.

77. Tague RG. Fusion of coccyx to sacrum in humans; prevalence, correlates, and effect on pelvic size, with obstetrical and evolutionary implications. Am J Phys Anthropol. 2011;145:426–37.

78. Thompson JR, Gibb JS, Genadry R, et al. Anatomy of pelvic arteries adjacent to the sacrospinous ligament: importance of the coccygeal branch of the inferior gluteal artery. Obstet Gynecol. 1999;94(6):973–7.

79. Tubbs RS, Levin MR, Loukas M, et al. Anatomy and landmarks for the superior and middle cluneal nerves: application to posterior iliac crest harvest and entrapment syndromes. J Neurosurg Spine. 2010;13(3):356–9.

80. van Wingerden JP, Vleeming A, Snijders CJ, et al. A functional-anatomical approach to the spine-pelvis mechanism: interaction between the biceps femoris muscle and the sacrotuberous ligament. Eur Spine J. 1993;2:140–4.

81. Vleeming A, Pool-Goudzwaard AL, Hammudoghlu D, et al. The function of the long dorsal sacroiliac ligament: its implication for understanding low back pain. Spine (Phila Pa 1976). 1996;21(5):556–62.

82. Vleeming A, Pool-Goudzwaard AL, Stoeckart E. The posterior layer of the thoracolumbar fascia. Its function in load transfer from spine to legs. Spine (Phila Pa 1976). 1995;20(7):753–8.

83. Vleeming A, Snijders CJ, Stoeckart R. The sacrotuberous ligament: a conceptual approach to its dynamic

role in stabilizing the SI-joint. Clin Biomech. 1989;4:201–3.

84. Vleeming A, Stoeckart R, Volkers AC, et al. Relation between form and function in the sacroiliac joint. Part I: clinical anatomical aspects. Spine (Phila Pa 1976). 1990;15:130–2.

85. Vleeming A, van Wingerden JP, Snijders CJ, et al. Load application to the sacrotuberous ligament; influences of sacroiliac joint mechanics. Clin Biomech. 1989;4(4):204–9.

86. Vleeming A, van Wingerden JP, Snijders CJ, et al. Mobility in the sacroiliac joints in the elderly: a kinematic and radiological study. Clin Biomech. 1992;7:170–6.

87. Waikakul S, Chandraphak S, Sangthongsil P. Anatomy of L4 to S3 nerve roots. J Orthop Surg. 2010;18(3): 352–5.

88. Waldrop JT, Ebraheim NA, Yeasting RA, Jackson WT. The location of the sacroiliac joint on the outer table of the posterior ilium. J Orthop Trauma. 1993; 7(6):510–3.

89. Walheim GG, Olerud S, Ribbe T. Motion of the pubic symphysis in pelvic instability. Scand J Rehabil Med. 1984;16:163–9.

90. Weisl H. The articular surfaces of the sacro-iliac joint and their relation to the movements of the sacrum. Acta Anat. 1954;22:1–14.

91. Weisl H. The movements of the sacro-iliac joint. Acta Anat. 1955;23:80–91.

92. Willard FH, Vleeming A, Schuenke MD, et al. The thoracolumbar fascia: anatomy, function, and clinical considerations. J Anat. 2012;221:507–36.

93. Xu R, Ebraheim NA, Yeasting RA, Jackson WT. Anatomic considerations for posterior iliac bone harvesting. Spine (Phila Pa 1976). 1996;21(9): 1017–20.

94. Yin W, Willard F, Carreiro J, et al. Sensory stimulation-guided sacroiliac joint radiofrequency neurotomy: technique based on neuroanatomy of the dorsal sacral plexus. Spine (Phila Pa 1976). 2003;28:2419–25.

Bruce E. Dall, Sonia V. Eden, Brandon Bucklen,
Mark Moldavsky, and Robert W. Mcnutt

Introduction

The normal range of motion (ROM) of the sacro-iliac joint (SIJ) has been measured in various ways and has been found to be minimal under normal conditions [1–4]. There are clinical situations where the SIJ has been "out of alignment" or has been "realigned" by the clinician based on external anatomical clinical findings. Controversy continues to exist regarding SIJ ROM in terms of stability in both clinical and surgical situations.

This chapter discusses what happens to the ROM of the SIJ when the posterior supporting ligament structures are sequentially transected after which adjacent joint (L5–S1) stabilization is performed. Clinical relevance is then discussed based on these findings.

Hypothesis

The working hypothesis for this experiment was that, after defining the ligament intact SIJ ROM in cadaver specimens, which is estimated to be between 2 and 6° based on the literature [1–4], the ROM would increase significantly with each successive posterior ligament transection and that a further increase in SIJ ROM would occur in this posterior ligament injured joint with the addition of L5–S1 fixation.

Materials and Methods

Specimen Preparation

Seven fresh human lumbar spines from L3 to the pelvis were used in the study (4M, 3F; 53 ± 11 years old). Specimens were stored in double plastic bags at −20 °C. After thawing overnight, the spines were dissected by carefully removing paravertebral musculature while avoiding disruption of spinal ligaments, joint capsules, joints, and intervertebral disks. The spines were

B.E. Dall, M.D. (✉)
Neurosurgery of Kalamazoo, Borgess Brain and
Spine Institute, Orthopedic Spine Division, Western
Michigan University Medical School, Kalamazoo,
MI, USA
e-mail: dall.bruce@yahoo.com

S.V. Eden, M.D.
Department of Neurological Surgery,
Borgess Brain and Spine Institute, Western Michigan
University Medical School, Kalamazoo, MI, USA

B. Bucklen, Ph.D. • M. Moldavsky, B.S., M.S.
Globus Medical Inc., 2560 General Armistead Ave.,
Audubon, PA 19403, USA
e-mail: bbucklen@globusmedical.com;
mmoldavsky@globusmedical.com

R.W. Mcnutt, B.S., M.S.
Statistical Consulting Center, Western Michigan
University, Kalamazoo, MI 49008, USA
e-mail: robert.w.mcnutt@wmich.edu

B.E. Dall et al. (eds.), *Surgery for the Painful, Dysfunctional Sacroiliac Joint,*
DOI 10.1007/978-3-319-10726-4_4, © Springer International Publishing Switzerland 2015

fixed proximally at L3 and distally at the pelvis, in a three-to-one mixture of bond auto body filler and fiberglass resin (Bondo MarHyde Corp, Atlanta, GA). The sacrum and pubic symphysis were free to move. Saline (0.9 %) was used throughout testing so the specimens remained moist and retained their viscoelastic properties.

Flexibility Testing

The spines were placed on a custom built six degree-of-freedom testing machine and held in place with high-powered magnets. Pure unconstrained bending moments were applied in flexion–extension, lateral bending, and axial rotation using a multidirectional flexibility protocol [5–7]. The six degree-of-freedom machine applies unconstrained loading through three cephalad stepper motors located in each of the three physiological rotation axes [8–12]. Moreover, the supports are mounted on air bearings to provide near frictionless resistance to the natural kinematics of the spine, which allows the spine to be unconstrained during load application. To account for the viscoelasticity of tissue, data was taken from the third cycle. A load control protocol with servomotors applying a pure moment at L3 at a rate of $1.5°$ per second to a maximum moment of ± 8.5 Nm, in all three planes, was performed (Fig. 4.1).

Range of Motion

Plexiglass markers, each having three infrared light-emitting diodes, were secured rigidly to L3, L4, L5, sacrum, left iliac crest, and right iliac crest via bone screws to track motion using the Optotrak Certus (NDI, Inc., Waterloo, Canada) motion analysis system. The location of the markers (denoting a rigid body) is aligned approximately sagittal along the curvature of the spine. The Optotrak Certus software superimposes the coordinate systems of two adjacent vertebral bodies in order to inferentially determine the relative Eulerian rotations in each of the three planes.

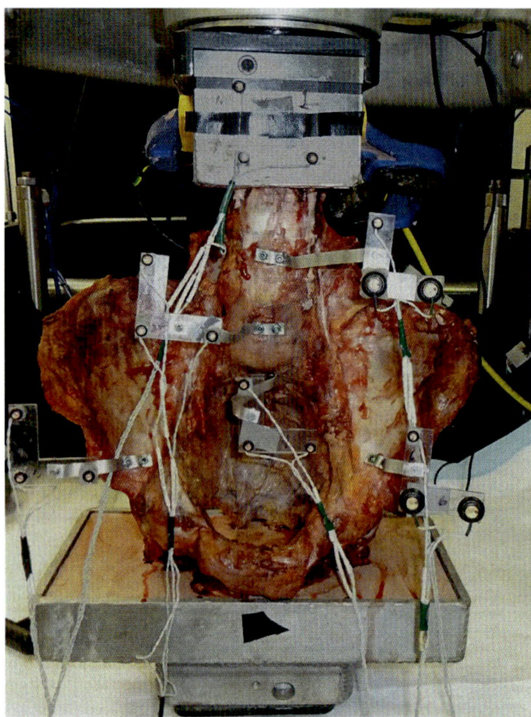

Fig. 4.1 Specimen mounted on six degree-of-freedom spine tester with rigid body markers for motion tracking

Surgical Reconstruction Groups

All specimens were tested intact with no damage to ligaments or bones. The REVERE® Stabilization System (Globus Medical Inc., Audubon, PA) was used for the 5.5 mm-diameter rigid titanium rod construct. Each of the seven specimens were tested in the following order: (1) intact; (2) left side sacrotuberous ligament (cephalad portion) injury (L-STL cut); (3) left side dorsal sacroiliac and interosseous ligaments injury (L-DSIL + L-IL cut), with the cumulative injury resulting in a transection of the entire left posterior ligament complex (L-PL complex cut); and (4) L5–S1 rigid instrumentation (L5–S1 rigid) placed adjacent to the posterior ligament injured SIJ. L-STL cut construct was performed by carefully dissecting the cephalad portion of the sacrotuberous ligament at a point just below the posterior superior iliac spine. Rongeur and a scalpel were used to completely transect the ligament (Fig. 4.2).

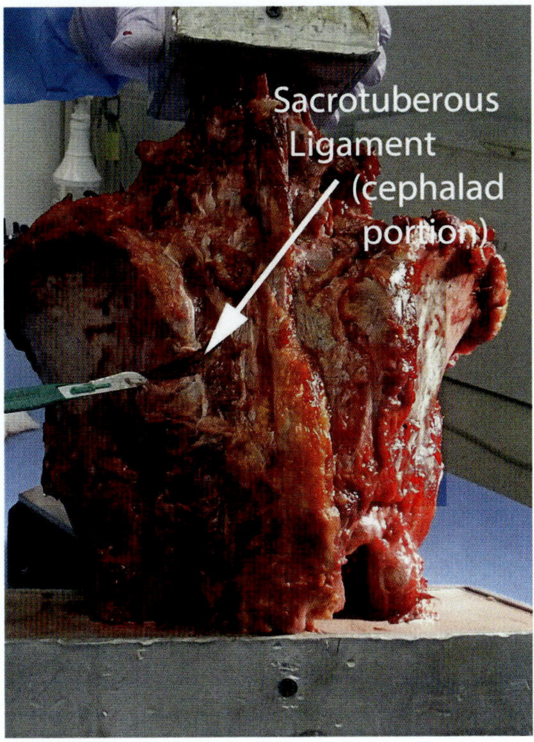

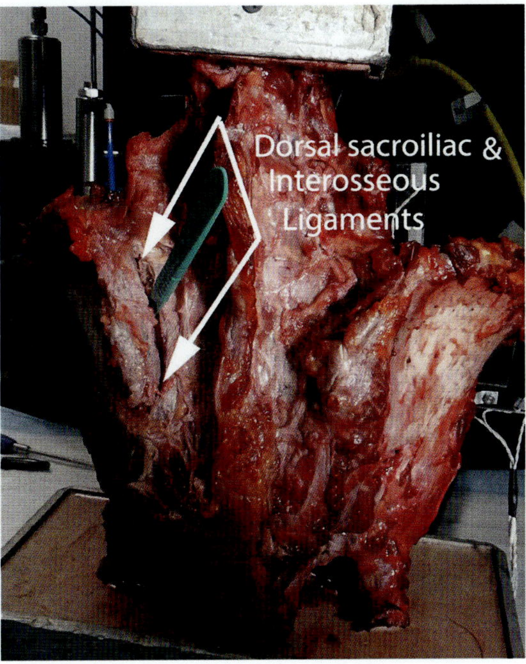

Fig. 4.2 Specimen with transected posterior sacrotuberous ligament (cephalad portion)

Fig. 4.3 Specimen, with previous transection of the posterior sacrotuberous ligament, now with the additional transection of the dorsal sacroiliac ligament and the interosseous ligament. This constitutes a transection of the entire posterior supporting ligament structure for the SIJ

The L-PL complex cut construct was created by inserting the scalpel into the entire junction of the posterior iliac crest and sacrum from its most cephalad to its most caudal borders transecting all of dorsal sacroiliac and interosseous ligaments down to the joint (Fig. 4.3).

Statistical Analysis

The data points include one range of motion measurement per specimen, under uniform stresses, for three different directions. These measurements were taken at each of the ten stages mentioned above, including intact, simulated injuries and stabilization constructs. For raw data, see Appendix B.

To test the hypotheses, analysis involved paired comparisons of range of motion measurements between each of the first four successive measurements. The Shapiro–Wilks normality test was applied to the measurements for each stage to check assumptions of the paired t-test. While more than half of the individual samples were found to diverge significantly from normality, it is acknowledged that the power of any such test is rather limited for such a small sample size. Therefore, the Wilcoxon sign test was also implemented. Note the agreement of significance (at $\alpha = 0.05$) between the two tests in Table 4.1.

Small sample sizes leave a question of power in the ability to detect differences. Using the average sample standard deviations over three directions, e.g.,

$$S_{\text{intact}\to\text{ISL cut}} = \left(S_{\text{F/E:intact}\to\text{ISL cut}} + S_{\text{lateral bend:intact}\to\text{ISL cut}} + S_{\text{axial rotation:intact}\to\text{ISL cut}} \right)/3$$

Table 4.1 Comparisons of range of motion measurements

Flexion–extension	Intact → STL cut	STL cut → PLC cut	PLC cut → L5–S1 rods
Change in ROM tested	Increase	Increase	Increase
t-stat (*p*-val)	0.0258	0.0316	0.0082
W-sgn (*p*-val)	0.0391	0.0078	0.0078
Significance	Yes	Yes	Yes
Lateral bend	Intact → STL cut	STL cut → PLC cut	PLC cut → L5–S1 rods
Change in ROM tested	Increase	Increase	Increase
t-stat (*p*-val)	0.6321	0.0518	0.7157
W-sgn (*p*-val)	0.7693	0.0574	0.7081
Significance	No	No	No
Axial rotation	Intact → STL cut	STL cut → PLC cut	PLC cut → L5–S1 rods
Change in ROM tested	Increase	Increase	Increase
t-stat (*p*-val)	0.5539	0.0283	0.1849
W-sgn (*p*-val)	0.6238	0.018	0.3057
Significance	No	Yes	No

The power curves are shown in Figs. 4.4 and 4.5.

Variables with Statistical Significance

The following statistically significant ($p < 0.05$) results were found:

- SIJ ROM in F/E increased with each successive posterior ligament (STL + DSIL and IL) transection.
- SIJ ROM in axial rotation increased only after all posterior ligaments (STL + DSIL and IL) were transected.
- SIJ ROM in F/E increased in the posterior ligament injured joint with the addition of L5–S1 posterior fixation.

Conclusions Verses Hypothesis

The average SIJ ROM with intact ligaments was very small and in ranges of 1° or less. With the transection of the STL, ROM increased in only

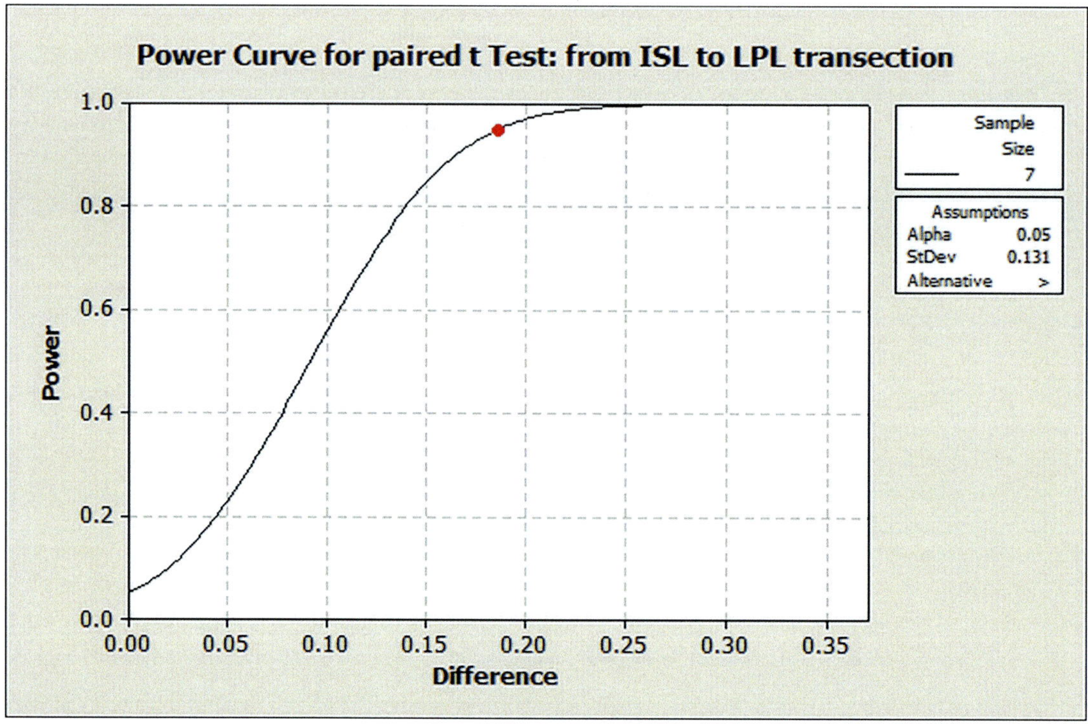

Fig. 4.4 Power curve for paired *t*-test: from ISL to L-PL transection

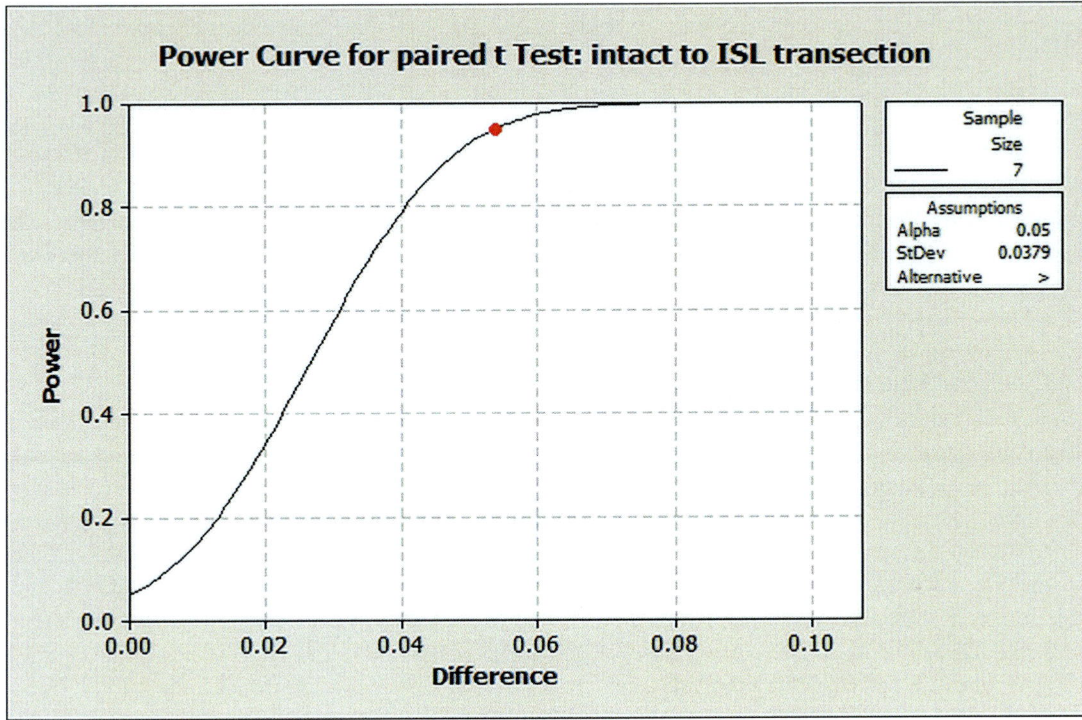

Fig. 4.5 Power curve for paired *t*-test: intact to ISL transection

the F/E plane, and with the subsequent transection of the DSIL and IL, ROM increased for the first time in axial rotation and further in F/E. Only one specimen increased its ROM past 2° (Chap. 18, Appendix two) despite posterior ligament transection and adjacent joint fixation. Thus, the larger "grossly destabilizing" ROMs hypothesized after transecting the posterior supporting ligaments were not realized. With the addition of L5–S1 pedicle screw and rod fixation, there did occur a further increase in the ROM of the posterior ligament injured SIJ in only the F/E plane and not in lateral bend or axial rotation.

Clinical Importance of Study Conclusions

The ROM of the SIJ is very minimal, even in its posterior ligament injured state, with ROMs averaging overall in the 1–2° range. These findings agree with our ROM findings in surgery when performing a posterior SIJ fusion after all the posterior ligaments are removed, as in this experiment, to access the joint in a patient who is asleep and paralyzed (Chap. 9). Given this knowledge, one must question what is really happening on a gross clinical level when this joint is "out of alignment" or the clinician has "put the joint back in place" in the absence of significant clinical trauma.

The transection of the posterior ligaments, the major known posterior stabilizers for the SIJ, did not render the SIJ grossly unstable (no measures > 2°) resulting in the need to further reflect on the importance of these structures in SIJ stability and if such small resulting changes in ROM are of clinical importance.

The addition of lumbosacral fixation does increase the F/E ROM of the posterior ligament injured SIJ. This result is in line with papers published on increased stresses on joints adjacent to rigidly fixated joints in the lumbar spine and increased changes in the SIJ with adjacent lumbosacral fusions [13–17].

Discussion

We know that the SIJ can become severely symptomatic with pain as a result of gross dislocation secondary to significant trauma and also in some patients with ligament stretching and/or tears secondary to the hormonal changes in late term pregnancy and/or vaginal delivery [18–22]. We also know that this joint can be rendered asymptomatic by subsequent rigid fixation [1, 23–25] and with the healing effects of the postpartum time period during which stiffening of the SIJ ligaments occurs. One of these results in the theoretical succession of motion and the other does not.

Increased motion and/or increased instability of the SIJ has been inextricably tied to the production of or the cause of the painful, symptomatic SIJ. Therefore, with the current knowledge base in place, it is difficult to consider that the fairly "stable" SIJ, as in the diagnosis of the dysfunctional SIJ, should hurt to the point where it not only becomes disabling but also requires treatments that would include fusion of the joint.

The purpose for this study and placing it in this textbook is to challenge the existing concept of "increased motion" = "increased pathology" = "increased symptoms." If one considers all the conditions that exist as the primary pathological causes for severe SIJ pain (Chap. 5), they are all conditions where in the SIJ ROM is minimal. With each of these types of "symptomatic stable pathology," the SIJ pain was either eliminated or significantly decreased using a surgical procedure to theoretically stop the motion of the SIJ. The question then becomes: Is it the *increased ROM* that is in some way tied to the symptomatology of the SIJ or is it a consequence of how the *existing ROM* is transferred through the SIJ? This study suggests that, even with significant gross transection of posterior ligaments, SIJ ROM does not increase very much. This finding has been corroborated many times over in surgery by one of the authors (BED) while doing the posterior midline open approach to the SIJ (Chap. 9). Because our experience is that stopping the ROM, regardless of its amount, in a symptomatic SIJ frequently significantly reduces or eliminates pain, ROM is a factor, to some degree, in the symptomatic dysfunctional SIJ. What might be considered is if it is the manner in which the existing ROM affects the joint structures themselves, and in which planes it is occurring, that influences pain production. The answers to these questions are currently unknown.

Conclusion

This in vitro cadaver study shows that overall motion in the SIJ is minimal and increases only slightly with transection of key posterior ligament structures. It opens the door to questioning what is really happening clinically with "realignment" procedures and why pain should be so dramatically relieved in severely disabled patients with a dysfunctional SIJ by simply stopping a few degrees of motion through the joint, if that is indeed what we are truly doing with SIJ fixation devices. It also raises the question as to what is really causing the pain in such a relatively stable joint. Future studies will need to consider how existing motion in the SIJ contributes to symptomatology in certain pathological conditions and why. From what this study shows us, and our own clinical experiences with the dysfunctional, essentially stable, SIJ, it does not seem to rely only on increasing ROM and gross instability.

References

1. Buchowski JM, et al. Functional and radiographic outcome of sacroiliac arthrodesis for the disorders of the sacroiliac joint. Spine J. 2005;5:520–8. discussion 529.
2. Foley BS, Buschbacher RM. Sacroiliac joint pain: anatomy, biomechanics, diagnosis, and treatment. Am J Phys Med Rehabil. 2006;85:997–1006.
3. Katz V, Schofferman J, Reynolds J. The sacroiliac joint: a potential cause of pain after lumbar fusion to the sacrum. J Spinal Disord Tech. 2003;16:96–9.
4. Walker JM. The sacroiliac joint: a critical review. Phys Ther. 1992;72:903–16.
5. Wilke HJ, Wenger K, Claes L. Testing criteria for spinal implants: recommendations for the standardization of in vitro stability testing of spinal implants. Eur Spine J. 1998;7(2):148–54.

6. Goel VK, et al. Test protocols for evaluation of spinal implants. J Bone Joint Surg Am. 2006;88 Suppl 2:103–9.

7. Panjabi MM. Hybrid multidirectional test method to evaluate spinal adjacent-level effects. Clin Biomech (Bristol, Avon). 2007;22(3):257–65.

8. Agarwala A, et al. Do facet screws provide the required stability in lumbar fixation? A biomechanical comparison of the Boucher technique and pedicular fixation in primary and circumferential fusions. Clin Biomech (Bristol, Avon). 2012;27(1):64–70.

9. Beutler WJ, et al. A biomechanical evaluation of a spacer with integrated plate for treating adjacent-level disease in the subaxial cervical spine. Spine J. 2012;12(7):585–9.

10. Durrani A, et al. Could junctional problems at the end of a long construct be addressed by providing a graduated reduction in stiffness? A biomechanical investigation. Spine (Phila Pa 1976). 2012;37(1):E16–22.

11. Lee JK, et al. In vitro biomechanical study to quantify range of motion, intradiscal pressure, and facet force of 3-level dynamic stabilization constructs with decreased stiffness. Spine (Phila Pa 1976). 2013;38(22):1913–9.

12. Majid K, et al. The biomechanical effect of transverse connectors use in a pre- and postlaminectomy model of the posterior cervical spine: an in vitro cadaveric study. Spine (Phila Pa 1976). 2011;36(26):E1694–701.

13. Frymoyer JW, Howe J, Kuhlmann D. The long term effects of spinal fusion on the sacroiliac joints and ilium. Clin Orthop. 1978;134:196–201.

14. Onsel C, Collier BD, Kir KM, Larson SJ, et al. Increased sacroiliac joint uptake after lumbar fusion and/or laminectomy. Clin Nucl Med. 1992;17(4):283–7.

15. Schoenfeld AJ. Adjacent segment degeneration after lumbar spinal fusion: risk factors and implications for clinical practice. Spine J. 2011;11(1):21–3.

16. Kim TH, Lee BH, Moon SH, Lee SH, Lee HM. Comparison of adjacent segment degeneration after successful posterolateral fusion with unilateral or bilateral pedicle screw instrumentation: a minimum 10-year follow-up. Spine J. 2013;13(10):1208–16.

17. Radcliff KE, Kepler CK, Jakoi A, Sidhu GS, Rihn J, Vaccaro AR. Adjacent segment disease in the lumbar spine following different treatment interventions. Spine J. 2013;13(10):1339–49.

18. Kharrazi FD, Rodgers WB, Kennedy JG, Lhowe DW. Parturition induced pelvic dislocation: a report of four cases. J Orthop Trauma. 1997;11(4):277–81.

19. Vleeming A, Buyruk HM, Stoeckart R, Karamursel S, Snijders CJ. An integrated therapy for peripartum pelvic instability: a study of the biomechanical effects of pelvic belts. Am J Obstet Gynecol. 1992;166(4):1243–7.

20. Zelle BA, Gruen GS, Brown S, George S. Sacroiliac joint dysfunction: evaluation and management. Clin J Pain. 2005;21(5):446–55.

21. Albert H, Godskesen M, Westergaard J. Prognosis in four syndromes of pelvic related pain. Acta Obstet Gynecol Scand. 2001;80(6):505–10.

22. Berg G, Hammar M, Moller-Nielsen J. Low back pain during pregnancy. Obstet Gynecol. 1998;71(1):71–5.

23. Waisbrod H, Kraninick JU, Gerbergshagen HU. Sacroiliac joint arthrodesis for chronic lower back pain. Arch Orthop Trauma Surg. 1987;106:238–40.

24. Belanger TA, Dall BE. Sacroiliac arthrodesis using posterior midline fascial splitting approach and pedicle screw instrumentation: a new technique. J Spinal Disord. 2001;14:118–24.

25. Wise CL, Dall BE. Minimally invasive sacroiliac joint arthrodesis: outcomes of a new technique. J Spinal Disord Tech. 2008;21:579–84.

Bruce E. Dall and Arnold Graham Smith

Introduction

The following chapter will discuss the pathological conditions and diagnoses that were present preoperatively in patients that subsequently were satisfied with their results, long term, after having a sacroiliac joint (SIJ) fusion. The importance of a correct diagnosis will be emphasized as well as considerations for the differential diagnosis. The reader should keep in mind that frequently pathology in the SIJ causing chronic debilitating pain does not stand-alone. Many times the same pathology affecting the SIJ can be present in other joints as well to include the lumbar spine. This is certainly true with some arthritic conditions. This particularly applies to inflammatory arthritis, which will be discussed as showing mixed results with SIJ fusion procedures. This is not a complete list, and other pathological conditions do exist and will need to be added as experience with them

B.E. Dall, M.D. (✉)
Neurosurgery of Kalamazoo, Borgess Brain
and Spine Institute, 1541 Gull Road, Kalamazoo,
MI 49048, USA

Orthopedic Spine Division, Western Michigan
University Medical School, Kalamazoo, MI USA
e-mail: dall.bruce@yahoo.com

A.G. Smith, M.D., P.A.
Orthopaedic Surgery, Baptist Medical
Center – South, 9191 R.G. Skinner Pkwy #103,
Jacksonville, FL 32256, USA
e-mail: backchap2@aol.com

develops. The three types of pathology that will not be discussed in this chapter are acute trauma, active infection, and conditions involving tumors. These are acute and frequently unstable conditions that fall more in the category of trauma surgery. The pathology discussed in this chapter involves essentially stable SIJs in a chronic pain setting.

Importance of an Accurate Diagnosis

In Chap. 6, the algorithm for the diagnosis and treatment of the dysfunctional SIJ will be discussed. It is important here, however, to cover a few of these points when considering painful pathology of the SIJ. When a patient presents with low back pain (LBP) and they point to a spot just over and slightly caudal to the posterior superior iliac spine (PSIS) (Fortin Finger Test [1–3]), it is mandatory that the clinician considers the SIJ in the differential diagnosis (Chap. 6). An agreement in the literature, which has been fully upheld at our institution, is that SIJ pain is rarely found clinically cephalad to the L5–S1 disk space [4, 5]. So, if a patient also has pain at L5 or more cephalad, the pathology of the lumbar spine must also be in the differential diagnosis. Our experience is that both the lumbar spine and the SIJ can be painful in the same patient and each possibly contributing to that patient's disability. If a patient has groin pain, it is possible for it to be emanating from the upper lumbar spine (lateral foraminal stenosis), the hip joint, the SIJ, or

B.E. Dall et al. (eds.), *Surgery for the Painful, Dysfunctional Sacroiliac Joint*,
DOI 10.1007/978-3-319-10726-4_5, © Springer International Publishing Switzerland 2015

multiples of these. We have found that at times a foraminal stenosis of the L4–L5 or L5–S1 can mimic SIJ pain. These concepts and more on diagnosis will be covered in detail in the chapter on the algorithm for diagnosis and treatment (Chap. 6), but, as one is encountering the various pathological states that can exist in the SIJ, it is important not to wear blinders and focus only on the SIJ.

Pathologic Conditions That Responded Positively to Fusion

These conditions will be discussed from a clinical perspective that a surgeon or therapist would encounter in the office when evaluating a patient. It is important to remember that the exact cause of the pain in all of these pathological conditions causing chronic pain in the SIJ is currently unknown. All that can be said at this time is that each of these diagnostic pathological conditions has been associated with the diagnosis of a dysfunctional SIJ and a fusion of that joint resulted in satisfactory relief of that pain at long-term follow-up. The only exceptions are the mixed results with inflammatory arthritis, which will be discussed.

Pathological conditions which can cause a SIJ to be chronically painful:

- Degenerative osteoarthritis
- Inflammatory arthritis
- Postpartum SIJ dysfunction
- Sacral osteoporosis
- Aggressive iliac bone graft harvest
- Overstressing joint with adjacent lumbosacral (LS) fusion
- Association with certain types of lumbosacral transitional vertebrae (LSTV)
- Failed attempt at previous SIJ fusion
- Idiopathic pain in normal-appearing SIJ

Degenerative Osteoarthritis (OA)

The degenerative form of osteoarthritis (OA) is a multifactorial disease in its primary state and an acquired multifactorial condition in its secondary state. For the clinician, these two states in which OA can occur have implications when evaluating the dysfunctional SIJ. If it is primary OA, there

may be a strong possibility that it may involve other joints as well. The same OA that is found in the SIJ is usually the same as is found in the lumbar spine. The hip joint itself also needs to be considered, as primary OA in the SIJ represents an "axial" presentation in large joints, which might include the hip joint. The message here is that the pain the patient is having could be originating from one, two, or all three of these anatomic sites. The secondary state of OA develops usually as a residual of some type of significant insult to the joint. It may result from a fall, secondary impacts such as breaking with a straight leg in a front-end automobile collision, a previous infection, a prior healed fracture of the joint or pelvis, and postradiation syndrome, and the list goes on. With secondary OA, the SIJ may be the only joint involved though thought should be given to the possibility of other pain-generating sites. With both types of OA, the SIJ is usually "relatively" stable and may or may not enhance on a bone scan. If there is abnormal enhancement on a bone scan [6], one should give serious consideration for this joint being a pain generator (Figs. 5.1 and 5.2).

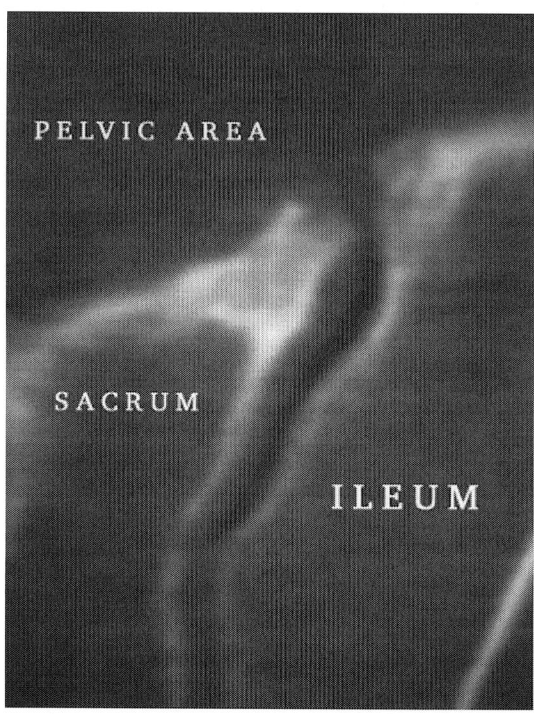

Fig. 5.1 Osteoarthritis of the sacroiliac joint demonstrating spurring, sclerosis, joint widening, and vacuum sign

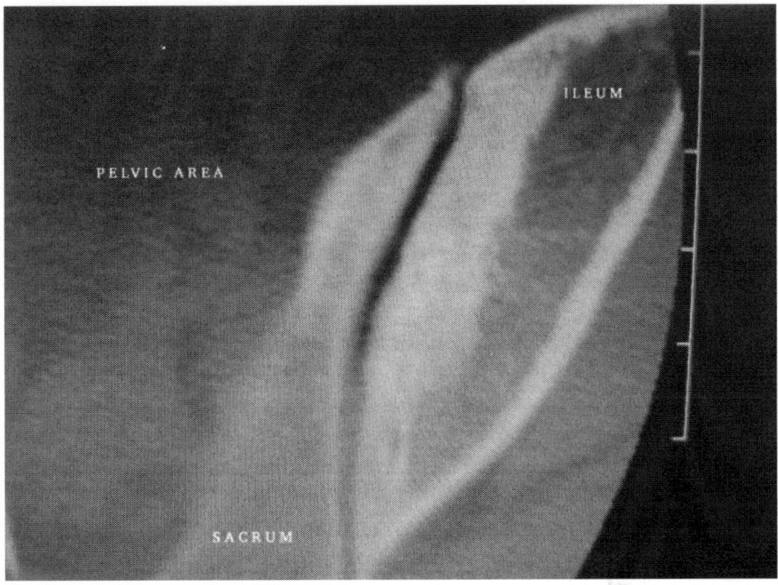

Fig. 5.2 Advanced osteoarthritis of the sacroiliac joint involving entire joint with resultant increase in bone density on both the iliac and sacral sides

Inflammatory Arthritis

This type of arthritis in the SIJ may arise from both a seropositive and seronegative inflammatory disease process. The conditions that have resulted in a successful fusion at our institution were rheumatoid arthritis (RA), the non-joint fusing form of HLA-B27-positive ankylosing spondylitis in a young female, Reiter's syndrome, and idiopathic sacroiliitis. These inflammatory types of arthritis in the SIJ can cause severe pain, both in the acute and chronic phases, and the delay in diagnosis can be excessive. The affected SIJs can be stable or demonstrating a microtype of instability secondary to the ligament–bone attachments being affected by the inflammatory process (enthesopathy). It is important to be in consultation with a rheumatologist when working with these patients (Fig. 5.3).

Case Example of RA Affecting the SIJ

The first patient to have a SIJ fusion at BBSI presented to us in 1991. She was 74 years old and unable to stand or put weight on her right leg secondary to severe pain and the feeling of instability. Her bone scan was significantly enhanced over the right SIJ, and her CT showed typical signs of joint erosions, surrounding osteoporosis, and an obvious separation of the joint margins. She had been suffering with this condition for several years, had seen countless doctors, and was confined to a wheel chair. Due to the current surgical standard being simply placing two screws across the joint into her osteoporotic sacrum, and her suggesting death as her next option, we devised a posterior midline approach to fuse and instrument her SIJ. This procedure allowed for better screw to bone fixation. There was no readily available instrumentation for this at that time so a bone plate (used for long bones) crossing the joint posteriorly fixated with large cancellous screws in the S1 pedicle and the ilium along with autogenous iliac bone graft were used. Due to the fixation being quite rigid, she was allowed to weight bear as tolerated in the first postoperative week and continued to ambulate with a walker, without significant pain, for nine years until her death from other causes. The result from this patient was the beginning of our understanding that the SIJ can cause severe disabling pain and that a fusion is a viable option in some patients (Fig. 5.4).

Our experience with fusing patients with inflammatory arthritis has been mixed. It contains some of our very best and also some of our worse results. Currently, our feeling is that

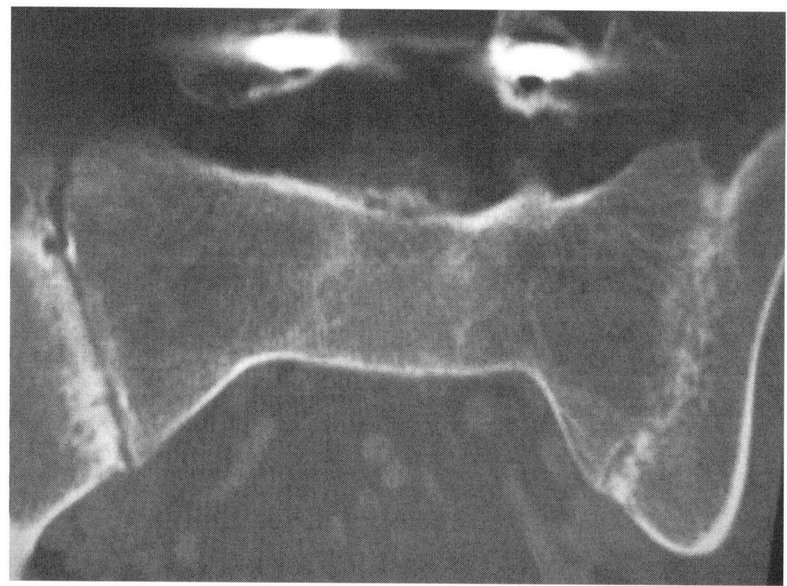

Fig. 5.3 Bilateral inflammatory joint changes showing, as you look at the image, a fusion on the right (asymptomatic) and an incomplete fusion on the left (symptomatic). Note the narrowing, sclerosis, and subchondral bone erosions on the unfused side. Also note the screws from the lumbosacral fusion that failed to resolve this patient's low back pain

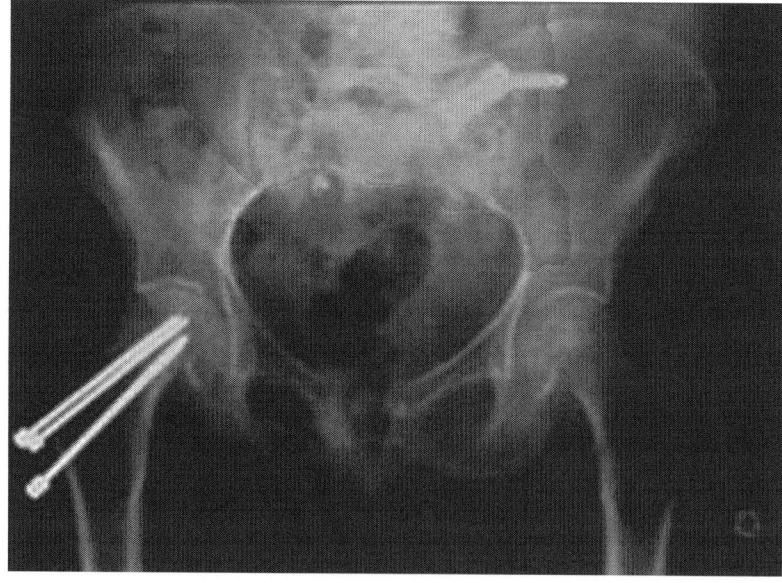

Fig. 5.4 Nine-year follow-up of elderly patient with severe rheumatoid arthritis and osteoporosis after fusion of her sacroiliac joint using a plate and cancellous screws

if it involves one joint and the patient does not have other systemic problems arising from their inflammatory arthritis diagnosis, they seem to respond the best to the surgery. If their condition is bilateral and they suffer with pain from multiple other sites related to the inflammatory process, caution should be taken when considering surgery. This situation is illustrated in the case shown in Fig. 5.5. Although some cases of inflammatory arthritis have done very well with fusion procedures others have not. Much more research and experience are needed in patients with this diagnosis to fully understand which subgroups would be the most appropriate for fusion surgery. A rheumatologist might be able to manage their condition as a better option to surgery (Fig. 5.5).

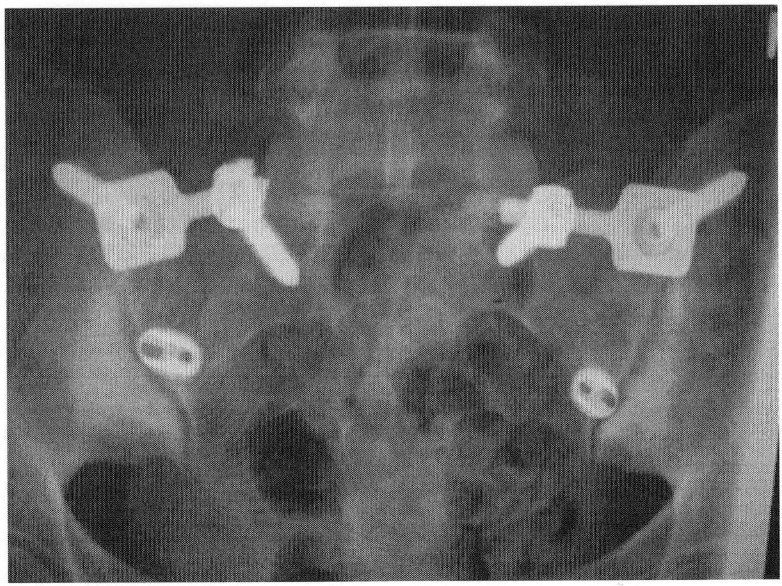

Fig. 5.5 Middle-aged female with severe bilateral sacroiliitis after a bilateral posterior midline fusion using custom instrumentation (Medtronic). Note that the cages are not approved for this purpose by the FDA and they are used as custom devices without label. Although initially successful, her pain returned after several months with no loosening of hardware on CT noted. Screws and rods were removed without improvement of pain

Postpartum SIJ Dysfunction

The obstetrics and gynecology literature has recognized for decades the abuse that the SIJs endure as a result of carrying the baby during the final weeks of pregnancy and as a result of a vaginal labor and delivery [7–11]. In most cases, the endogenous factors that allow for the laxity and occasional injury to the ligaments surrounding the SIJ during labor and delivery reverse themselves, and the pain that was associated with this event subsides. In a small number of cases, the pain does not resolve, and the patient continues on with chronic pain. Typically, this pain is endured and possibly alters activities or lifestyle. Occasionally, it becomes progressively severe and begins to cause increasing levels of disability. These types of patients frequently populate chronic pain clinics and get repeated injections into the SIJ for short-term relief. It has only been recently that such a patient is being referred for possible surgery. It is usually the primary care doctor, the patient's physical therapist, or a collaboration of both that sends this type of patient for a possible surgical solution. These patients are usually very frustrated and often depressed when they present to the surgeon for consultation. As a group, they also have the fewest findings on any imaging test. CT and the bone scan may be essentially normal. It will be the history that offers the clues to the etiology and the injection (Chap. 6) that ultimately solidifies the diagnosis.

Case Example

A patient, having a greater than 10-year follow-up at our institution, suffered from postpartum SIJ dysfunction. She also had a secondary diagnosis of HLA-B27-positive non-fusing ankylosing spondylitis. After the birth of her first child during her mid-20s, her pain slowly and steadily increased to a point of being very disabling. By the time we evaluated her in her late 40s, she had reached a point of constant pain and progressive inability to bear weight on her right leg and was having progressively more dyspareunia, receiving only short-term relief with injections, and becoming increasingly frustrated with her condition. After failing years of appropriate conservative treatments, she underwent a posterior SIJ fusion. At an 11-year follow-up, she was still having significant pain relief and increased functional ability. Her dyspareunia improved significantly as well. She remains very satisfied with her outcome and would do it again for the same result. This patient has gone on to council other patients with chronic SIJ dysfunction (Figs. 5.6 and 5.7).

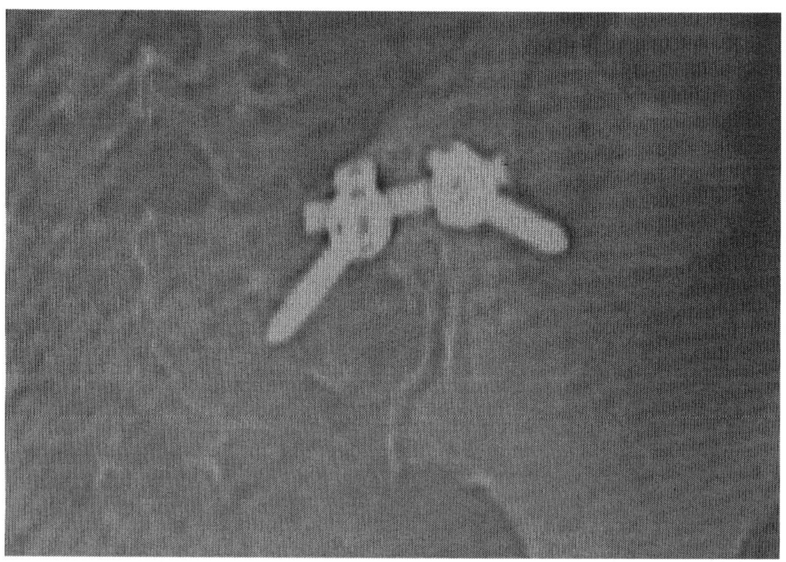

Fig. 5.6 Greater than 10-year follow-up AP X-ray of a right posterior midline sacroiliac joint fusion

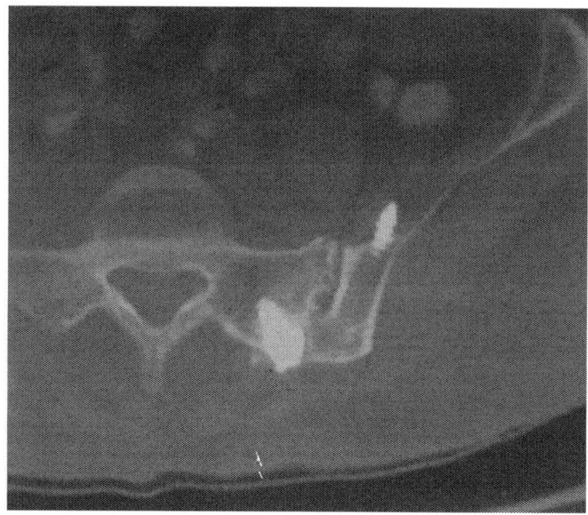

Fig. 5.7 Axial CT scan showing a solid sacroiliac joint fusion at greater than 10 years after a posterior midline sacroiliac joint fusion. Note the tip of the iliac screw in the iliacus muscle. This did not cause a problem and may have strengthened the stabilization with the cortical fixation of the medial iliac wall

Sacral Osteoporosis

This can be a very challenging condition, which can present to the clinician in various ways. We have encountered painful, dysfunctional SIJs adjacent to healed sacral insufficiency fractures due to osteoporosis, in RA, lupus, and Reiter's syndrome with their associated osteoporotic states, and after sacroplasties, which inadvertently injured the SIJ. Osteoporosis becomes very important for the surgeon to understand when considering the quality of the bone-instrumentation interface available in a patient needing a SIJ fusion. The sacrum, which consists of primarily cancellous bone, may have very little fixation potential for laterally based fusion systems. In these patients, it is important to consider other fixation points such as the S1 pedicle, placing the iliac screw between the cortical layers of the ilium allowing for more cortical bone surface area capture or considering posterior lateral into or obliquely crossing the longitudinal axis of the joint fixation where there might be more of a stronger subchondral cortical bone available in the osteoporotic patient (Fig. 5.8).

Aggressive Iliac Bone Graft (IBG) Harvesting

Harvesting IBG is becoming less frequent in modern spine and orthopedic surgeries as more bone is being harvested locally and being combined with bone growth proteins or other bone-enhancing factors to achieve a fusion. With the harvesting of bone from the posterior iliac crest

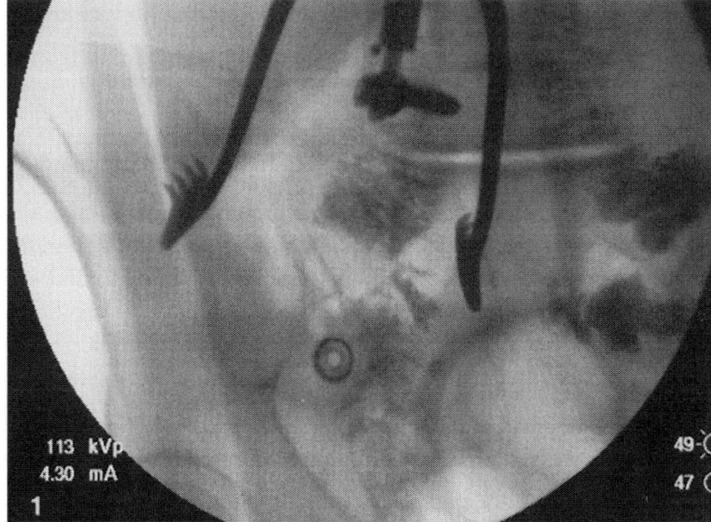

Fig. 5.8 Placing a cage into the sacroiliac joint as part of a posterior midline sacroiliac joint fusion. The sacroplasty, done elsewhere, entered the sacroiliac joint causing joint damage and resultant chronic pain. The fusion procedure relieved this iatrogenically caused pain

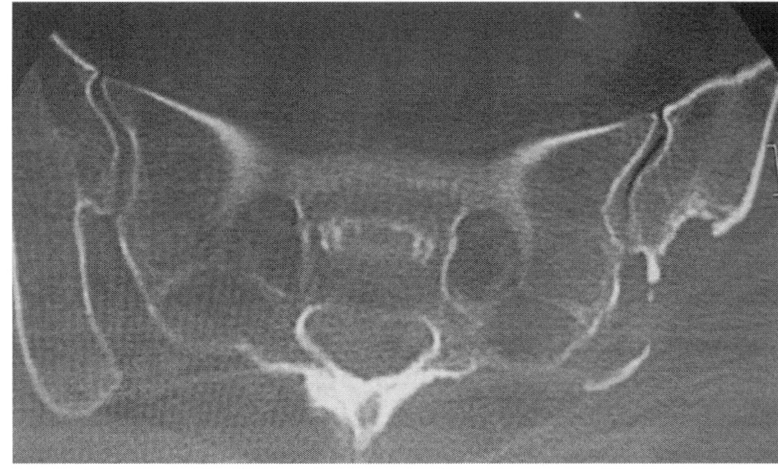

Fig. 5.9 Axial CT scan showing chronic changes in the sacroiliac joint adjacent to an aggressive iliac bone graft harvest. Note that the medial wall of the ileum is essentially removed and the presence of a vacuum sign in the sacroiliac joint. Comparison is made with the contralateral side

area, there are two potential ways to damage the SIJ. An indirect way is to cut the cephalad attachment of the posterior sacrotuberous ligament, located just posterior and slightly caudal to the PSIS. This is a major posterior stabilizer for the SIJ. Although this is a theoretical concept, we feel that we have seen such instabilities, resulting from aggressive stripping during IBG harvesting in our own hands, where the SIJ has gone on to become arthritic and painful secondary to subsequent iatrogenic micro instability and eventually require fusion. A more direct way to injure the SIJ is to remove so much bone that the joint is injured directly by the instruments involved.

When too much bone is removed, this may also injure supporting ligament structures allowing for increasing instability and possible joint degeneration [12, 13] (Fig. 5.9).

LSTV and the SIJ

In one type of LSTV, Castellvi type II (a and b), the pseudo joint of the LSTV, which is known to be a potential pain generator, is anatomically in intimate contact with the SIJ [14, 15]. Although the possibility of the SIJ being a pain generator in these types of patients is theoretical, we feel that

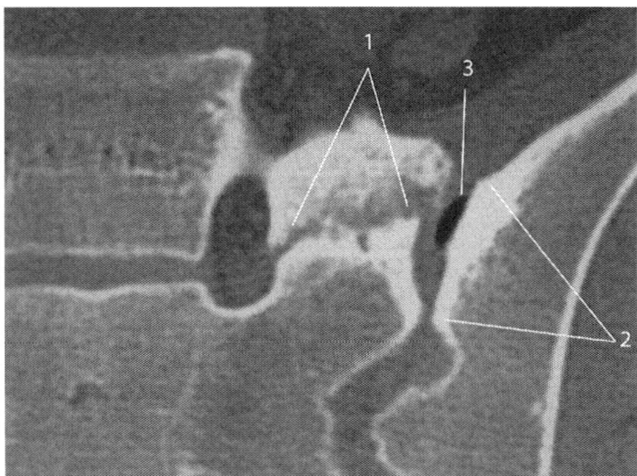

Fig. 5.10 Axial CT scan showing a Castellvi type IIa lumbosacral transitional vertebrae. 1. Shows the arthritic "pseudo joint" of the LSTV. 2. Shows the close proximity of the "pseudo joint" to the synovial margins of the sacroiliac joint. 3. Shows a vacuum sign in the sacroiliac joint. With this combination, the source of LBP might be confusing

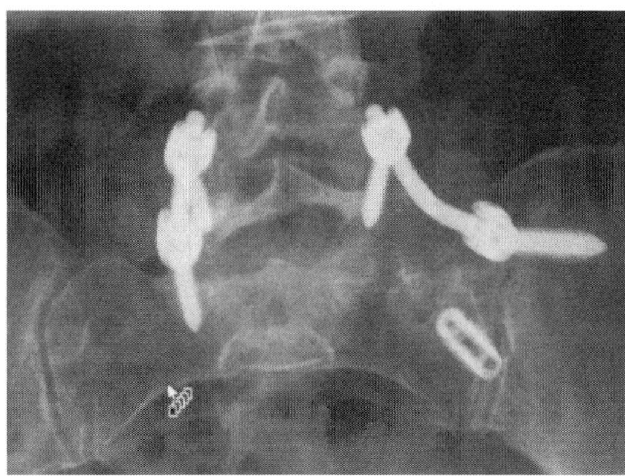

Fig. 5.11 AP X-ray showing a combined fusion of the LSTV and the SIJ using the posterior midline approach

we have encountered two patients where it was most likely the case. Further research is needed to prove that both the pseudo joint of the LSTV and the SIJ can be pain generators in the same patient, on the same side, and at the same time. At the time of this writing, we feel it appropriate to simply say that the possibility could exist and that the clinician should be aware that both of these anatomical entities should be thoroughly evaluated and, where appropriate, treated when making a diagnosis in such a patient (Figs. 5.10 and 5.11).

LS Fusion, Especially with Instrumentation

There have been several publications demonstrating the development of pain in the SIJ after a LS fusion [6, 16, 17]. BBSI has been involved in cadaver research, which has demonstrated an increase in the range of motion in the SIJ resulting from L5 to S1 fixation (Chap. 4). If an IBG was harvested during the LS fusion, it is possible that the SIJ posterior ligament structure might have been damaged setting up the joint for potential micro instability and injury, as discussed in a previous section. It is felt by many spine surgeons, who have a good understanding of the SIJ, that many of the "failed LS fusion" procedures are due to new, old, or exacerbated pain emanating from the SIJ. Those surgeons who understand this and go the extra mile to make the diagnosis of a dysfunctional SIJ may have the opportunity to turn a failure into a success (Fig. 5.12).

Failed Attempt at Previous SIJ Fusion

SIJ fusion procedures are on the rise, especially in the United States. This is due to several factors to include the increased awareness of the SIJ as a pain generator and the creation of several new systems with which to fuse the joint. Each type of surgery for fusing the SIJ is also capable of failing to do so, thus necessitating a salvage surgery. There are also those previous trauma patients whose SIJs have been stabilized by trauma surgeons, using the two screws across the joint method, and who are continuing to have significant pain, as a true fusion was never accomplished. Patients who have had a failed attempt to surgically treat the SIJ can be complicated to evaluate and treat for several reasons. They are fearful, as they have already had one or more attempts to fuse the joint. Long lateral incisions may have been utilized, which could have cut cluneal nerves resulting in secondary pain, which will persist after any further surgery. The type and placement of previously used instrumentation

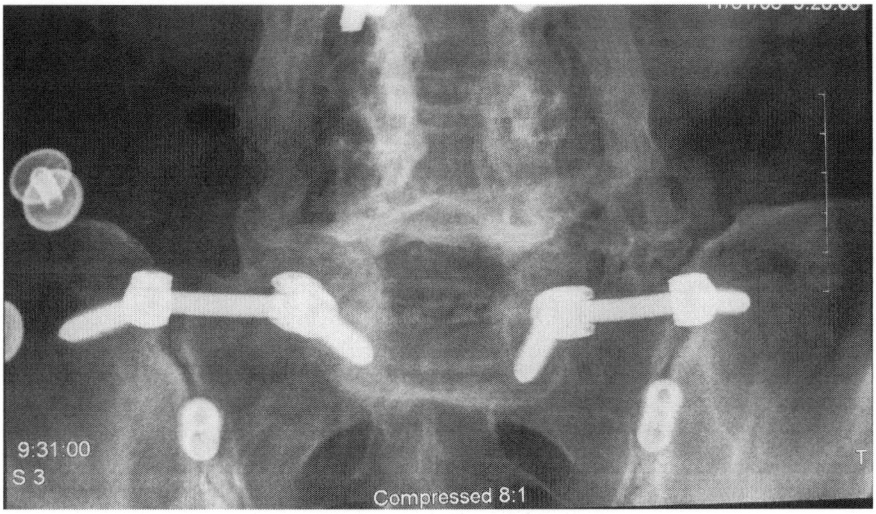

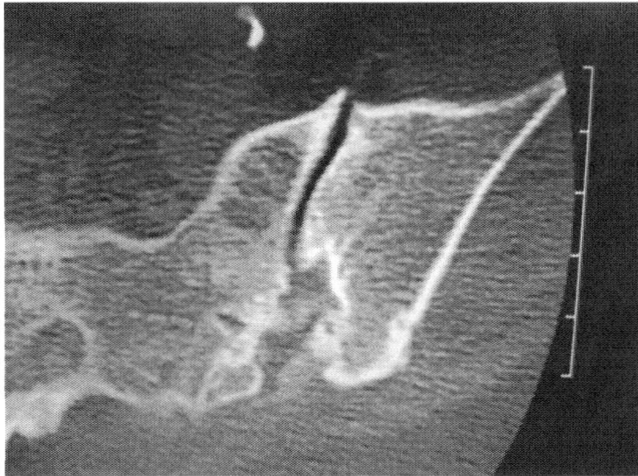

Fig. 5.12 AP X-ray showing bilateral sacroiliac joint fusions using the posterior midline approach. This patient also required an extension of her lumbosacral fusion up to the lower thoracic spine. Both were accomplished with one posterior midline incision. She went from a VAS of 8 to 2 at her 4-year follow-up

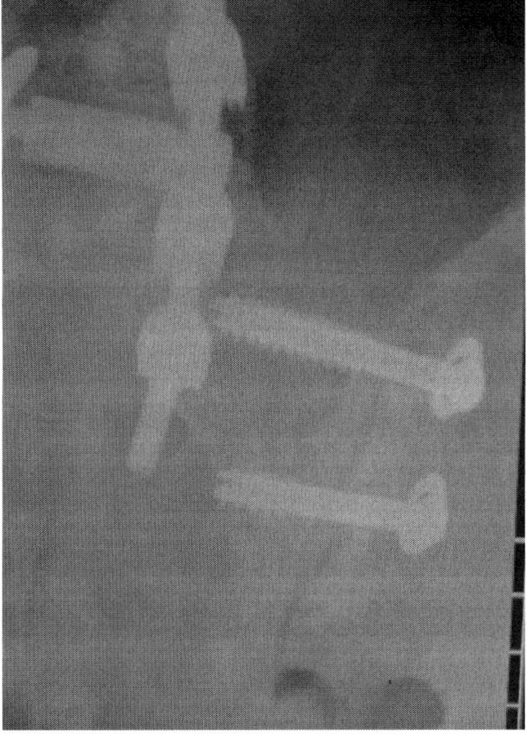

Fig. 5.13 Axial CT scan demonstrating a failed direct posterior bone grafting of the sacroiliac joint. Note that the fusion attempt was in the posterior ligamentous region of the joint, all the bone graft has been reabsorbed, and there is a persistent vacuum sign in the true synovial portion of the joint

may be difficult to remove or to work around. When any type of revision SIJ fusion surgery is being considered, it ups the ante on what is needed in the knowledge base of the treating surgeon. More than just the standard "cookbook," lateral approach might be required to salvage the joint (Figs. 5.13, 5.14, and 5.15).

Fig. 5.14 AP X-ray showing a failed fusion attempt for the sacroiliac joint using two lateral screws for fixation. This patient also presented with a long lumbosacral fusion

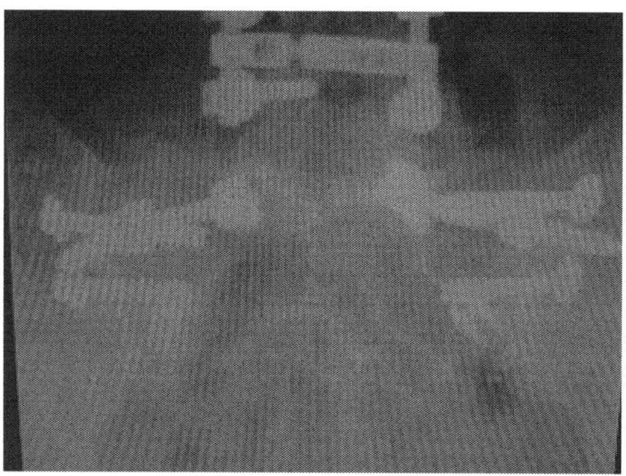

Fig. 5.15 Using the posterior midline approach. The new instrumentation was able to be placed in a plane approximately 90° to the failed hardware on both sides. Iliac bone was used for grafting. This patient went on to a solid fusion bilaterally with a satisfactory result in the long term

Idiopathic Pain in the Normal-Appearing SIJ

Some type of detectable change in or around the joint characterizes the above pathological conditions. These are seen in X-ray images, CT scans, other types of imaging, blood work, and other objective evidence that the SIJ is not normal. It is much more confusing when a patient has an injection verified painful and dysfunctional SIJ and all the imaging and blood work are normal. If we look for analogies elsewhere, we can look at the patient with a chronically painful sprained ankle that is causing significant disability. Although the images of the ankle may be normal and the clinical exam shows no instability, we still have a patient with a chronically painful ankle joint. If conservative treatment for it fails, they either live with it in a disabling lifestyle or the intuitive surgeon does something about it. In reference to the SIJ, think of a patient who falls directly on their buttock and suffers a severe sprain to that joint. The images and blood tests are normal, but every time the patient rolls over bed or gets up from a sitting position the sprained joint hurts just like the sprained ankle hurts with its provocative movements. Over time, this condition can become chronically more painful and begin to result in worsening disability. There are protocols for the chronically sprained ankle, which is causing disability, and when the conservative treatments do not work there are well-described surgeries to address this situation. We are now entering a phase of medical and surgical understanding to begin offering the same types of treatment considerations for the "normal looking" chronically painful and disabling "sprained" SIJ [18, 19].

Conclusion

This chapter examined the types of pathological conditions that existed in patients who subsequently, after failure of conservative treatments, went on to have successful SIJ fusion surgeries followed long term. The complexities associated with the pathological diagnosis of inflammatory arthritis were discussed. It also examines those patients who had normal imaging and laboratory studies associated with their dysfunctional SIJ that likewise had successful surgical results. This list of pathological conditions will expand as this subject receives more focus, and more patient experiences are recorded. As time goes on, we will also find better ways to objectively examine the SIJ with improved science so that the number of "normal looking" chronically painful SIJs decreases and we are able to provide an identifiable diagnosis instead.

References

1. Dreyfuss P, Michaelsen M, Pauza K, McLarty J. The value of medical history and physical in diagnosing sacroiliac joint pain. Spine. 1996;21:2594–602.
2. Fortin JD, Dwyer AP, West S. Sacroiliac joint pain referral maps upon applying a new injection/arthrography technique, part I. Spine. 1994;19:1475–82.
3. Fortin JD, Aprill CN, Ponthieux B. Sacroiliac joint pain referral maps upon applying a new injection/arthrography technique, part II. Spine. 1994;19:1483–9.
4. Schwarzer AC, Aprill CN, Bogduk N. The sacroiliac joint in chronic low back pain. Spine. 1995;20:31–7.
5. Dreyfuss P, Dreyer S, Cole A, Mayo K. Sacroiliac joint pain. J Am Acad Orthop Surg. 2004;12(4):255–65.

6. Onsel C, Collier BD, Kir KM, Larson SJ. Increased sacroiliac joint uptake after lumbar fusion and/or laminectomy. Clin Nucl Med. 1992;17(4):283–7.

7. Kharrazi FD, Rodgers WB, Kennedy JG, Lhowe DW. Parturition induced pelvic dislocation: a report of four cases. J Orthop Trauma. 1997;11:277–82.

8. Vleeming A, Buyruk HM, Stoeckart R, Karamursel S, Snijders CJ. An integrated therapy for peripartum pelvic instability: a study of the biomechanical effects of pelvic belts. Am J Obstet Gynecol. 1992;166:1243–7.

9. Zelle BA, Gruen GS, Brown S, George S. Sacroiliac joint dysfunction: evaluation and management. Clin J Pain. 2005;21:446–55.

10. Albert H, Godskesen M, Westergaard J. Prognosis in four syndromes of pelvic related pain. Acta Obstet Gynecol Scand. 2001;80:505–10.

11. Berg G, Hammar M, Moller-Nielsen J. Low back pain during pregnancy. Obstet Gynecol. 1988;71:71–5.

12. Ebraheim NA, Elgafy H, Semaan HB. Computed tomographic findings in patients with persistent sacroiliac pain after posterior iliac graft harvesting. Spine. 2000;25:2047–51.

13. Frymoyer JW, Hanley E, Howe J. Disc excision and spine fusion in the management of lumbar disc disease: a minimum ten year follow-up. Spine. 1978;3:1–6.

14. Konin GP, Walz DM. Lumbosacral transitional vertebrae: classification, imaging findings and clinical relevance. AJNR Am J Neuroradiol. 2010;31(10):1778–86. doi:10.3174/ajnr.A2036. A review article. Electronic publication.

15. Castellvi AE, Goldstein LA, Chan DP. Lumbosacral transitional vertebrae and their relationship with lumbar extradural defects. Spine. 1984;9:493–5.

16. Katz V, Schofferman J, Reynolds J. The sacroiliac joint: a potential cause of pain after lumbar fusion to the sacrum. J Spinal Disord Tech. 2003;16:96–9.

17. Frymoyer JW, Howe J, Kuhlmann D. The long-term effects of spinal fusion on the sacroiliac joint and ilium. Clin Orthop. 1978;134:196–201.

18. Fortin JD. Sacroiliac joint dysfunction: a new perspective. J Back Musculoskelet Rehabil. 1993;3:31–43.

19. LeBlanc KE. Sacroiliac sprain: an overlooked cause of back pain. Am Fam Physician. 1992;46:1459–63.

Algorithm for the Diagnosis and Treatment of the Dysfunctional Sacroiliac Joint

Bruce E. Dall, Sonia V. Eden, Michael D. Rahl, and Arnold Graham Smith

Introduction

This chapter looks in depth at an organized methodical approach for diagnosing and treating the dysfunctional SIJ. The Borgess Brain and Spine Institute (BBSI) created it based on years of diagnosing and treating patients with this condition [1]. Since that time, further editing of this algorithm has occurred with input from Arnold Graham Smith, MD, Jacksonville, Florida, and Michael Rahl, DPT, trained at the University of Connecticut. This algorithm is meant to be a general guide for the clinician, providing a simple, reliable path through the process of diagnosing and treating the painful, stable SIJ. It is not meant to be an exhaustive review of all the literature that has contributed to its creation. Although this algorithm has worked well for our patients at the BBSI, it is only one concept as to how clinicians might proceed. As time passes, some of the steps in this algorithm are expected to change due to increasing knowledge and experience. There are three main principles that allow this algorithm to remain straightforward and easy to reproduce. The simplest treatments are discussed first, moving into the more complex treatments as needed. The least invasive measures are used at the beginning reserving the more invasive ones for later if necessary. Lastly, the least expensive treatments are used before moving into the increasingly more costly procedures.

B.E. Dall, M.D. (✉)
Neurosurgery of Kalamazoo, Borgess Brain and Spine Institute, Orthopedic Spine Division, Western Michigan University Medical School, Kalamazoo, MI, USA
e-mail: dall.bruce@yahoo.com

S.V. Eden, M.D.
Department of Neurological Surgery, Borgess Brain and Spine Institute, Western Michigan University Medical School, Kalamazoo, MI, USA

M.D. Rahl, P.T., D.P.T., O.C.S., C.S.C.S.
Full Potential Physical Therapy, 286 Hoover Boulevard, Holland, MI 49423, USA
e-mail: michael@fullpotentialpt.com

A.G. Smith, M.D., P.A.
Orthopaedic surgery, Baptist Medical Center – South, 9191 R.G. Skinner Pkwy #103, Jacksonville, FL 32256, USA
e-mail: backchap2@aol.com

Philosophy for this algorithm:
- Diagnosis and treatment >>> Simple to complex
- Degree of invasiveness >>> Minimal to major
- Overall cost >>> Least to most

It is also important to keep in mind that the definitive diagnosis of a dysfunctional, painful, stable SIJ does not need to be made at the start of treatment. At first, it is treated like common low

B.E. Dall et al. (eds.), *Surgery for the Painful, Dysfunctional Sacroiliac Joint*, DOI 10.1007/978-3-319-10726-4_6, © Springer International Publishing Switzerland 2015

back pain (LBP) with the hope that traditional LBP treatment measures will make a positive difference in the pain level. It is when more invasive treatment measures are being considered that a definitive diagnosis must be made, and how that can be accomplished will be explained in this chapter. It also must be understood that the average surgeon seeing a patient for the first time, who has been in extensive treatment prior, will possibly present with an injection verified diagnosis of a dysfunctional SIJ. In these circumstances, it is important for the physician to be sure all the appropriate steps in the algorithm up to injection have been covered and no useful conservative measures for treatment have been overlooked.

The Algorithm

First Things First

The algorithm begins by first helping the clinician decide whether or not the SIJ might be a significant pain generator. We know from the literature that between 15 and 22 % of patients presenting with LBP will have some or all of the pain emanating from the SIJ [2–5]. When a patient presents with a SIJ problem, they will have historical information and specific location pain complaints, which will help to differentiate potential SIJ, pain from the usual LBP. It is important for the clinician to understand that even if they suspect the SIJ to be a pain generator, all pain in the area of the SIJ should be considered as coming from the lumbar spine until proven otherwise. So the clinician must understand the location of and the radiating nature of pain originating from a compressed lumbar nerve, spinal stenosis, a degenerative lumbar disk, degenerative facet joints, and spinal instability. These diagnoses are covered extensively in the literature and in multiple other textbooks and will only be alluded to in this chapter. The other caveat to consider is whether the pain is acute or chronic. If the pain is acute (<12 weeks duration), pain in the SIJ is treated like all acute forms of LBP. This algorithm begins when the clinician can reliably state that the potential for pain coming from the SIJ is greater than that of the lumbar spine.

This is usually after a lumbar MRI, plain flexion extension films of the lumbar spine, and possibly a CT scan and/or a bone scan have ruled out the above-stated lumbar pathologies as sources for the pain. If these tests show significant pathology that could account for the pain in the area of the SIJ, then treatment needs to proceed in those directions first according to current standards until those pain sources are eradicated, always keeping in mind that pain from the SIJ can coexist with pain originating from the lumbar spine.

> • Has the Lumbar Spine Been Ruled Out as a Pain Generator?

Diagnosis

Certain historical facts, which are well documented in the literature [6–15], have a high correlation with pain originating from the SIJ. A female patient may recall the pain starting just before, during, or just after a vaginal delivery and steadily worsening over time. In others, there may have been a significant fall directly on the buttock sometimes severe enough to be associated with bruising or even a fracture of the sacrum or pelvis. A patient may have had a previous lumbosacral fusion, with or without instrumentation that is thought to increase stresses through the SIJ. A bone graft may have been harvested from the iliac crest on the same side as a patient's pain complaints. A classic means of injuring the SIJ is during a head on collision in an automobile when the patient brakes with a straight leg upon impact, transferring the stress directly to the ipsilateral SIJ. They may have a history of scoliosis with a pelvic obliquity or leg length discrepancy, causing malalignments, which might overstress the joint. Previous trauma patients may have had a pelvic disruption that injured the SIJ directly or indirectly. There may be a history of inflammatory arthritis with associated painful sacroiliitis present. A history of having a gait abnormality might suggest a problem with the SIJ. When these facts surface in the patient's history, it is important to consider the possibility of a painful dysfunctional SIJ.

Historical facts that may indicate SIJ pain:
- Pain continuing after vaginal delivery
- Fall directly on the buttock
- Previous lumbosacral fusion
- Braking for a front-end automobile collision
- Bone graft harvest ipsilateral side
- Previous pelvic disruption
- Inflammatory arthritis
- Gait abnormality
- Scoliosis
- Leg length discrepancy

There are three symptoms about which the clinician should question each patient when suspecting a dysfunctional SIJ. The first is about sitting. They will usually admit that sitting is difficult, they have trouble sitting through dinner or church, and they frequently favor sitting on the contralateral side. This differs from some other types of lumbar pathology where sitting might provide some relief of symptoms. The second is about sleeping. Usually the patient with a painful SIJ has no problem getting to sleep, but the problem occurs when rolling over during sleep. This can actually wake them up. If awake, they sometimes have to manually help the ipsilateral leg in the effort to roll over. Many patients with chronically painful SIJs are sleep deprived. The third symptom to ask about is stumbling. Sharp pain in the SIJ seems, at times, to be felt by the "whole leg," and a "give way" can occur causing the patient to stumble. In extreme cases, this results in a fall. Due to this feeling of whole leg weakness and instability, stairs can be a problem. The patient may relate that climbing stairs must be taken one at a time leading with the good non-painful side.

Three suggestive symptoms:
- Painful sitting on affected side
- Ipsilateral pain standing on one leg
- Frequent stumbling due to "give way" of affected leg

A Word on Dyspareunia

For the sexually active female with a painful dysfunctional SIJ, dyspareunia (pain occurring with intercourse) can be a very disabling symptom both physically and emotionally. This usually does not get talked about unless the clinician asks the question. The supine position with legs abducted and forceful penetration all expose the SIJ to forces that can both injure the SIJ or exacerbate current SIJ symptomatology. In a study published in 2008 using a posterior minimally invasive approach for SIJ fusion, dyspareunia was evaluated as part of the prospective protocol. With long-term follow-up, this symptom improved to a significant degree ($p = 0.0028$) after SIJ fusion [16]. Many types of organic pathology can contribute to the cause of dyspareunia, but it is important to consider the SIJ as a possible cause when presented with this condition and to ask about dyspareunia when dealing with a painful SIJ.

Clinical Exam

At this time, the literature would suggest that no physical examination test is reliable in diagnosing the painful SIJ [4, 5]. Many practitioners who see large numbers of patients with SIJ pain, and surgeons who successfully fuse SIJs in patients with pain, will attest that a very reliable clinical sign that pain may be coming from the SIJ is a positive "Fortin Finger Test" [17–21]. This is where the patient points with his or her index finger to the area just below the posterior superior iliac spine (PSIS) as the area of maximum pain (Fig. 6.1).

A literature review would suggest that if the pain is below the level of the L5 vertebral body, and there are no dural tension signs (i.e., positive SLR), then the pain generator might be the SIJ [4, 20].

At this point, with strong suspicion that the pain might be coming from the SIJ, some clinicians would want to verify the diagnosis by injection before continuing with treatment knowing that the injection itself would potentially start the treatment process. The down side of doing an injection at this point is that if the SIJ

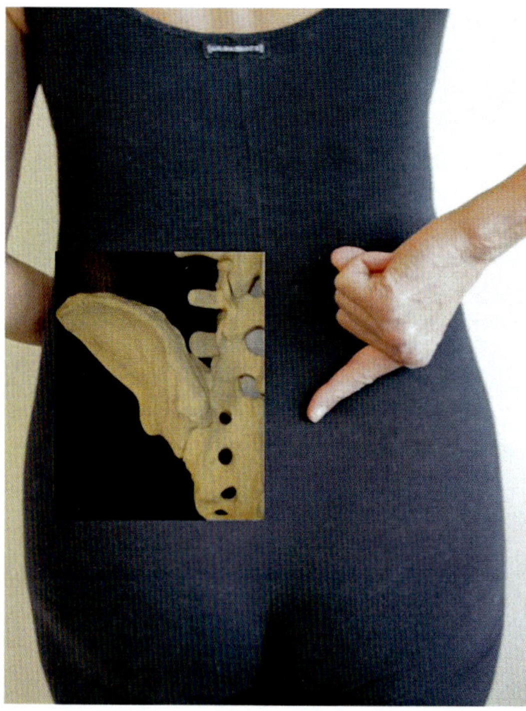

Fig. 6.1 Patient is pointing to a point at or just caudal to the posterior superior iliac spine, the most usual site for sacroiliac joint pain (Fortin Finger Test). If a patient points to this spot, the clinician must rule out the sacroiliac joint as a potential pain generator. *Copyright Borgess Health*

is a normal joint and not the pain generator, an injection could possibly cause changes that might render the joint other than normal. More study is needed to validate this concern. Most practitioners would do some conservative treatment measures first that might work and avoid any invasion into the joint if successful. The algorithm allows for both options depending on the judgment and the training of the provider.

Treatment

Now, it is time to begin treatment. It is here that many clinicians become confused and lost about where to start, how long to do something, and what to do next. Again, the treatment process should start simple, using less-invasive measures, and cost the least. If these do not work, then it is time to move up to more complex and invasive treatments.

Types of conservative treatment:
- Basic measures for low back pain prior to imaging studies
- Imaging studies followed by, if appropriate, manipulation
- Formal physical therapy
- Injections

Conservative Treatment Prior to Imaging or Injections

Treatment begins with anti-inflammatory medications, the possible use of a brace (sacral belt), and an alteration of activities. Anti-inflammatory medications can, in some patients, produce miraculous results from the start suggesting that there is a significant inflammatory component to the SIJ pain. When anti-inflammatory medication does not work or the effects are not enough, then the addition of a sacral belt might make a significant difference in the pain. The sacral belt is worn to control symptoms as much or as little as the patient determines is necessary. There is no known negative effect on the muscles by wearing a sacral belt on a continuous basis, as the back muscles are not being unloaded by this brace. One complication from wearing a sacral belt is trochanteric bursitis due to direct pressure on this region, which, if occurs, may necessitate discontinuing the sacral belt. The main activities that patients tend to avoid to reduce symptomatology are sitting, standing long periods on the ipsilateral leg, laying on the affected side, and, in women, sexual intercourse with abducted legs. Avoiding these activities as a way to control symptoms can be challenging as many are required for activities of daily living or needed for human relationships.

Imaging Studies

If the conservative measures thus far have not significantly decreased pain, it is at this point that we would recommend obtaining imaging studies of the SIJ and surrounding areas. Keep in mind that all the necessary imaging for suspected lumbar-related pain has already been done prior to starting this algorithm. If the usual "red flags" for a trauma, infection, or tumor had surfaced before this time (e.g., rapid weight loss, night pain, recent severe trauma, etc.), X-rays would have been done at the first consultation. It is important now to rule out hip joint pathology, sacral stress fracture, tumor, infection, or other causes that might need to be treated in specific ways other than with this algorithm. This is when a diagnosis of sacroiliitis might be made and a referral to a rheumatologist recommended. The X-rays we would recommend would be an AP of the pelvis to include both hips and specific oblique X-rays of the SIJs. A CT scan or an MRI would remain optional at this time only to further clarify an abnormality or suspicion found on the plain films. It should be remembered that there is no correlation in the literature between how a SIJ looks on imaging and how it feels in the patient in the absence of a fracture, tumor, or infection [4, 5, 21, 22].

Manipulation

Manipulation is the next treatment that should be considered if the more conservative measures have not helped and nothing alarming is found on X-ray. The neuromuscular and physiological effects of thrusting maneuvers have been found, in our experience at BBSI, to be the most beneficial in the treatment of SIJ pain at this stage in the algorithm. Chiropractors, osteopaths, or physical therapists trained in these treatment modalities should be the ones providing these treatments. Manipulation can be one of the most successful conservative treatment measures for the painful dysfunctional SIJ and should be done prior to moving into more complex, expensive, and invasive treatments. If manipulation efforts, lasting no longer than 6–12 weeks, result in no lasting improvement, a formal physical therapy evaluation and treatment program is recommended [2].

Physical Therapy

Physical therapists will evaluate and treat the entire thoracolumbar, pelvic, and lower extremity anatomy. Interventions will be utilized to stretch, strengthen, and stabilize all of the musculoskeletal structures that have an effect on the SIJs. This will be done in an effort to promote structural and force symmetry through and around the SIJs. Also, the therapist can utilize modalities such as ice, heat, ultrasound, etc. to optimize outcomes. This chapter will not discuss the seemingly end-less ways that these methods can be accomplished by the physical therapist. Chapter 14 covers the post-fusion rehabilitation by physical therapy.

Injections

Injections can be done at different points within this algorithm based on the experience of each individual patient and surgeon. It is placed here in the algorithm due to the fact that in a new patient being diagnosed and treated for the first time for a dysfunctional SIJ, an injection is not really needed in the treatment regimen until now. It is realized by the authors that this is a controversial statement, and in reality, our usual patient is referred to us having already had one or more diagnostic and/or therapeutic SIJ injections. It then becomes our job to be sure that all the necessary algorithm steps up to this one have been satisfied before moving on through the algorithm. If 6–12 weeks of physical therapy is not improving the patient, then more invasive and more costly measures are introduced. These start with injections if they have not already been performed. If a SIJ injection has not been done up to this point, then this injection is both diagnostic and potentially therapeutic [5, 20]. Injections should be performed using fluoroscopy with contrast dye to verify that a long-acting anesthetic agent and a steroid preparation have indeed entered the SIJ. The patient's spine surgeon, physiatrist, anesthesiologist, interventional radiologist, or pain physician routinely performs the injections (Fig. 6.2).

A Two-Way Street

The process of performing SIJ injections requires communication between both the physician performing the injection and the patient receiving the injection. It is mandatory that the physician thoroughly understands exactly where the patient's pain is primarily felt and where it radiates. Since the injection is the clinician's way of making an accurate diagnosis of a dysfunctional SIJ, and it is frequently also the primary way of making a diagnosis of facet syndrome, symptomatic foraminal stenosis that might respond to decompression, and primary discogenic pain, it is paramount that the clinician has from the beginning a clear idea of where the patient's pain might be coming from. It is only through constant

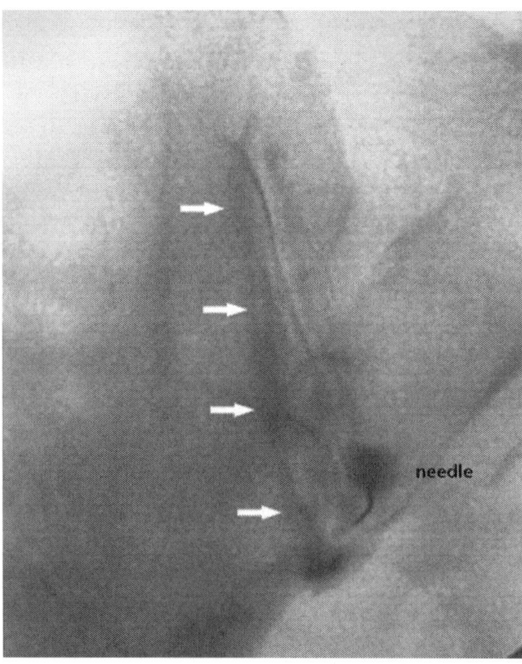

Fig. 6.2 Oblique image showing the needle at the most caudal portion of the joint with dye outlining the entire joint

dialogue with the patient before, during, and after the injection(s) that the best accurate information about the patient's pain can be obtained. The process of "honing in" on the diagnosis through repeated injections and injections into other areas can therefore be very complex and requires a dedicated physician to ultimately make the correct diagnosis or multiple diagnoses as the case may be.

Injections and Radiating Leg Pain

One of the confusing symptoms in patients with a dysfunctional SIJ is the presence of radiating leg pain. With the advent of injecting the SIJ with dye, to confirm that the medication being injected is indeed going into the joint, the dye has been visualized "leaking" out of the joint, through tears in the joint capsule. This leaking is verification that whatever else is in the joint (e.g., synovial fluid, lysozymes, etc.) can leak out and come in contact with surrounding tissues. Many of these tissues are nerve roots or a plexus of nerves. If whatever contacting the nerve tissue is irritating the nerve, the result might be the generating of an impulse in the nerve, thus creating referred pain down the leg. It is our experience that an EMG in such a patient is usually normal as there has been no nerve compression or permanent nerve tissue injury (Fig. 6.3).

The Injection Specialist

The injection specialist may or may not be the surgeon who will ultimately make the decision to operate on a SIJ. Many of us participating in the writing of this textbook did at one time do our own injections, and one or two still do. The propagation of injection specialist within the "pain management" segment of medicine now enables surgeons to send their patients to such specialists for these injections. Suffice it to say that the injection specialist has a formidable job to make an accurate diagnosis by using their injection abilities, as has been stated earlier, but it is beyond the scope of this textbook to provide teaching on the specifics of how to become an expert in the injection field.

Intra- Versus Extra-articular Injections

It should be understood that there are both intra-articular SIJ pain generators and extra-articular ones as well. The literature suggests that both intra-articular and extra-articular injections can be of benefit for both diagnosis and potential treatment in patients with painful, dysfunctional SIJs [16, 23–28]. Fluoroscopy should be used for the extra-articular injections as well. Our current institutional standard at BBSI is to perform an intra-articular injection and to consider an extra-articular injection only if the intra-articular injection was negative and the clinician has a very high suspicion that the pain is SIJ related and no lumbosacral pathology has been found.

Diagnostic Part of the Injection

Occasionally, the pain generators can be coming from both the SIJ and the lumbar spine (e.g., facet joints, foraminal stenosis), and injections become the only way to diagnose them accurately and potentially treat them. The diagnostic portion of the SIJ injection occurs by evaluating the patient's pain level for up to 2 h postinjection while the long-acting anesthetic agent is working. If the patient has significant relief during this time, it is assumed that the SIJ is the pain generator. We feel that significant pain relief is equal to or greater than a 70 % reduction in pain. It is then hoped that the steroid that was injected with the anesthetic agent will successfully cause pain relief within 24–48 h and last for weeks to months. If an injection successfully diagnoses the

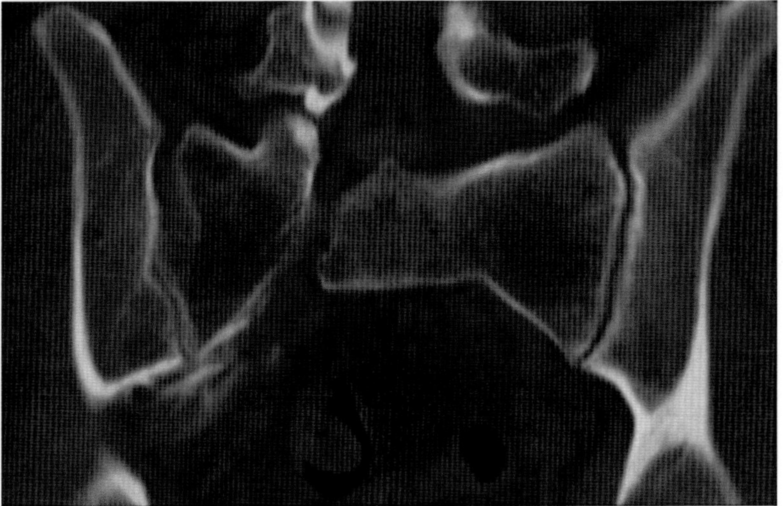

Fig. 6.3 Dye leaking out of the caudal portion of the SIJ joint capsule coming in potential contact with nerve tissue, which can result in radiating pain

SIJ as the pain generator and the pain is relieved for a long period of time, then another injection can be done if the pain returns to its previous pre-injection level. If the injection was diagnostic but did not provide long-lasting relief, then there is no reason to repeat the injection unless a diagnostic block is once again required or the clinician is considering an extra-articular source of the SIJ pain and wishes to perform an extra-articular injection. At any time that the patient's response to the injections results in questioning the SIJ as being the pain generator, the lumbar spine should be reevaluated as a possible source of the pain.

When Injections Are Enough

If the injections are able to reduce the pain levels to 3–4/10 on the visual analog scale (VAS) or less on a long-term basis, then all the aspects of the algorithm up to this point that have been relatively successful can be used over and over with judicious use of injection therapy to maintain the patient at a functional level.

More Invasive, Complex, and Costly Treatments
Alternative Treatments

It is at this juncture that the clinician can consider procedures, which are available but have not had consistent success in the literature for treating the painful, stable SIJ. These would be considered "alternative" treatments at this time and would include prolotherapy, neuroaugmentation, visco-supplementation, radiofrequency ablation, and acupuncture. All of these treatment modalities have had some success, but not enough to become mainline treatments for the painful SIJ. Please read the references pertaining to these alternate methods for further information [29–35].

Fusion

It is only when all of the treatments in the algorithm thus far have failed, to include any of the "alternate" treatment methods that may have been tried, the injection(s) has definitively diagnosed the SIJ as the pain generator, and the patient is continuing to live with constant chronic pain, which limits their ability to perform activities of daily living, that a fusion procedure might be considered. The role of the fusion to treat the chronic dysfunctional painful SIJ has been controversial at best. Recently, there has been resurgence in the literature supporting the role of fusion for the painful dysfunctional SIJ (Chap. 2). Surgeons interested in the SIJ have primarily been orthopedic surgeons, orthopedic surgeons with spine or trauma fellowships, and neurosurgeons who have had exposure to the SIJ by orthopedic surgeons. Most surgeons feel that a fusion of this joint should be kept as the last form of treatment after all else has failed. The patient should have chronic pain (>6 months), be disabled from activities of daily living, failed all reasonable conservative treatments, and be mentally capable of having goal direction and reasonable expectations concerning the surgery and the potential outcomes. At this point in time, there is no standard way to fuse the SIJ. The type of surgery done is

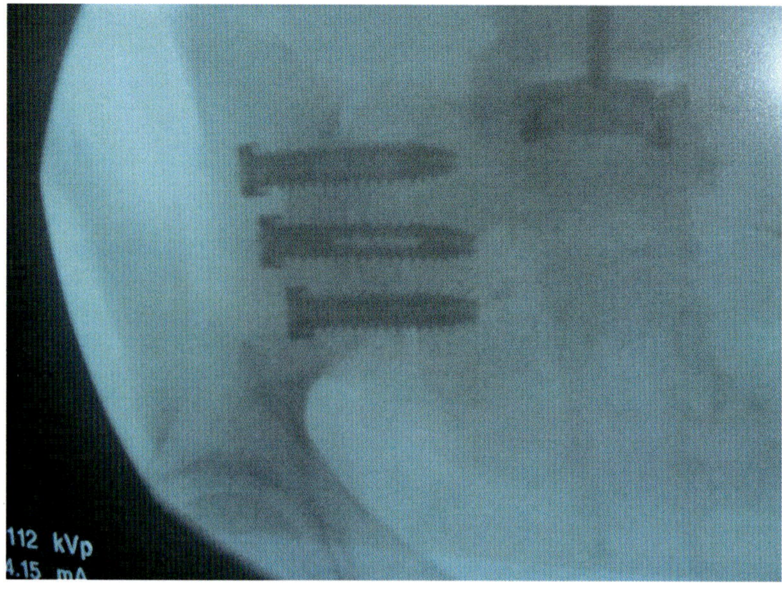

Fig. 6.4 AP image in surgery demonstrating the final positioning of the instrumentation (Globus Medical, SI-LOK) at BBSI using a lateral minimally invasive approach. This approach is currently the most utilized approach for sacroiliac joint fusion (Chap. 8)

totally dependent on the training and experience of the treating surgeon. The joint may be approached anteriorly, laterally, posterior laterally, and posteriorly, with some of these options being done minimally invasively (Fig. 6.4).

> Criteria for considering a fusion for the dysfunctional SIJ:
> - Must be an adult with mature pelvis
> - Have chronic pain lasting >6 months
> - Be disabled from all activities of daily living
> - Have failed all reasonable forms of conservative treatment
> - Had a "valid" diagnostic SIJ injection
> - Be mentally capable of goal direction and appropriate expectations postsurgery

There is considerable variety in how the surgery is performed and how the patient is treated during their recovery (e.g., type of brace and duration, postoperative weight bearing, etc.), but one single fact appears to be quite clear in the literature to date concerning the result of such surgery. If a fusion is done successfully, in the appropriate patient for all the appropriate reasons, and the patient is appropriately rehabilitated, then success rates are very high (80 % range) for relieving pain and improving function (Chap. 2). In some instances, the most conservative treatment method for patients being treated chronically for pain might be a fusion procedure [36].

A Word About Postoperative Narcotics in the "Chronic Pain Patient"

It should be noted that even in the best circumstance where treatment has significantly reduced or relieved the patient's pain, it may take some time to wean the patient from some of the high-dose narcotic medication that many of them have been using for long periods, possibly years, to treat pain and to remain functional. The physician who has had them on long-term pain management would be the most logical person to help the patient wean from the narcotics after successful surgical treatment of their SIJ. At BBSI, we consider chronic narcotic use prior to surgery as a separate diagnostic entity and work to ensure that the patient is being appropriately followed postsurgery to adequately address this issue.

Restrictions After Fusion of the SIJ

If the patient has experienced significant pain relief as a result of the surgery, the patient is then encouraged to resume all activities as tolerated. Restrictions are reserved for patients having residual symptoms in the SIJ not completely controlled by treatment or if pathology and pain in

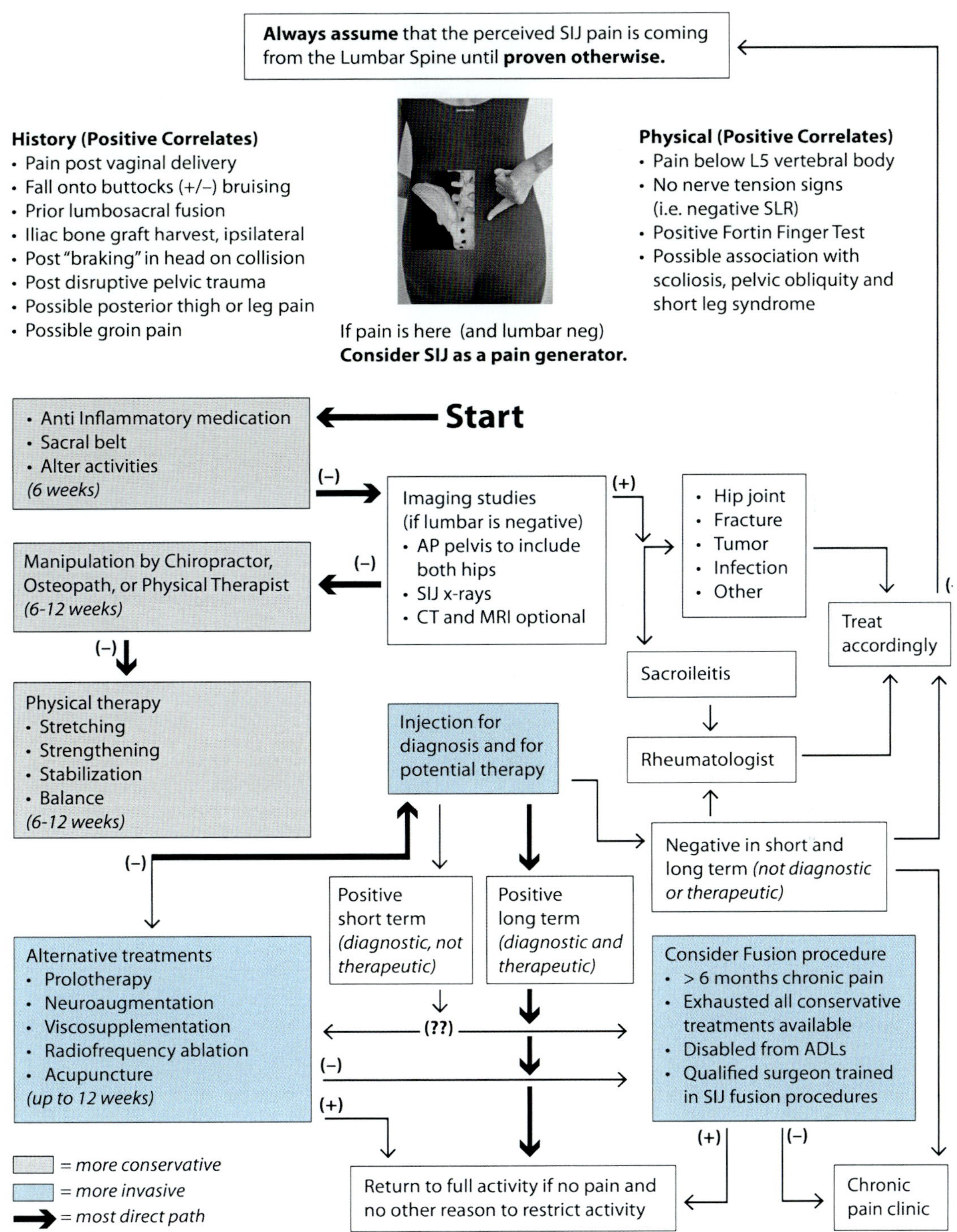

Fig. 6.5 Illustration showing the recommended steps in the algorithm for the diagnosis and treatment of the dysfunctional sacroiliac joint. *Copyright Borgess Health*

the lumbar spine require them. A single SIJ treated successfully with fusion usually does not require restrictions.

Chronic Pain Management

If a patient fails all the steps of the algorithm that are appropriate for them, a referral to, or back to, a chronic pain management institution is appropriate.

Conclusion

This algorithm was developed to assist the surgeon and other clinicians in their attempt to diagnose and treat the patient with pain possibly originating from the SIJ. It is assumed that this algorithm will undergo much change as more is learned about this very complex joint in terms of anatomy, diagnosis, and treatment options (Fig. 6.5).

References

1. Dall BE, Eden SV, Brumblay H. Algorithm for the diagnosis and treatment of the dysfunctional sacroiliac joint. 2010. http://www.borgess.com/files/bbsi/pdf/si_joint_white.pdf
2. Zelle BA, Gruen GS, Brown S, George S. Sacroiliac joint dysfunction: evaluation and management. Clin J Pain. 2005;21:446–55.
3. Bernard TN, Kirkaldy-Willis WH. Recognizing specific characteristics of non-specific low back pain. Clin Orthop. 1987;217:266–80.
4. Schwarzer AC, Aprill CN, Bogduk N. The sacroiliac joint in low back pain. Spine. 1995;20:31–7.
5. Maigne JY, Aivaliklis A, Pfefer F. Results of the sacroiliac joint double block and value of sacroiliac provocation tests in 54 patients with low back pain. Spine. 1996;21:1889–92.
6. Schuit D, McPoil TG, Mulesa P. Incidence of sacroiliac joint malalignments in leg length discrepancies. J Am Podiatr Med Assoc. 1989;79:380–3.
7. Herzog W, Conway PJ. Gait analysis of sacroiliac joint patients. J Manipulative Physiol Ther. 1994;17:124–7.
8. Schoenberger M, Hellmich K. Sacroiliac dislocation and scoliosis. Hippokrates. 1964;35:476–9.
9. Katz V, Schofferman J, Reynolds J. "The sacroiliac joint" a potential cause of pain after lumbar fusion to the sacrum. J Spinal Disord Tech. 2003;16:96–9.
10. Ebraheim NA, Elgafy H, Semaan HB. Computed tomographic findings in patients with persistent sacroiliac pain after posterior iliac graft harvesting. Spine. 2000;25:2047–51.
11. Albert H, Godskesen M, Westergaard J. Prognosis in four syndromes of pregnancy-related pelvic pain. Acta Obstet Gynecol Scand. 2001;80:505–10.
12. Berg G, Hammar M, Moller-Nielsen J. Low back pain during pregnancy. Obstet Gynecol. 1988;71:71–5.
13. Daly JM, Frame PS, Rapoza PA. Sacroiliac subluxations: a common treatable cause of low back pain in pregnancy. Fam Pract Res J. 1991;11:149–59.
14. Bollow M, Braun J, Hamm B. Sacroiliitis: the key symptom of spondyloarthropathies. 1. The clinical aspects (German). Rofo. 1997;166:95–100.
15. Cush JJ, Lipsky PE. Reiter's syndrome and reactive arthritis. In: Koopman WJ, editor. Arthritis and allied conditions: a textbook of rheumatology, vol. 1. 14th ed. Philadelphia, PA: Lippincott Williams & Wilkins; 2001. p. 1324–44.
16. Wise CL, Dall BE. Minimally invasive sacroiliac arthrodesis: outcomes of a new technique. J Spinal Disord Tech. 2008;8:579–84.
17. Dreyfuss P, Michaelsen M, Pauza K, McLarty J. The value of the medical history and physical examination in diagnosing sacroiliac joint pain. Spine. 1996;21:2594–602.
18. Fortin JD, Dwyer AP, West S. Sacroiliac joint pain referral maps upon applying a new injection/arthrography technique, part I. Spine. 1994;19:1475–82.
19. Fortin JD, Aprill CN, Ponthieux B. Sacroiliac joint pain referral maps upon applying a new injection/arthrography technique, part I. Spine. 1994;19:1483–9.
20. Dreyfuss P, Dreyer S, Cole A, Mayo K. Sacroiliac joint pain. J Am Acad Orthop Surg. 2004;12:255–65.
21. Prather H. Sacroiliac joint pain: practical management. Clin J Sport Med. 2003;13:252–5.
22. Bernard TN, Cassidy JD. The sacroiliac joint syndrome: pathophysiology, diagnosis, and management. In: Frymoyer JW, editor. The adult spine: principles and practice. New York: Raven; 1991. p. 2107–30.
23. Maugars Y, Mathis C, Berthelot JM, Charlier C, Prost A. Assessment of the efficacy of sacroiliac corticosteroid injections in spondyloarthropathies: a double-blind study. Br J Rheumatol. 1996;35:767–70.
24. Braun J, Bollow M, Seyrekbasan F. Computed tomography guided corticosteroid injection of the sacroiliac joint in patients with spondyloarthropathy with sacroiliitis: clinical outcome and follow-up by dynamic magnetic resonance imaging. J Rheumatol. 1996;23:659–64.
25. Luukkainen R, Nissila M, Asikainen E. Periarticular corticosteroid treatment of the sacroiliac joint in patients with seronegative spondyloarthropathy. Clin Exp Rheumatol. 1999;17:88–90.
26. Luukkainen R, Wennerstrand PV, Kautiainen HH. Efficacy of periarticular corticosteroid treatment of the sacroiliac joint in non-spondyloarthropathic patients with chronic low back pain in the region of the sacroiliac joint. Clin Exp Rheumatol. 2002;20:52–4.
27. Belanger TA, Dall BE. Sacroiliac arthrodesis using a posterior midline fascial splitting approach and pedi-

cle screw instrumentation: a new technique. J Spinal Disord. 2001;2:118–24.

28. Borowsky CD, Fagen G. Sources of sacroiliac region pain: insights gained from study comparing standard intra- and peri-articular injection. Arch Phys Med Rehabil. 2008;89:2048–56.

29. Klein RG, Edk BC, Delong WB, Mooney V. A randomized double blind trial of dextrose-glycerine-phenol injections for chronic low back pain. J Spinal Disord. 1993;6:23–33.

30. Calvillo O, Esses SI, Ponder C, D'Agostino C, Tanhui E. Neuroaugmentation in the management of sacroiliac joint pain: a report of two cases. Spine. 1998;23:1069–72.

31. Yin W, Willard F, Carreiro J, Dreyfuss P. Sensory stimulation-guided sacroiliac joint radiofrequency neurotomy: technique based on neuroanatomy of the dorsal sacral plexus. Spine. 2003;28:2419–25.

32. Buijs EJ, Kamphuis ET, Groen GJ. Radiofrequency treatment of sacroiliac joint-related pain aimed at the first three sacral dorsal rami: a minimal approach. Pain Clin. 2004;16:139–46.

33. Ferrante FM, King LF, Roche EA. Radiofrequency sacroiliac joint denervation for sacroiliac syndrome. Reg Anesth Pain Med. 2001;26:137–42.

34. Gevargez A, Groenemeyer D, Schirp S, Braun M. CT-guided percutaneous radiofrequency denervation of the sacroiliac joint. Eur Radiol. 2002;12:1360–5.

35. Srejic U, Calvillo O, Kabakibou K. Viscosupplementation: a new concept in the treatment of sacroiliac joint syndrome: a preliminary report of four cases. Reg Anesth Pain Med. 1999;24:84–8.

36. Ackerman SJ, Polly DW, Knight T, Schneider K, Holt T, Cummings J. Comparison of the costs of nonoperative care to minimally invasive surgery for sacroiliac joint disruption and degenerative sacroiliitis in a United States Medicare population: potential economic implications of a new minimally-invasive technology. Clinicoecon Outcomes Res. 2013;5:575–87.

Bruce E. Dall

Introduction

During my own educational process spanning medical school, orthopedic residency, and a spine surgery fellowship, I never learned much about the sacroiliac joint (SIJ) in terms of functionality and pain generation. I certainly did not learn that people could become functionally disabled with chronic severe pain from a stable appearing SIJ or that fusion surgery could be performed with, at times, almost miraculous results. It was not until I was faced with such a patient that I realized how unequipped I was to both diagnose and treat this problem. As the years past, I began to realize that most surgeons, except for trauma surgeons, were in the same boat as me. Due to the increase in diagnosis of the dysfunctional SIJ and now having surgical instrumentation dedicated to fusing the joint that is all changing. This chapter discusses a few of the urgent considerations for a surgeon embarking on becoming a fuser of the SIJ. These tips have no particular order and will be discussed in various ways throughout this book. I chose to put a chapter together discussing

B.E. Dall, M.D. (✉)
Neurosurgery of Kalamazoo, Borgess Brain
and Spine Institute, 1541 Gull Road,
Kalamazoo, MI 49048, USA

Orthopedic Spine Division, Western Michigan
University Medical School, Kalamazoo, MI USA
e-mail: dall.bruce@yahoo.com

them as a group in hopes that none would be missed from the book altogether as I feel each is important to at least consider.

The Borgess Brain and Spine Institute Experience

Borgess Brain and Spine Institute (BBSI) has been diagnosing and treating the dysfunctional SIJ patient for over two decades and has become an international referral center for this condition. As an institution dedicated to spinal surgery for more than 40 years, it has published many peer-reviewed articles on both the spine and the SIJ. Original research has lead to the creation of an algorithm (Chap. 6) to diagnose and treat the dysfunctional SIJ, new approaches for fusing the joint (Chaps. 9 and 10), and new devices to assist in the fusion process. As a result of the following hundreds of post-fusion patients, a very large database for patients with this diagnosis has been created. Multiple publications are currently in the process of formulation based on outcomes from these patients. It is by understanding this data and the core aspects of the dysfunctional SIJ patient that we can make suggestions to a surgeon who now wants to learn more about the surgical treatment of these patients. It is important for the reader to understand that opinions concerning the following paragraphs are primarily the author's and are based on vast personal experience. Other experts might have opposing views.

B.E. Dall et al. (eds.), *Surgery for the Painful, Dysfunctional Sacroiliac Joint*,
DOI 10.1007/978-3-319-10726-4_7, © Springer International Publishing Switzerland 2015

Important Considerations When Operating on the Dysfunctional SIJ

Although the considerations confronting the surgeon who is going to operate on the SIJ are seemingly countless, we have found that the following deserve special mention here.

Important items a surgeon new to the SIJ should understand:

- Three-dimensional orientation of the joint
- Considerations when imaging in the anterior–posterior plane
- Location and importance of the cluneal nerves, sciatic nerve, and superior gluteal artery
- Osteopenia and Osteoporosis ramifications
- Patient demographics and their ramifications for results
- Should the joint be "realigned" before fusion surgery?
- Bilateral fusion considerations
- Fusing both lumbar spine and SIJ at same setting, considerations
- The morbidly obese patient
- Why rehabilitate?
- Different approaches for different surgeons

Three-Dimensional Orientation of the Joint

With the SIJ located nearly equidistant from anterior to posterior in the sagittal plane and angled obliquely with its undulating shape, it is very difficult to conceptualize its place in space when examining or operating on a patient. Being located in the midst of the pelvic bones also makes it challenging to image the entire joint in one plane. When using fluoroscopy in surgery to visualize the joint from posterior, there always seems to be two joint images making it a guessing game for the surgeon (Fig. 7.1).

There is a basic fact about the orientation of the joint that has been relatively constant and if well understood can help the surgeon. When viewing the dorsal aspect of the patient, the general overall orientation of the joint is approximately a 20–30° angulation from posteromedial to anterolateral. If, however, the

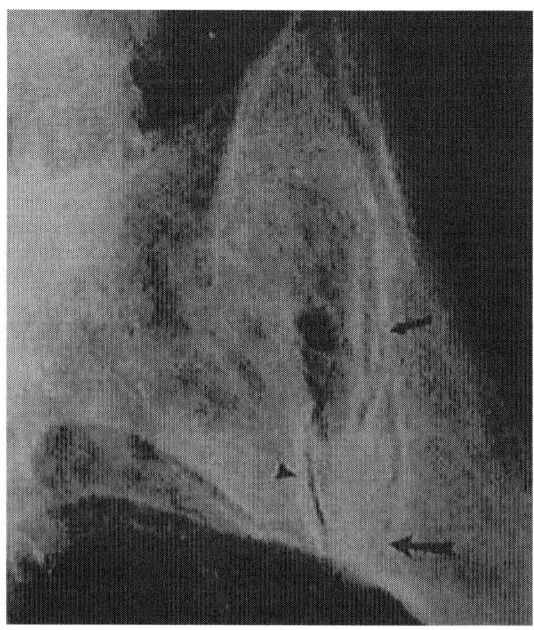

Fig. 7.1 AP intraoperative image of sacroiliac joint showing two "confusing" joint lines

joint is analyzed in sections, again from the dorsal aspect, there exists an angular difference between them. The cephalad portion basically maintains the 20–30° oblique angle from posteromedial to anterolateral, whereas the caudal portion is almost in a line perpendicular to the floor and may even angle slightly anteromedial (Fig. 7.2).

This is why those injecting into the joint do so at the caudal end where, when visualized posterior to anterior in the coronal plane under fluoroscopy with some slight oblique medial or lateral angulation, this joint becomes one joint line allowing for accurate joint injection (Fig. 7.3).

This knowledge is useful when using image to place a cage from posterior into the longitudinal axis of the joint in its caudal portion. It is in this section of the joint that the ilium is closest to the sacrum and has less posterior ligament mass. It is in this caudal section that the best fusions can occur when approached posteriorly. Interestingly, the subchondral bone of the true SIJ is also where some of the thickest and strongest cortical bone exists for screw or cage fixation. Instrumentation placed in this section has a better chance of firmly connecting the ilium to the sacrum.

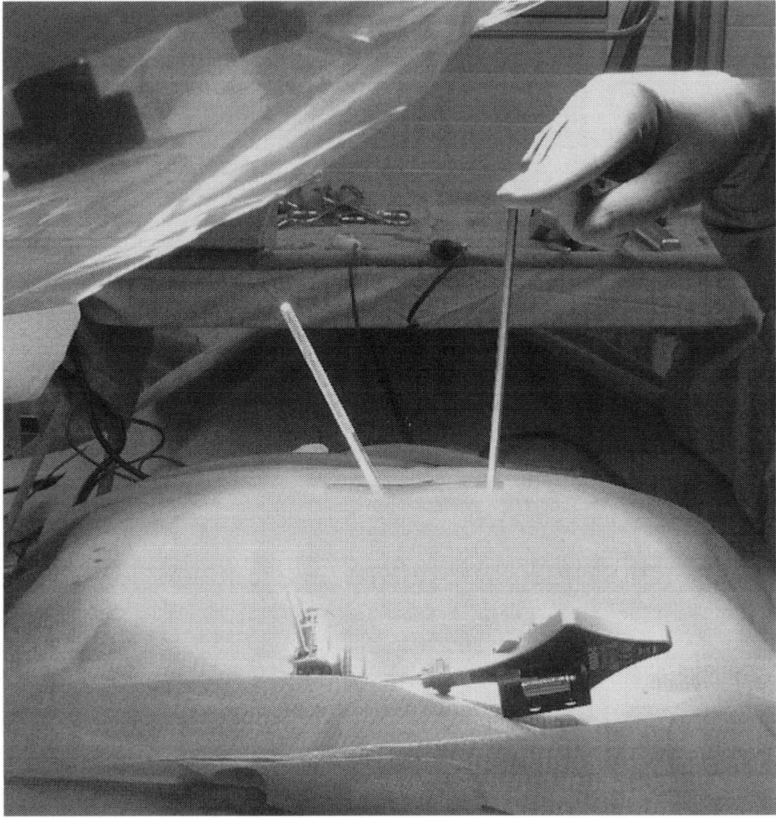

Fig. 7.2 Intraoperative photo showing two K-wires. The vertical wire is in the longitudinal axis of the caudal portion of the sacroiliac joint and the angled wire is in the cephalad portion of the joint

Considerations When Imaging in the Anterior–Posterior Plane

Imaging the patient in the lateral plane is very straightforward, has been discussed in the literature for decades, and will be covered in detail in the Chap. 8 discussions on the minimally invasive lateral approach. What is less familiar for the surgeon is understanding the anatomical details in the patient being imaged using the anterior–posterior (AP) plane in the various angles ranging from 30° cephalad (outlet view) to 30° caudad (inlet view). In relation to the SIJ orientation in the prone position, each of these angles views the joint in very different ways. When using AP image to perform posterior lateral screw or cage insertion, these various angles must be clearly understood for successful instrumentation. Starting with the straight AP image view (Figs. 7.4 and 7.5), note the location of the S1 pedicle, the S1 foramen, and the posterior superior iliac spine (PSIS), as these are the landmarks that will be most obvious as they change position when angling the image in this plane. The value of the straight AP image is to assure that the spine and pelvis are symmetrically oriented in the coronal plane with the spinous processes in the centerline and the sacrum and iliac wings appearing equal bilaterally. This view also shows the most prominent portion of the PSIS the best in an area just lateral and cephalad to the S1 pedicle and foramen.

When the AP view is moved to the 30° cephalad position, what is being imaged is the "outlet" view (Figs. 7.6 and 7.7). Note again the location of the S1 pedicle, the S1 foramen, and the PSIS. These change in location dramatically with this angular change in the image. This image is very valuable when instrumenting as it gives the best view of the S1 pedicle and the S1 and S2 foramina.

The third AP angle we will consider is the 30° caudal, or "inlet" view. This represents a 60° angular change in viewing of the AP anatomy

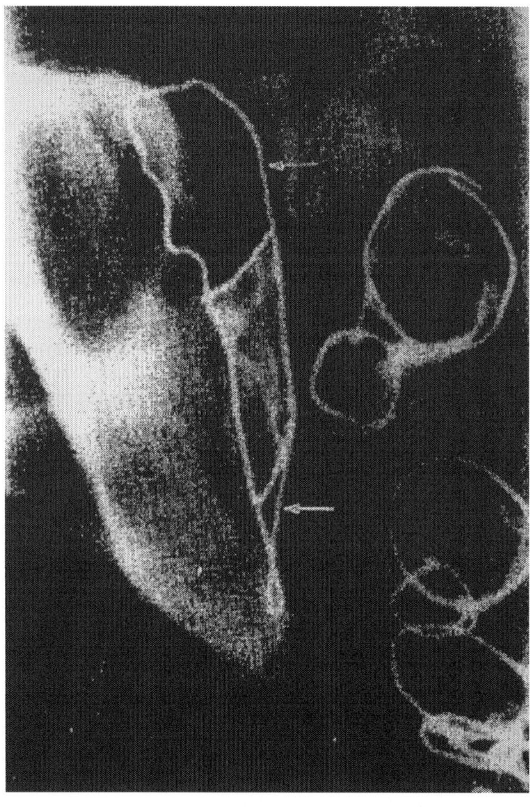

Fig. 7.3 Image showing the outline of the sacroiliac joint (*arrows*) from posterior demonstrating its "propeller-like" configuration

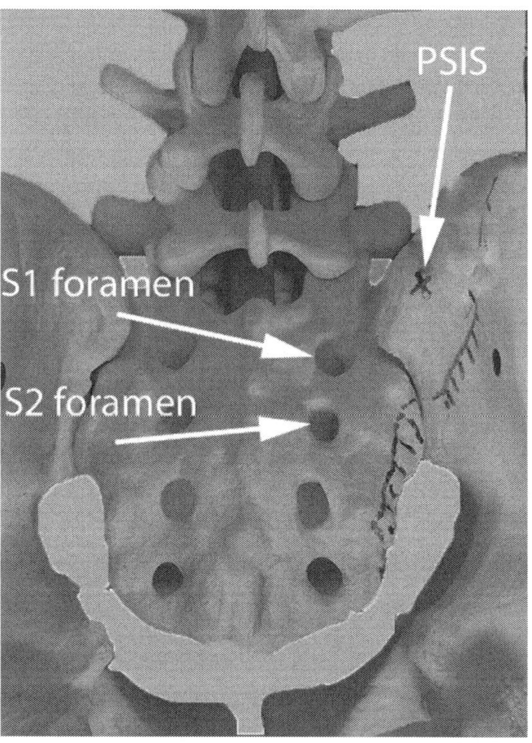

Fig. 7.5 Shows skeletal anatomy with AP image. Note that the PSIS is cephalad to the S1 foramen and possibly at the level of the L5–S1 disk space

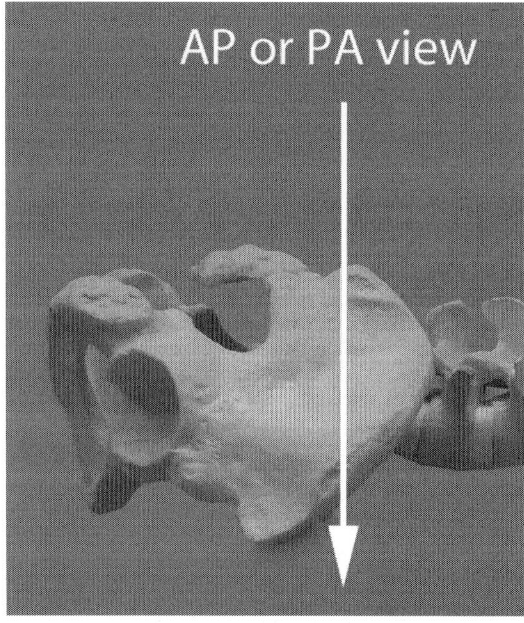

Fig. 7.4 Shows AP or PA plane for imaging for pelvis

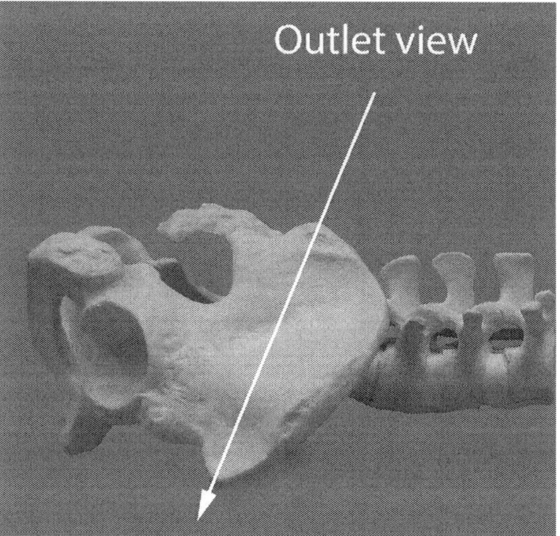

Fig. 7.6 Shows 30° (approximate) cephalad plane of AP imaging for pelvis, the "outlet" view

compared to the 30° cephalad view. The primary value of this view is to visualize the anterior arch of the sacrum, which consists of the anterior

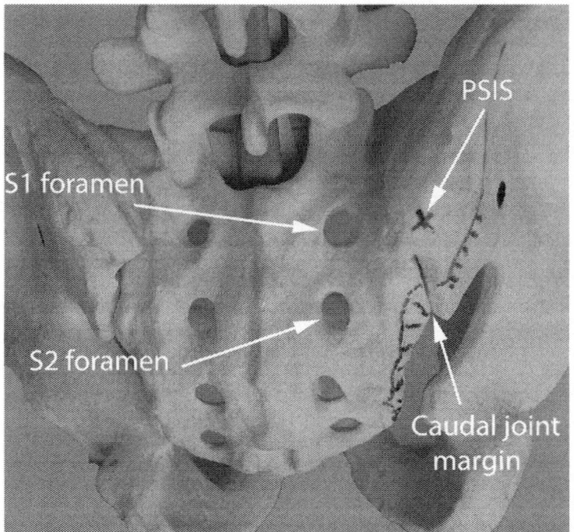

Fig. 7.7 Demonstrates the "outlet" pelvic view which shows the PSIS as being directly lateral to the S1 foramen and the lowest part of the joint margin directly lateral to the S2 foramen (this can vary according to individual)

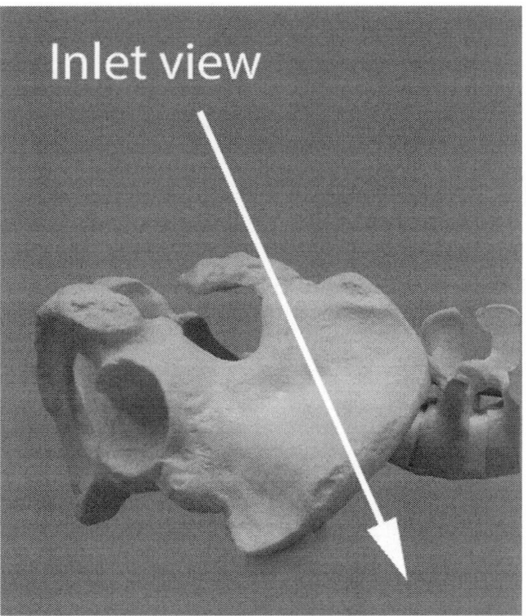

Fig. 7.8 Shows 30° (approximate) caudal plane of AP imaging for pelvis, "inlet" view

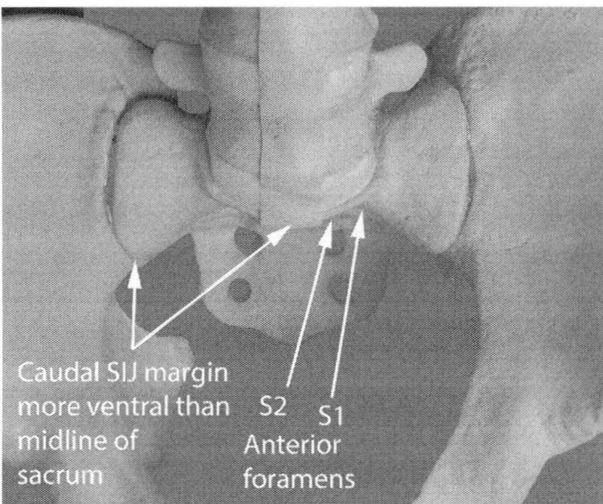

Fig. 7.9 Demonstrates the "inlet" pelvic view, which shows the anterior margin of the sacrum. This view helps to avoid anterior penetration of the sacrum into the pelvis when placing instrumentation

elements of the sacral alae and both the S1 and S2 exiting foramina. Just caudal to the S2 foramen, the sacrum usually angles in a caudal direction and severs its joint connection with the ilium. This caudal portion of the sacrum acts more like an apophasis serving no weight-bearing structural function but is an attachment for multiple ligaments and muscles forming the pelvic sling. This 30° caudal inlet angular view of the sacrum is the primary one used for assuring that no instrumentation goes anterior to the sacrum into the pelvis. It should always be checked as one of the final images after any of the instrumented approaches (Figs. 7.8 and 7.9).

When imaging using the various angles in the AP plane, the surgeon must be fully knowledgeable of the anatomical landmarks present and how they change in relation to one another as the angle of the image changes. From anyone of these three AP angles, there is also the ability to angle obliquely either medial or lateral to further define a location. There frequently is a "learning curve" to understanding what is actually being seen and what the surgeon is expecting to see during these surgeries. If at any time the surgeon becomes confused by the image, it is imperative to return to a known image angle or to move the image "live," for the shortest period of time possible, until the anatomy in the image is fully understood. If there is still confusion, the question of aborting the current plan comes into play.

Location and Importance of the Cluneal Nerves, Sciatic Nerve, and Superior Gluteal Artery

The subject of cluneal nerves has been discussed in Chap. 3 on anatomy, but a few facts concerning these nerves deserve further dialogue. The cluneal nerves enter the posterior gluteal space approximately 8–12 cm cephalad and lateral to the PSIS along the rim of the ilium to fan out over the buttock (see Figs. 3.10 and 3.14). These nerves access the superficial deep fascial layer, which extends from the midline of the spine laterally over the gluteal musculature. When these sensory nerves are cut, they form neuromas on their transected ends, which can become a source of chronic pain for various different reasons. Hutchinson published how to reflect the cluneal nerves safely out of harms way when using the posterior midline fascial splitting approach to harvest iliac bone graft [1]. He presented dramatic results in significantly decreasing or eliminating the chronic pain occurring from cluneal nerve injury with this method. The potential for injury to the cluneal nerves should be on the surgeon's mind as he/she considers where to make the incision for exposure to the SIJ. The literature illustrates several techniques where the incision is along the entire arch of the ilium or long straight incisions placed posterolaterally that certainly cross into cluneal nerve territory. Three incision types do, in general, avoid the cluneal nerves. The first type is the posterior midline incision and fascial splitting approach discussed by Hutchinson. The second type are those incisions used for posterior lateral minimally invasive approaches, which essentially are located at, lateral, or inferior to the PSIS and extending for 2 in. or less. The third type is the lateral minimally invasive approach (Fig. 7.10).

The superior gluteal artery is a branch off of the internal iliac artery that quickly exits the pelvis through the sciatic notch (see Figs. 3.12 and 3.14). It angles cephalad, anterior, and lateral as it branches out between the gluteal muscle layers to provide blood supply to those muscles. Injury to this artery has been implicated as a potentially disastrous complication in the harvesting of the iliac bone graft [2]. Considering that its path literally crosses over the ilium where the SIJ can be superimposed, it is at potential risk with any direct lateral instrumentation effort. If transected, it can retract back inside the pelvis, and if a significant hematoma should occur, be advised that this may need extreme measures to treat. It is possible that interventional radiology might be needed to clot off the bleeder or that an open procedure might be required. At this point, one should also be reminded that the distance from the sciatic notch (see Figs. 3.6 and 7.11), where both the superior gluteal artery and the sciatic nerve exit, is only a few centimeters from the insertion point of the most posterior caudal fixation device using the minimally invasive straight lateral approach. Great caution is advised probing this area while using image in attempting to secure the point of placement for the subsequent drilling and insertion of instrumentation as pushing the probe into the sciatic notch is very possible and can result in neurologic or vascular trauma.

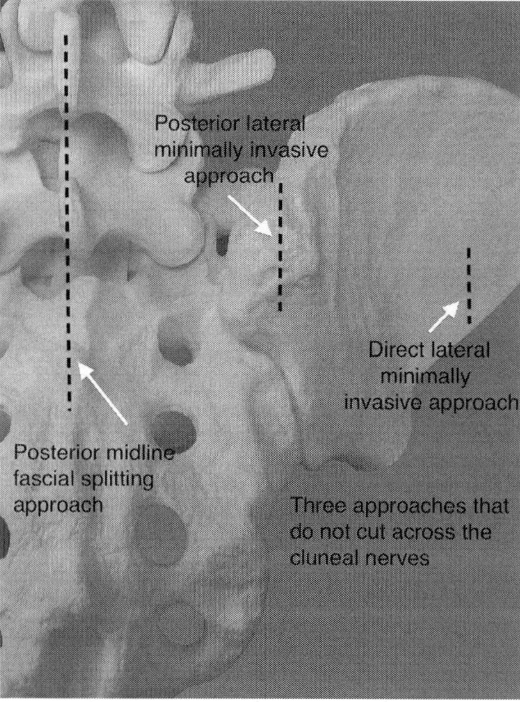

Fig. 7.10 Various posterior and lateral incisions to approach the sacroiliac joint with *arrows* pointing to those which are less likely to injure the cluneal nerves

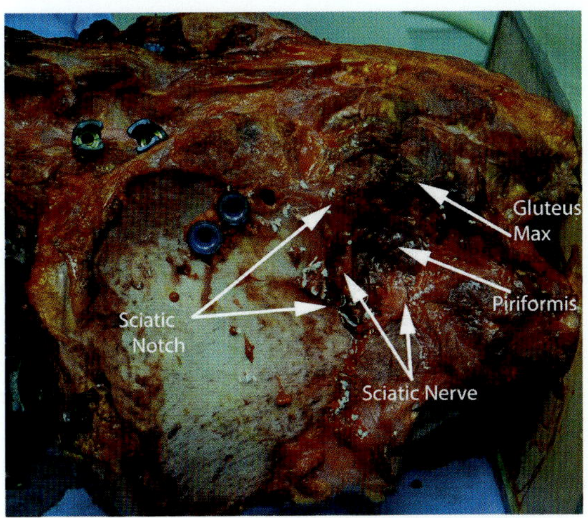

Fig. 7.11 Photo of instrument placement location in lateral ileum of cadaver. Note the proximity of the most caudal drill hole to the sciatic notch, which contains both the sciatic nerve and the superior gluteal artery. *Courtesy Globus Medical, Inc. Audubon, PA*

Osteoporosis and Its Ramifications

Decreased bone density continues to be the harbinger of potential complications for surgeons inserting instrumentation for fusions. We are now in an era when many of the patients presenting to us at risk have had a bone density test. It is not unusual for such a patient to be on some type of bone density enhancer. Currently, there are no specific standard bone density numbers, which preclude the possibility of inserting instrumentation. Most of these types of patients are either avoided secondary to a significant history of fracture or they are found out intraoperatively. Should SIJ surgery be performed on a patient having known osteoporosis? Due to the body of the sacrum along with the sacral ala being areas where some of the earliest and most extensive decreases in bone density occur, the wisdom of using a direct lateral approach in these patients might be questioned. Our first dysfunctional SIJ fusion patient was elderly and had a long history of rheumatoid arthritis. By definition today, she had osteoporosis. Because it was felt that surgery needed to be done and the only option at that time was placing two screws across the ilium into the osteoporotic sacrum, a posterior approach was devised. This approach (Chap. 9) utilized the S1

pedicle and the longitudinal cortical layers of the narrower portion of the ilium, which provided excellent fixation for 9 years and allowed her to ambulate with a walker until she died from other causes. We feel that when faced with known osteoporosis and it has been decided to proceed with SIJ surgery, the surgeon should be aware that the sacrum can be essentially hollow in some of these patients, and a search for the technique that has a higher likelihood of providing the strongest metal to bone interface should be used. As the procedures are discussed in this book, it would be beneficial to pay attention to the potential bone available and the usual quality of that bone for fixation with each technique.

Patient Demographics and Ramifications for Results

It has only been in the past few years that the basic profile for a patient with a dysfunctional SIJ has been defined by the BBSI. This data resulted from 100 consecutive patients over a 5-year period presenting with chronic SIJ pain, who eventually underwent a unilateral or bilateral SIJ fusion. Our findings suggest that the average SIJ fusion patient can be potentially complex and very challenging. Our average patient was female, middle aged, and had been receiving conservative treatment for their pain for an average of 4 years. During this time, they saw multiple doctors, to include orthopedic surgeons, neurosurgeons, anesthesiologists, and physiatrists, and had injections into their back for pain. Most were undiagnosed, despite the fact that many had had an injection into the SIJ, under fluoroscopy with more than 2 h of temporary relief. They were frequently disabled and depressed. More than two thirds were on chronic narcotic use for greater than 2 years, and many were dependent on the medications. Despite the fact that over one half of these patients were under current ongoing injection treatments in chronic pain clinics, they were most often referred not by their pain doctors but by their physical therapist or their primary care physician, or they found their way to the office via their own initiative and the Internet. They were generally desperate and for the most part still highly motivated. A few patients at our institution did have a more recent onset of pain and were quickly diagnosed and referred, but this was certainly not the norm. It is important for the surgeon to understand that these preoperative demographics might exist in their patients presenting with a dysfunctional SIJ. Their expectations could be unrealistic, and they might be carrying other emotional or psychological baggage that must be acknowledged. These patients require a lot of education concerning their diagnosis and the options for modern surgical treatment and for the potential results after surgery and rehabilitation. For those dependent on narcotics, the immediate postoperative treatment must include a pathway for continuing on these medications with a plan for weaning assuming that the surgery is successful. Many of these patients have other pain issues that will not be treated by a fusion of the SIJ alone, and these have to be considered during the preoperative education and postoperatively as well. The demographics of these patients are a product of our current medical system and the existing knowledge base among clinicians and surgeons in medicine today. This is rapidly changing and will continue to change over time as more and more clinicians and surgeons become educated on the dysfunctional SIJ, and it reaches a point where it is being taught in residency programs and in medical schools. Until then, however, anyone actively performing SIJ fusions for the dysfunctional joint is to be considered a tertiary center for that condition, and these are the types of patients that may be coming through the door.

Should the Joint Be "Realigned" Before Fusion Surgery?

First of all, the reader needs to bear in mind three things. This response is one surgeon's opinion, patients frequently want this done, and long after this book is finished, this will continue to be a controversial subject. The following is based on my observation of the SIJ as viewed through hundreds of posterior open surgeries to fuse this joint. Many of these patients had a history of being "realigned" by their physical therapist and chiropractors, frequently with great short-term pain relief, before finally ending up having a fusion surgery. During the posterior midline approach for fusing the SIJ (Chap. 9), the entire posterior ligament-supporting complex is effectively removed. At the same time, the patient is paralyzed with total muscle relaxation as the result of anesthesia. One would assume that under these circumstances, this joint, which previously needed realignment for being "displaced" and "out of line," would certainly demonstrate significant movement and instability. The truth is that it remains very stable with, at most, 1–2° of motion when attempting to move the joint using screws firmly fixed in the sacrum and ilium as levers. This was not what I was expecting to see, and it was a time to pause and reflect. Having this experience, I then arranged for a cadaver experiment at Globus Medical (Audubon, PA) to test this finding in a controlled situation. Using a machine to test range of motion in 6°, a pelvis, stripped of all muscle and only having ligament support, was tested. The normal range of motion of the SIJ averaged less than 1° in each of flexion and extension, axial rotation, and lateral bending in seven consecutive cadaver specimens. So, with the same ligaments transected as in surgery, the range of motion averaged less than 2° in all the cadaver specimens. This experiment can be reviewed in its entirety in Chap. 4. My opinion is that this joint is essentially a very stable joint in the patient with the diagnosis of a dysfunctional SIJ with the capability of almost imperceptible movement. Therefore, unless the preoperative CT scan shows significant displacement and instability, which is usually not the case, there is no scientific rationale for trying to put the SIJ somewhere else prior to fusion surgery. My suspicion is that this one paragraph might elicit more controversy than any other portion of the book.

Bilateral Fusion Considerations

Our experience is that approximately one third of patients presenting with the diagnosis of a dysfunctional SIJ are in need of a bilateral fusion. These patients frequently have had a previous lumbosacral fusion, or they have a degenerative

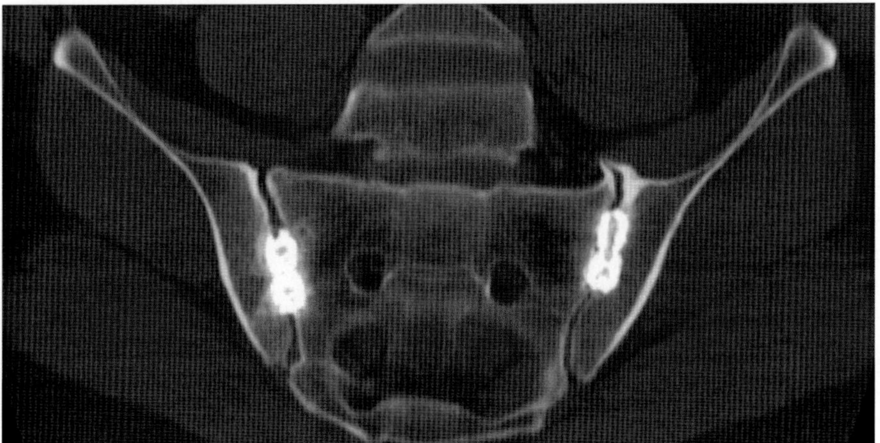

Fig. 7.12 Coronal CT scan showing long-term, clinically successful, follow-up of bilateral minimally invasive sacroiliac joint fusions

arthritis that attacks the large axial joints affecting the lumbar spine and the SIJs equally. We have reserved a bilateral fusion for the patient having essentially equal pain in each joint after all the steps in the algorithm (Chap. 6) have been accomplished. The two factors that weigh heavy on the decision to do a bilateral fusion are the potential incisions involved and the allowance for weight bearing after surgery. We have performed our bilateral fusions using either the posterior midline technique (Chap. 9) or the posterior lateral minimally invasive technique (Chap. 10). In the first instance, there is one midline incision through which both fusions are performed. In the second instance, there are two incisions, which are each less than 2 in. in length and cosmetically acceptable. With each of these procedures, using appropriate instrumentation, immediate postoperative full weight bearing is allowed, which helps to accelerate the rehabilitation process. We have found that there is no difference in outcomes at 4 years when one or both of the SIJs are fused. A trend which we are observing is that if a patient is symptomatic in both diagnosis-validated dysfunctional SIJs, but one joint is responsible for the bulk of the pain the patient suffers with, and only that joint is fused, there has been a very low chance of having to fuse the other joint during long-term follow-up. Several of these patients have been followed for more than 10 years. Studies addressing this issue will need to be done to determine whether this trend is scientifically valid. We have avoided doing bilateral SIJ fusions using the lateral minimally invasive techniques due to the postoperative limited weight-bearing issues. We expect this to change with time as more instrumentation companies are creating lateral fixation devices that will hold up to immediate weight bearing in the appropriate patient having adequate bone density. No such lateral device has yet allowed immediate postoperative full weight-bearing activity. We believe that the fixation is theoretically superior with the posterior and posterior lateral techniques, even in the patient with osteoporosis, due to greater advantage to connect with the more dense cortical and subchondral bone just adjacent to the joint margins. The success of a bilateral SIJ fusion seems to be largely dependent on creating minimal incisions, one midline incision, the least amount of instrumentation required for good contact with cortical bone and subsequent fusion, and immediate postoperative full weight-bearing status. Again, further research is needed to validate our findings (Fig. 7.12).

Fusing Both the Lumbar Spine and the SIJ: Considerations

Approximately one third of our SIJ fusions were performed in concert with a lumbar fusion. This is a very controversial issue, and the final word is not in concerning the right or wrong of this decision.

Our philosophy has been to first make a firm diagnosis of lumbar pathology using all the published criteria available in the literature to do so. Then, only when a dysfunctional SIJ is clearly in the differential diagnosis, and we work our way through the algorithm (see Chap. 6) to make a definitive diagnosis, do we consider performing a fusion of both areas at the same setting. This opinion has evolved over two decades influenced strongly by failed, perfectly good lumbosacral fusions, which subsequently had good outcomes after fusing the also painful SIJs. When we performed this type of combination surgery, which included either a unilateral or bilateral SIJ fusion, we used the single posterior midline technique and allowed immediate postoperative weight bearing in a thoracolumbosacral orthosis (TLSO) with a pantaloon attachment. In our 5-year review of 100 fusion patients, one third having both areas fused, there was no significant difference between those having an SIJ fusion alone or in combination with a lumbosacral fusion when looking at outcomes or complications. We have not found a down side using this procedural technique with our patients. It is our belief that further prospective research is needed to attest that this method is the correct one or not. At this time, such a prospective study is underway at our institution (Fig. 7.13).

The Morbidly Obese Patient

With our society steadily becoming more and more obese, the chance of encountering the morbidly obese patient with a dysfunctional SIJ is increasing as well. In a recent study of patients having successful SIJ fusions at BBSI, approximately one third of the patients were morbidly obese (Fig. 7.14).

All these patients, of course, receive extensive conservative care in hopes that surgery can be avoided, but, for those having surgery as their last hope and option, the surgeon is faced with multiple challenges. After consideration of the entire medical, anesthesia, and positioning factors that accompany any morbidly obese patient undergoing surgery, there are a few

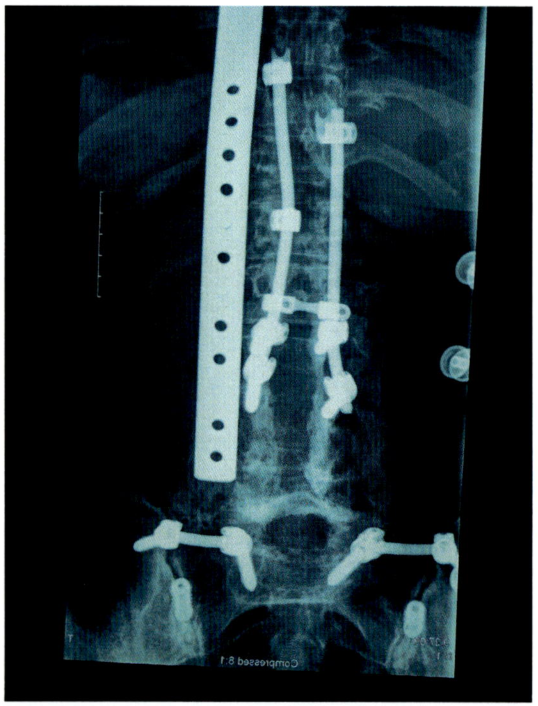

Fig. 7.13 Postoperative AP X-ray of bilateral sacroiliac joint fusions and extension of lumbar fusion using the posterior midline approach. This patient had a VAS of 1/10 at 4-year follow-up

special considerations for the surgeon fusing a SIJ in such a patient. Three of these factors, all overlapping, concern the approach, the type of instrumentation, and the weight-bearing status postsurgery. The approach is important in regard to the fluoroscopy that might be used during surgery. Images in the AP plane are usually better detailed than those in the lateral plane. This has to do usually with the amount of bone, muscle, and adipose tissue being far greater in mass when imaging through both hips and pelvic bones from side to side with the lateral approach compared to imaging from front to back or back to front using a posterior approach. Thus, a posterior or posterior lateral approach, minimally invasive if possible, might result in the best imaging possibility for placement of instrumentation (Fig. 7.15).

The second consideration is the type of hardware being used. This ties directly into the third consideration of potential weight bearing postoperatively. The type of hardware should, in the

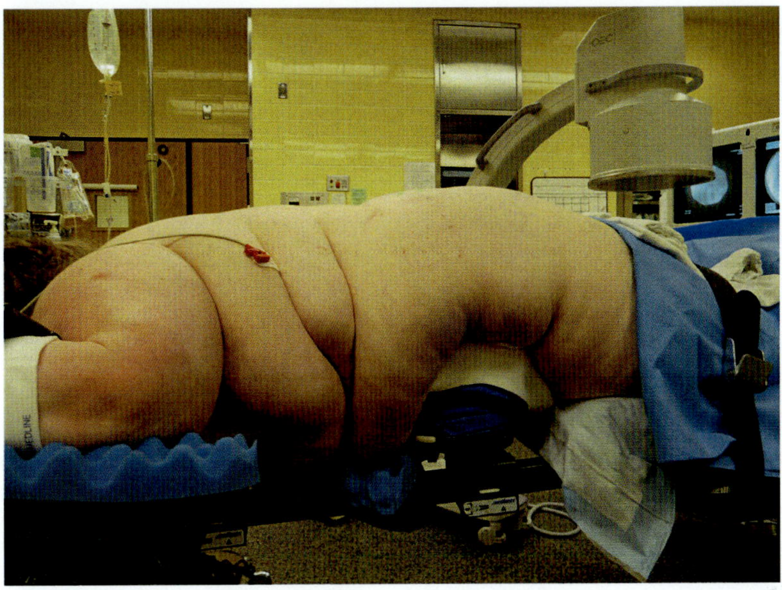

Fig. 7.14 Morbidly obese patient in prone position for a posterior lateral minimally invasive sacroiliac joint fusion

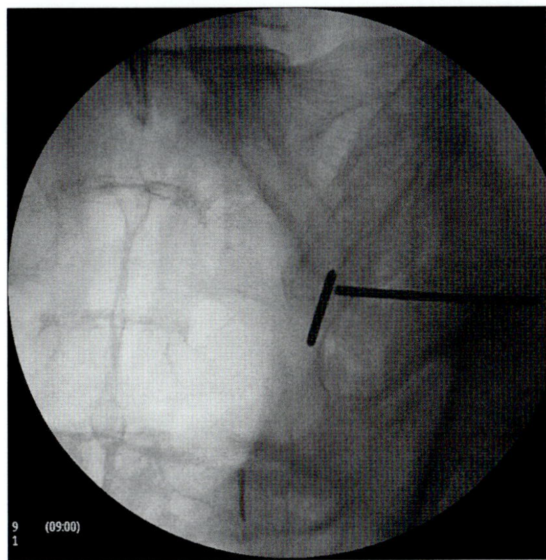

Fig. 7.15 Demonstrates very clear AP image visualization in the same morbidly obese patient using 30° cephalad "outlet" view which shows the PSIS (vertical pin) directly lateral to the S1 foramen. This patient also has a LSTV, consisting of sacral lumbarization, on the same side which can also be seen well with this view

on the affected side, a posterior or posterior lateral approach with rigid fixation, capturing as much of the denser cortical and subcortical bone as possible, is desired for allowing the patient to be up and into full rehabilitation as soon as possible. If this goal is attained, it can help tremendously to limit the myriad of potential postoperative complications that can befall the morbidly obese patient. When considering the success with the morbidly obese patient in achieving the goal of significantly decreasing their pain with this surgery, results varied according to how morbid their obesity was. In a recent review of our retrospective data, those morbidly obese patients with a BMI of >35 tended to have significantly less reduction of pain than those morbidly obese patients with a BMI <35 despite the fact that they all appeared to be solidly fused on CT scan. Again, further research is needed to prove the validity of these findings (Fig. 7.16).

Why Rehabilitate?

When considering the average type of patient we have operated on at our institution, it is apparent that many of these patients are in very poor physical condition going into this surgery.

morbidly obese patient, result in a very rigid fixation of the sacroiliac joint to allow for full weight bearing immediately postsurgery. Again, considering that at this point in time, all direct lateral approaches require limited weight bearing

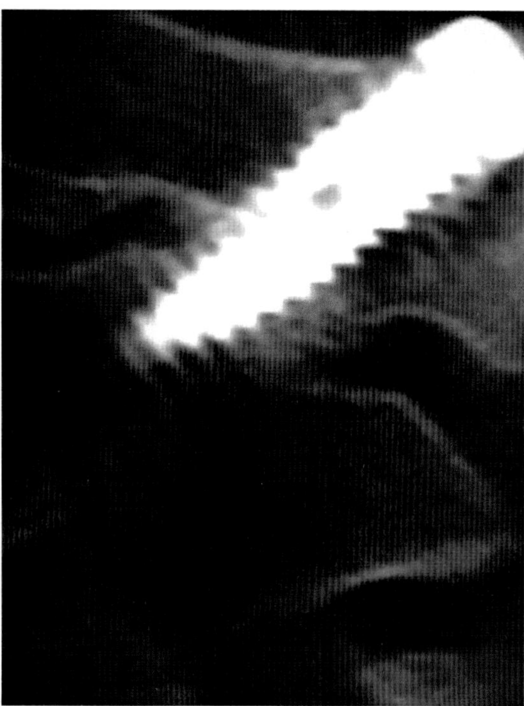

Fig. 7.16 Axial CT scan demonstrating bone fusing across joint in the same morbidly obese patient 6 months postsurgery (instrumentation Globus Medical, SI-LOK, Audubon, PA)

Without rehabilitating such a patient after surgery, they have a high likelihood of a poor outcome over time, as they will remain weak and deconditioned. Working with a physical therapist that understands the SIJ and the structures that surround it (Chap. 14) gives this type of postoperative patient the best chance for full recovery and maximum function. Frequently, it is the physical therapist that teaches the postoperative SIJ patient to have and reach appropriate goals after this surgery. Having a dedicated physical therapy staff for rehabilitating both the LS spine and the SIJ will definitely increase the chance for a successful outcome in these patients.

Different Approaches for Different Surgeons

The type of education and experience the surgeon has tends to influence the approach to the SIJ they will feel most comfortable with. For example, the orthopedic trauma surgeon has a greater affinity for the straight lateral approach due to the lateral femur, hip, and pelvic surgeries with which they are very familiar. It was this type of surgeon who first put, and still puts, lateral screws across the SIJ for acute pelvic trauma affecting that joint. They are comfortable with the lateral pelvic anatomy and have the knowledge base to deal with a complication from this approach. It is the orthopedic trauma surgeon who would most likely perform the rare anterior SIJ fusion in a patient with a dysfunctional SIJ. The orthopedic spine surgeon, who does not do pelvic trauma cases, is most at home with the posterior approaches to the SIJ. The deformity orthopedic spine surgeons have been posteriorly crossing the SIJ for decades in order to achieve iliac wing fixation to improve stability across the LS joint to decrease nonunions. Though they are very familiar with the posterior anatomy medial to the iliac wing, they have steered clear of the sciatic notch and anything much anterior to the lateral gluteal ridge. Neurosurgeons are also more familiar with the anatomy posteriorly, as they do not routinely perform any types of surgeries lateral to the ilium. Surgeons in each of the three specialties must learn about surgeries for the SIJ by reading the scant published literature and by being taught by another surgeon the ways that surgeon currently does this surgery resulting from their own experience. Fusions for the dysfunctional SIJ are currently not a section of education in any surgical society, and there is nothing on anyone's board reviews that offers questions concerning this type of surgery [3]. Again, trauma, infection, and tumors are discussed in great depth in the literature, but these are acutely unstable situations and are very different in terms of treatment than the painful, mostly stable, dysfunctional SIJ.

Conclusion

This chapter has focused on a few of the major areas that are both unique to the techniques of fusing the SIJ but also, if not well understood, can present the surgeon with potentially challenging situations and possibly poor patient results. The position and orientation of the SIJ within the pelvic structure and the vital anatomy surrounding it must be clearly understood by the surgeon in order to properly interpret the intraoperative images and perform the safest procedure for the patient. A surgeon who recognizes his/her own capabilities, understands rate-limiting factors for a given patient, and is not afraid to seek the advice of those having significant experience with these surgeries will be the most likely to have satisfied patients in the long run.

References

1. Hutchinson MR, Dall BE. Midline fascial splitting approach to the iliac crest for bone graft. A new approach. Spine. 1994;1:62–6.
2. Fowler BL, Dall BE, Rowe DE. Complications associated with harvesting autogenous iliac bone graft. Am J Orthop. 1995;12:895–903.
3. Dall BE. Someone needs to claim it! Spine J. 2009;2: 190–1.

Lateral Approach, Minimally Invasive

8

Sonia V. Eden

Introduction

This chapter will discuss the pertinent history regarding this approach and outline the surgical technique. General indications and contraindications to this procure as well as potential complications and previously documented outcomes associated with this approach will be addressed.

Literature Review

Several authors have published literature describing the successful use of a lateral approach to fuse the traumatic sacroiliac joint (SIJ) [1–4]. Al-Khayer first described the use of a percutaneous, lateral approach to fuse the nontraumatic SIJ in 2008 [5]. They reported the results of a percutaneous placement of a hollow modular anchorage (HMA) screw across the SIJ via a lateral approach. It was a retrospective analysis that reviewed the results of nine patients who underwent the procedure between August 2000 and August 2006. They concluded that this technique was a safe and effective treatment for nontraumatic SIJ pain in patients who had failed all conservative treatment options. Khurana subsequently published the results of 15 patients undergoing this same SIJ stabilization procedure and concluded that this was a satisfactory method to achieve SIJ fusion [6]. In 2012, Mason et al. published a prospective outcome study of 73 patients undergoing SIJ stabilization with the HMA screw. They found that the procedure was beneficial in pain-relief and functional improvement in the study patients [7]. Rudolf and Sachs also reported on a total of 51 patients undergoing lateral percutaneous placement of titanium implants across the SIJ in 2012 [8, 9]. They noted statistically significant improvement in pain function and low complication rates.

Indications and Current Uses

- This minimally invasive approach is FDA approved for SIJ disruptions and for degenerative sacroiliitis.

Since 2008, when the FDA issued the first 510 (k) for a direct lateral minimally invasive device to fuse the arthritic SIJ (Chap. 1), there has been a plethora of instrumentation devices being manufactured for fusion of the SIJ via this approach. As a result, the current most used approach for fusing/stabilizing the SIJ is the lateral minimally invasive approach. The volume of very recent literature concerning this approach is increasing at a rapid rate. However, there are no long-term

S.V. Eden, M.D. (✉)
Department of Neurosurgery, Borgess Medical Center, 1541 Gull Road, #200, Kalamazoo, MI 49048, USA
e-mail: soniaeden@borgess.com

B.E. Dall et al. (eds.), *Surgery for the Painful, Dysfunctional Sacroiliac Joint*, DOI 10.1007/978-3-319-10726-4_8, © Springer International Publishing Switzerland 2015

studies with these new instrumentations to guide the surgeon's decision making at the time of this writing.

Contraindications

- Significant osteoporosis.
- Morbid obesity.
- Presence of anatomical anomalies that make lateral imaging questionable.
- Full weight bearing postoperatively is required.
- Iliac wing is damaged or a part is missing (e.g., PSIS has been previously removed or a vigorous bone graft harvesting has been done).

This procedure is indicated for the painful, dysfunctional SIJ that has failed conservative treatment measures. Contraindications include significant osteoporosis, morbid or gross obesity limiting imaging capabilities, and unusual anatomy making landmarks unclear.

This procedure can be performed unilaterally or bilaterally. However, in the author's experience, patients who have undergone bilateral procedures have longer postoperative recovery time. This may be due to the inability to remove pressure from the buttocks with partial weight bearing in patients undergoing bilateral procedures. Because of this, we have elected to perform only unilateral procedures when using this approach at our institution. In some patients, once the most severe SIJ is stabilized, the contralateral SIJ symptoms might resolve. When they don't resolve, the procedure may be performed on the contralateral SIJ at a later date.

Lateral Minimally Invasive Approach, Step by Step

Step 1: Positioning

After the patient is placed under general anesthesia, the patient is positioned in the prone position on a radiolucent, frame-based spine table such as the Allen Table (Allen Medical) or the Jackson Table (Mizuho OSI). All pressure points should be carefully checked and padded, with special care to ensure that there is no pressure in the brachial plexi. Prophylactic antibiotics are administered within 1 h of the incision time.

Step 2: Intraoperative Image Planning

Once the patient is appropriately positioned, setting up the C-arm fluoroscope and obtaining excellent intraoperative imaging of the sacrum and pelvis is paramount. The three views used during this procedure are the pelvic inlet view, the pelvic outlet view, and the lateral view (Figs. 8.1, 8.2, and 8.3).

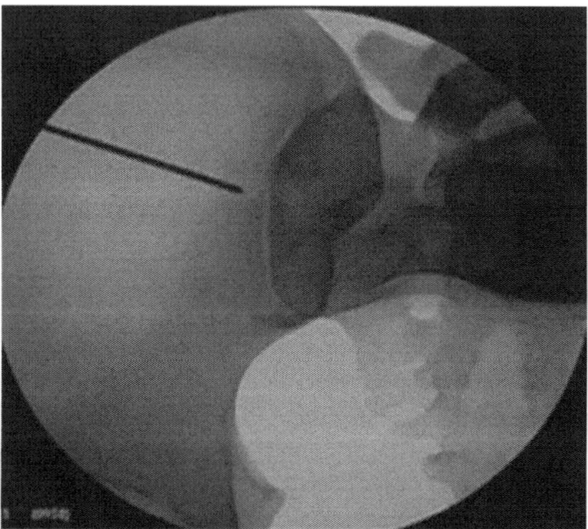

Fig. 8.1 Inlet view

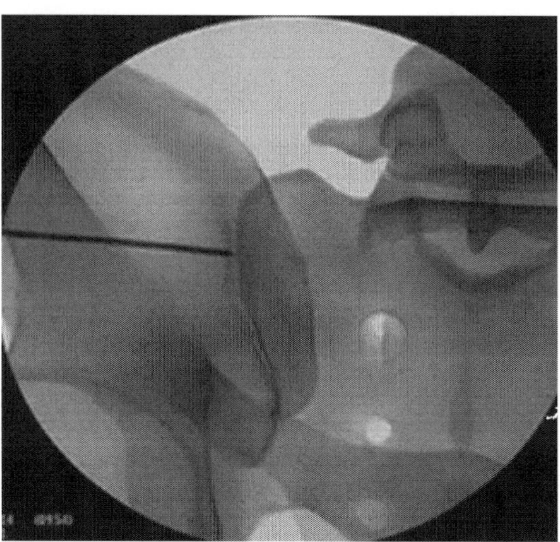

Fig. 8.2 Outlet view

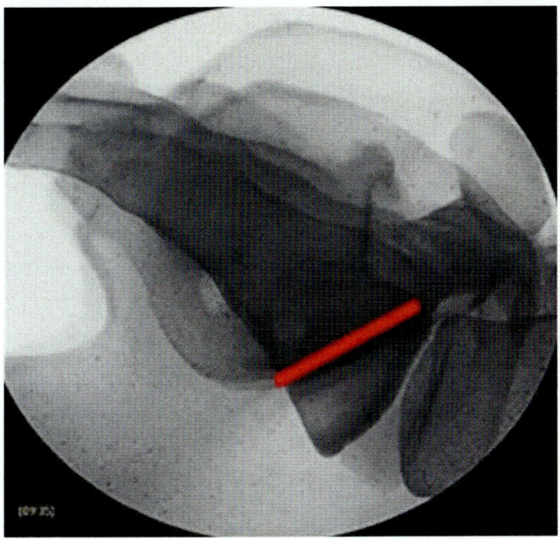

Fig. 8.3 Lateral view

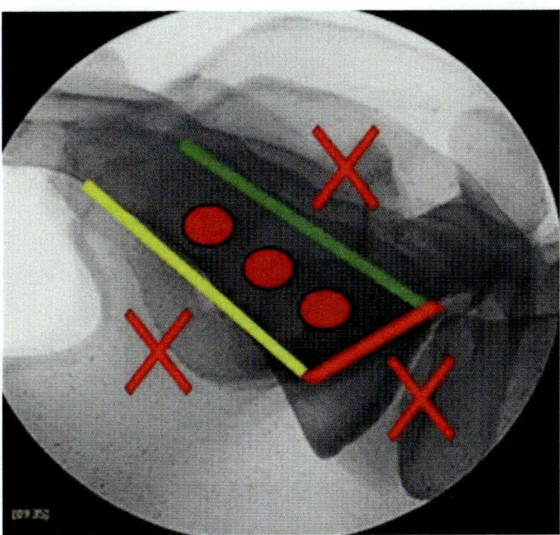

Fig. 8.4 Safe zones delineated on a lateral view

Pelvic Outlet View: This view is a cephalad projection of the sacrum [10]. This view is very important for bringing the neural foramina into view. The X-ray beam is typically perpendicular to the plane of the sacrum with the X-ray beam tilted approximately 25°–35° cephalad (Fig. 8.2).

Lateral View: The lateral view is a "true lateral" view through the sacrum and pelvis. The key to obtaining a true lateral is to wag the C-arm fluoroscope in a direction that results in aligning the sacral alae and iliac notches in the same plane (Fig. 8.3). The true lateral view helps define the "safe zones" for hardware placement during the lateral approach (Fig. 8.4).

Hardware should be placed within the sacrum with care to not breach the anterior sacral wall. Placement should not be too posterior within the sacrum to avoid entering the sacral canal. Also, the purchase is reduced with posteriorly placed hardware. There are several ligamentous structures along the dorsal wall of the sacrum, and placement among these structures would decrease the strength of the instrumentation. In addition, all hardware should be placed caudal to the sacral alae to maximize hardware purchase. This "safe zone" is outlined in Fig. 8.5.

Pelvic Inlet View: This view is the least utilized view in this surgical procedure. It is typically used to make sure that the hardware placed in the pelvis and sacrum does not breach

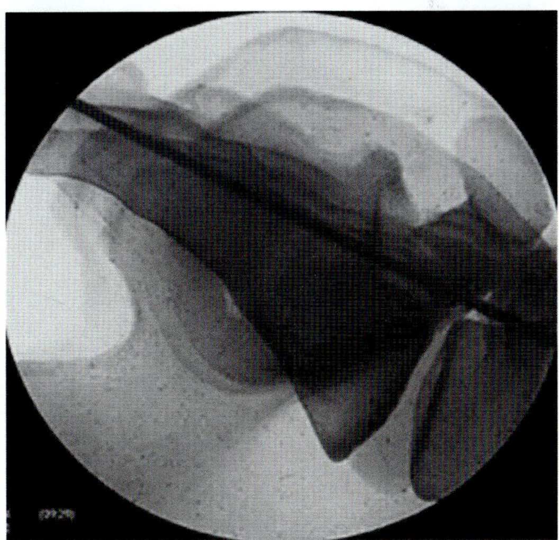

Fig. 8.5 Posterior wall, sacrum

the anterior sacral wall and enter the pelvis [10]. The fluoroscope is positioned for an AP view of the sacrum with the X-ray beam tilted approximately 25° caudally (Fig. 8.1).

Step 3: Skin Marking

Using the lateral view, the margins of the posterior wall of the sacrum and the sacral alae are outlined on the skin of the ipsilateral buttock using a marker (Figs. 8.6 and 8.7). A 3 cm incision is marked on the skin approximately 1–2 cm dorsal to the posterior sacral wall line.

Step 4: Guide Wire Placement

The skin is incised sharply. The guide wire is inserted into the incision with its tip on the cortical wall of the ilium. The ideal insertion point is then determined utilizing the lateral fluoroscopic view. The ideal starting point is 0.5–1 cm ventral to the posterior sacral wall and 1 cm caudal to the sacral alar line (Fig. 8.8).

The pelvic outlet view is then used to confirm that the trajectory of the guide wire crosses the SIJ and respects the neural foramina (Fig. 8.9).

Once these two views have confirmed a safe trajectory for the guide wire, the guide wire is either tapped or drilled across the SIJ (Fig. 8.10).

Please refer to Fig. 8.4 to see the "safe zone." The guide wires should be positioned such that they are all at least 1–2 mm lateral to the lateral border of the neural foramina in order to avoid injury to the neural elements (Fig. 8.10). Some surgeons may elect to place the screws that are just cephalad and caudal to the first sacral foramen deeper into the sacrum to obtain more bony purchase. We do not currently do this at our institution, as we have obtained adequate purchase with the shorter screws.

Step 5: Tubular Retractor Placement

Sequential dilators are placed over the guide wire. Following the last sequential dilation, the tubular retractor is inserted. This will serve as the working channel for the procedure (Fig. 8.11).

Step 6: Hardware Placement

Under fluoroscopic guidance, a light-hand high-speed drill is used to drill across the SIJ (Fig. 8.12).

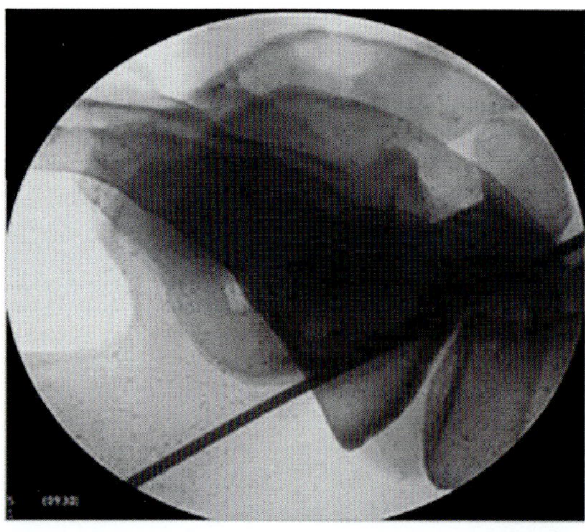

Fig. 8.6 Sacral ala

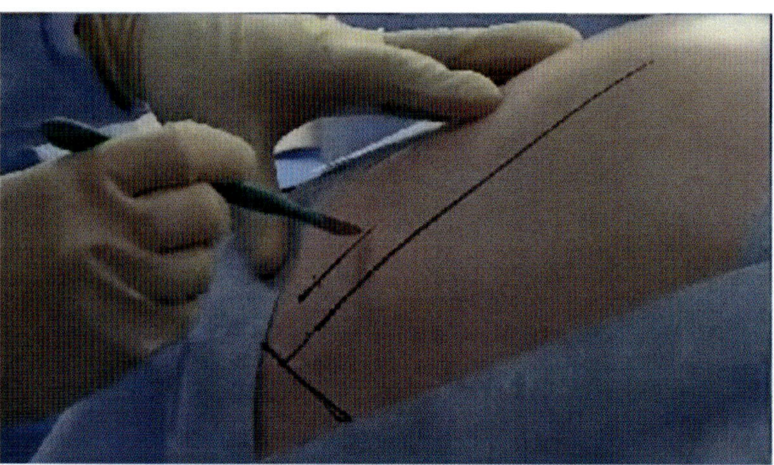

Fig. 8.7 Skin marking, 3 cm incision

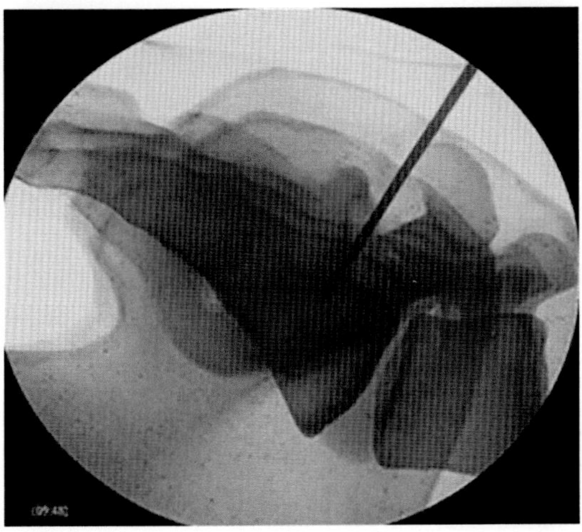

Fig. 8.8 Lateral view, initial placement and trajectory

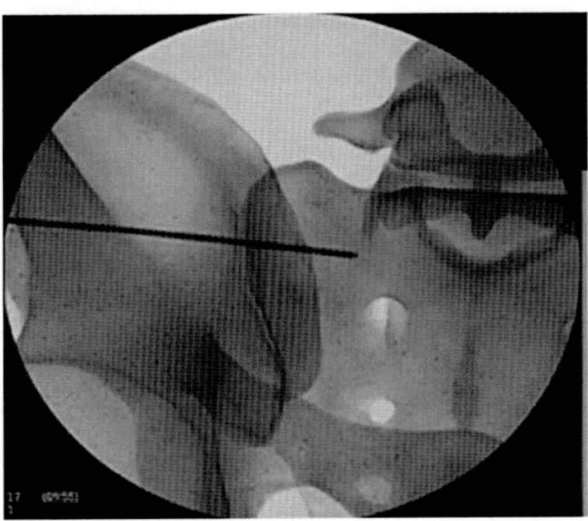

Fig. 8.10 Initial pin, final placement

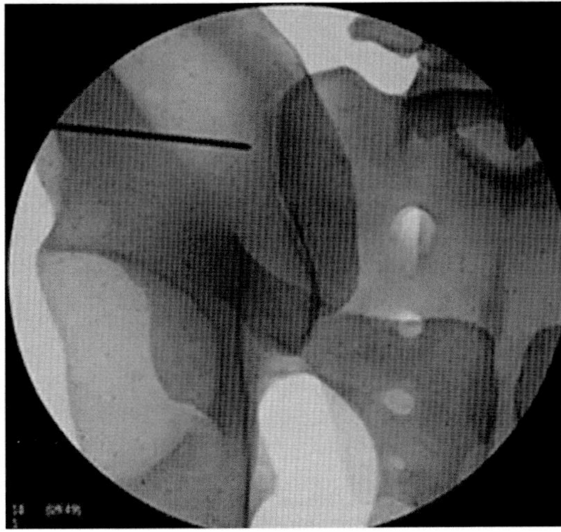

Fig. 8.9 Pelvic outlet view, initial pin placement and trajectory

Autograft bone can be harvested from the drill for later use, if indicated. The pelvic outlet and lateral views are used to ensure that drilling proceeds in a safe fashion. Once the trajectory has been drilled, the hardware of choice is placed over the guide wire across the SIJ (Fig. 8.13).

The tubular retractor is removed and the first guide wire is left in position.

Step 7: Additional Guide Wire Placement

The guide wire guide is placed over the first guide wire and the second guide wire is placed through the pin guide. Lateral and pelvic outlet views are used to confirm safe and appropriate positioning of the guide wire (Figs. 8.14 and 8.15).

The high-speed drill is used to drill across the SIJ over the second guide wire. Steps 5 and 6 are subsequently repeated. Final pelvic outlet, inlet, and lateral views are taken to confirm satisfactory hardware placement (Figs. 8.16, 8.17, and 8.18).

Typically, three implants are placed with the first being placed in line with the S1 pedicle. The second is typically placed adjacent to or above the S1 foramen. The third implant is usually between the S1 and S2 foramina (Fig. 8.16). Variations in patient anatomy may prevent the placement of three implants or alter the typical implant positions at times.

Step 8: Closure

Meticulous hemostasis is achieved. The wound is irrigated with antibiotic irrigation and closed in a layer fashion. Sterile dressings are applied.

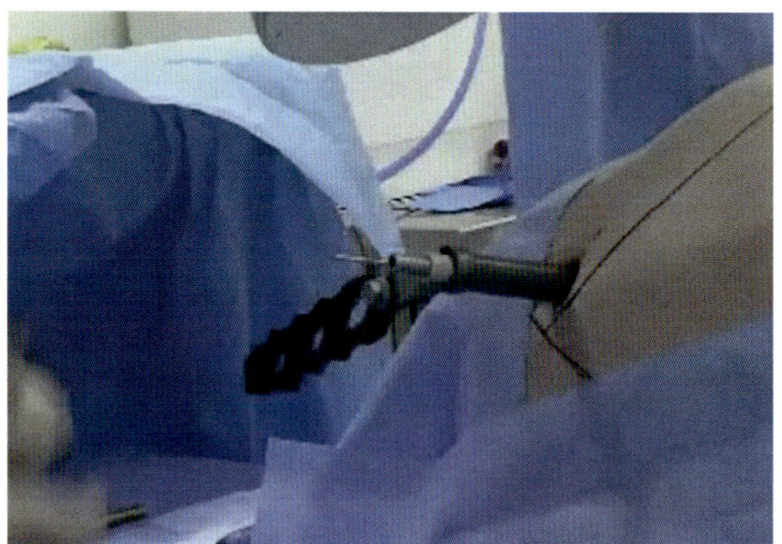

Fig. 8.11 Tubular retractor placement

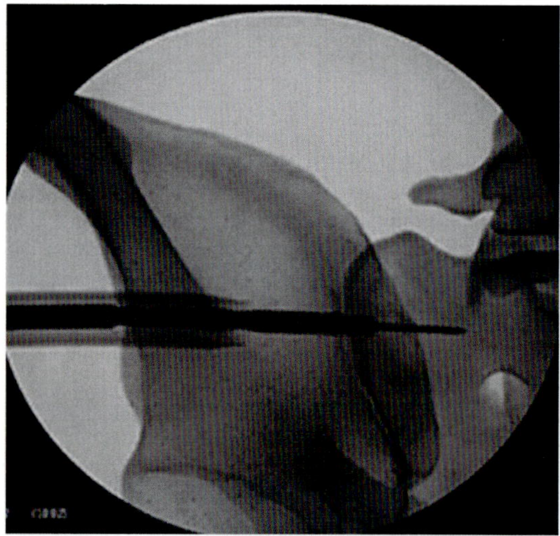

Fig. 8.12 Drilling for pin placement

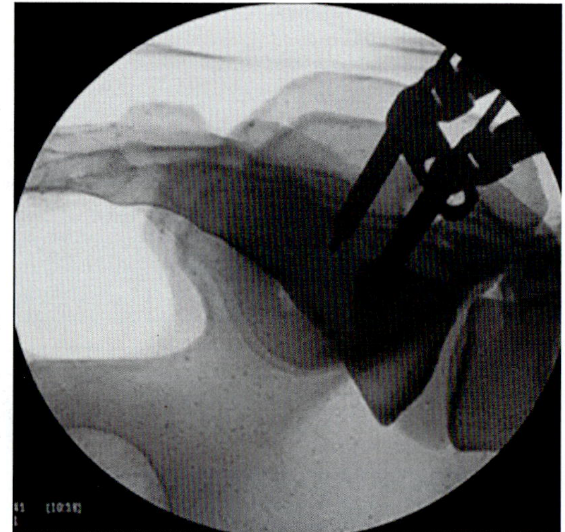

Fig. 8.14 Lateral view, second pin

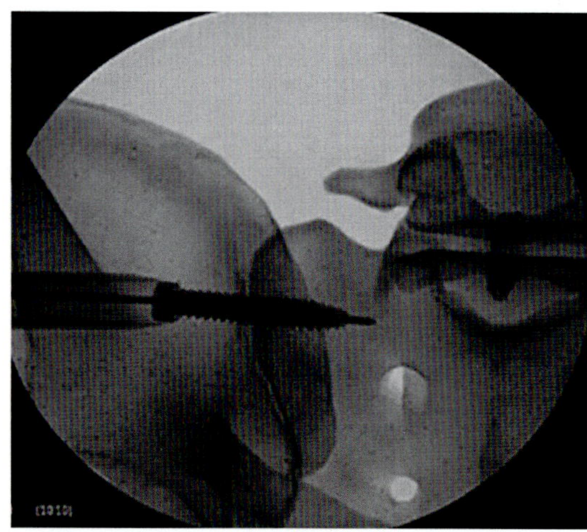

Fig. 8.13 Initial screw

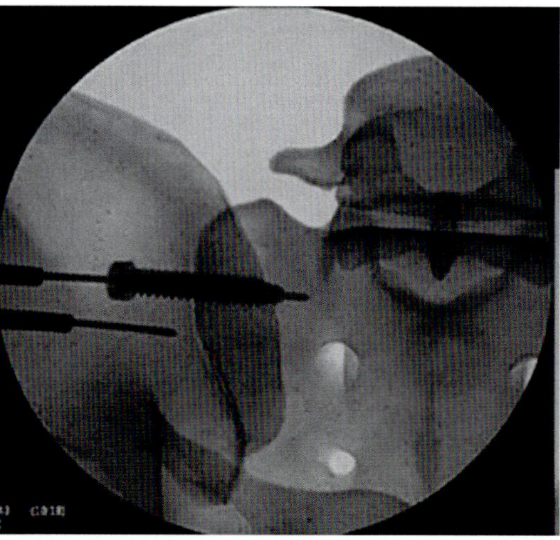

Fig. 8.15 Outlet view, second pin placement

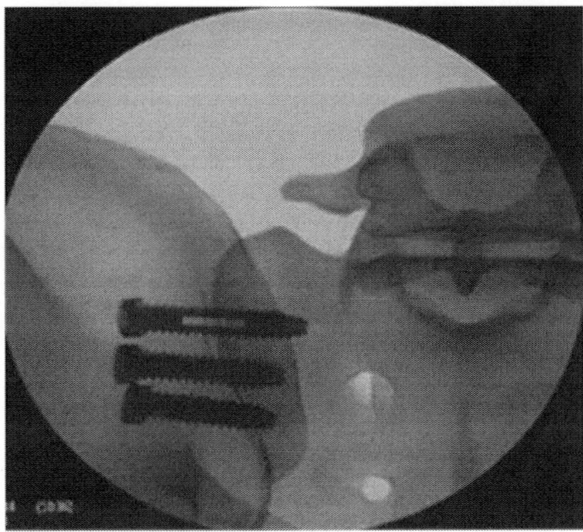

Fig. 8.16 Final outlet view

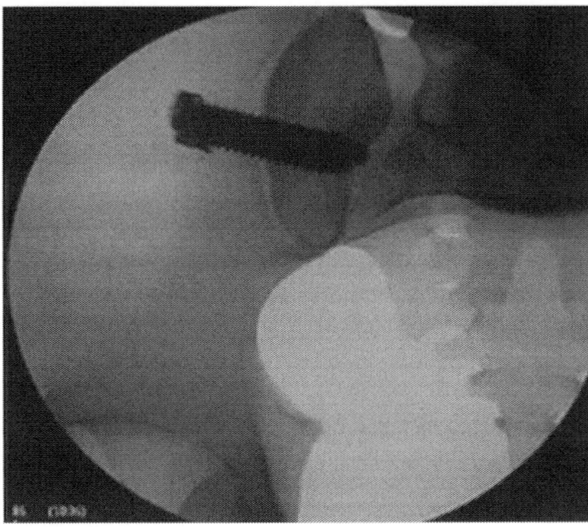

Fig. 8.17 Final inlet view

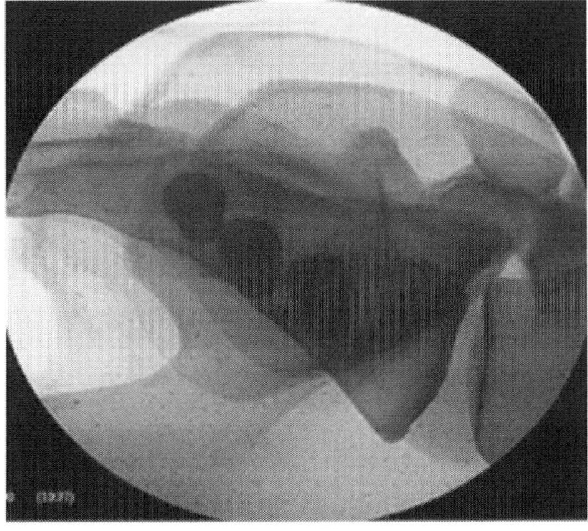

Fig. 8.18 Final lateral view

Postoperative Management

Following this procedure, patients are usually kept in the hospital overnight. They are allowed to ambulate with partial weight bearing on the operated side for approximately 4–6 weeks. Postoperative restrictions include no lifting greater than 15 pounds and avoidance of excessive bending or twisting for 12 weeks. At 6 weeks post-op, the patients are started in a course of postoperative physical therapy, and they are also released from their partial weight bearing restrictions. They are able to resume full activity levels without any restrictions at 12 weeks post-op, provided restrictions are not necessary because of continued pain.

Patients are followed in the office with postoperative X-rays at 6 weeks, 12 weeks, 6 months, and 1 year post-op. CT scans are typically performed only if patients don't demonstrate clinical improvement or there is a concern about the status of the fusion.

Complications and Reoperations

Potential complications that might result in further surgery:
- Superior gluteal artery injury.
- Sciatic nerve injury at point of sciatic notch.
- Fracture of ilium.
- Nerve root injury within sacral foramen.
- Malposition of hardware.
- Loosening of hardware in osteoporotic bone.
- Injury to intrapelvic structures.
- Wound infection.

Potential complications of this approach include injury to a branch of the superior gluteal artery. Since the approach traverses the gluteus medius and gluteus maximus via percutaneous access routes, there is always a potential for significant bleeding secondary to arterial injury. When this occurs, arterial embolization may be necessary to control the bleeding. Self-limited buttock hematomas have also been reported from vascular injury during this approach as well [8]. Additional reported complications have included superficial or deep wound infections and malpositioned implants resulting in nerve root pain or injuries requiring reoperation [5, 7, 8]. One non-displaced fracture of the ilium was reported in the Rudolf study [8]. The fracture did heal with conservative treatment measures. The reported overall reoperation rate for this lateral approach is 0.05 % [5–9].

Chapter Summary

Although this percutaneous lateral approach has been performed for the stabilization of the traumatic SIJ for years, it is relatively new to the literature for treatment of the painful, dysfunctional SIJ. This approach is a safe and satisfactory approach for treating the painful, stable dysfunctional SIJ. Proper patient selection is critical to ensure optimal patient outcomes, and in the appropriately selected patients, this procedure can be performed safely and result in pain-relief as well as functional improvement.

References

1. Bale RJ, et al. Stereotactic CT-guided percutaneous stabilization of posterior pelvic ring fractures: a pre-clinical cadaver study. J Vasc Interv Radiol. 2008; 19(7):1093–8.
2. Beaule PE, Antoniades J, Matta JM. Trans-sacral fixation for failed posterior fixation of the pelvic ring. Arch Orthop Trauma Surg. 2006;126(1):49–52.
3. Cherkes-Zade DI. Osteoplastic correction of the pelvic ring in old injuries of the sacroiliac and pubic joints aggravated by a large divergence of the pubic symphysis. Clin Orthop Relat Res. 1991;266:19–22.
4. Keating JF, et al. Early fixation of the vertically unstable pelvis: the role of iliosacral screw fixation of the posterior lesion. J Orthop Trauma. 1999;13(2): 107–13.
5. Al-Khayer A, et al. Percutaneous sacroiliac joint arthrodesis: a novel technique. J Spinal Disord Tech. 2008;21(5):359–63.
6. Khurana A, et al. Percutaneous fusion of the sacroiliac joint with hollow modular anchorage screws: clinical and radiological outcome. J Bone Joint Surg Br. 2009;91(5):627–31.
7. Mason LW, Chopra I, Mohanty K. The percutaneous stabilisation of the sacroiliac joint with hollow modular anchorage screws: a prospective outcome study. Eur Spine J. 2013;22(10):2325–31.
8. Rudolf L. Sacroiliac joint arthrodesis-MIS technique with titanium implants: report of the first 50 patients and outcomes. Open Orthop J. 2012;6:495–502.
9. Sachs D, Capobianco R. One year successful outcomes for novel sacroiliac joint arthrodesis system. Ann Surg Innov Res. 2012;6(1):13.
10. Clifford R. Wheeless, III, MD. Inlet and Outlet views, Wheeless' textbook of orthopaedics, Wheeless on line.com, 2012.

Bruce E. Dall

Introduction

This chapter will discuss the relevant history regarding this approach, the pertinent literature that defines it, and the various ways that this approach has been utilized for fusing the dysfunctional sacroiliac joint (SIJ). The general indications and contraindications will be discussed for the approach group as a whole, and if differences exist with the use of various hardware or technique variations, these will be outlined as those variances are discussed. The technique will then be explained step by step noting where options exist for variance depending on the instrumentation being used. The most common complications and outcomes for this approach will be discussed. Lastly, a brief discussion of ways to salvage a failed surgery using this approach will be explained.

B.E. Dall, M.D. (✉)
Neurosurgery of Kalamazoo, Borgess Brain
and Spine Institute, 1541 Gull Road, Kalamazoo,
MI 49048, USA

Orthopedic Spine Division, Western Michigan
University Medical School, Kalamazoo, MI USA
e-mail: dall.bruce@yahoo.com

Literature and Historical Review

The first publication using the posterior midline approach to fuse a dysfunctional SIJ was by Belanger in 2001 [1]. He explains that the basis for the approach stemmed from a 1994 article by Hutchinson [2], which described approaching the iliac crest for bone graft harvesting using a posterior midline incision. From the midline, the superficial thoracolumbar fascia, a caudal contribution of the latissimus dorsi, was defined and separated from the deep thoracolumbar fascia, a caudal and lateral contribution of the erector spinae, allowing for a blunt fascial splitting approach between these two layers to the ilium. Since the cluneal nerves were in the more superficial of the two fascial layers, they were elevated up and out of the way, while the iliac crest was approached with an incision along its ridge and careful subperiosteal dissection laterally. The harvesting of iliac bone graft (IBG) followed this. This technique also allowed for excellent fascia-to-fascia closure over the remaining iliac crest. By protecting the cluneal nerves and obtaining a tight closure, the clinical results in terms of decreased pain post-bone graft harvesting were dramatic (Fig. 9.1).

Belanger used this approach to access the iliac wing after which the posterior superior iliac spine (PSIS) was removed, the posterior aspect of the SIJ was curetted out, bone graft was placed into this space, an S1 pedicle screw was placed, a screw was placed between the inner and outer

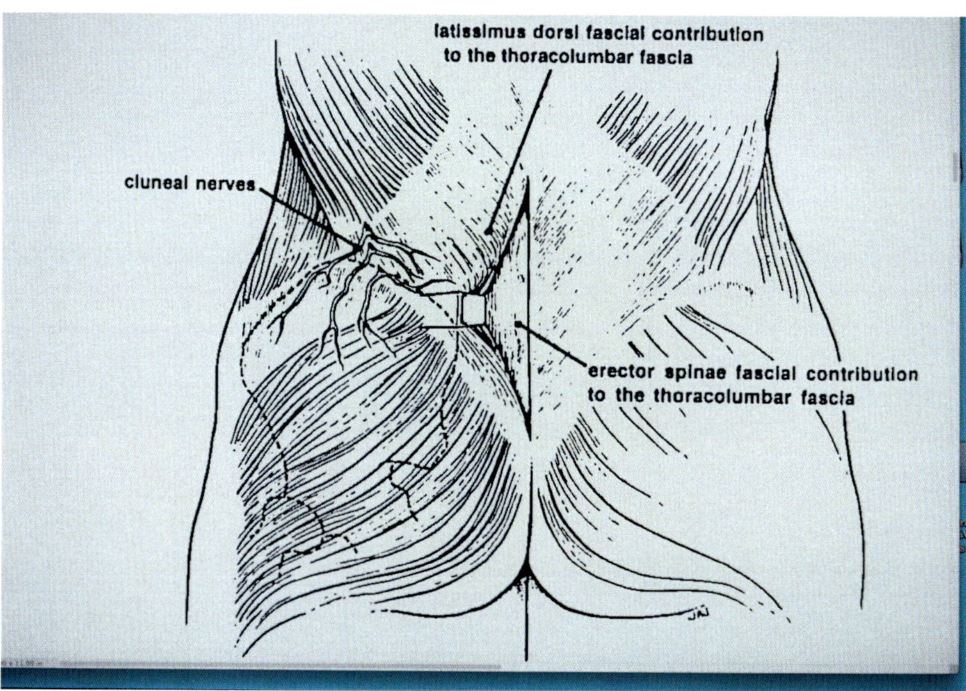

Fig. 9.1 Shows the muscle fascial contribution to the superficial and deep layers of the thoracolumbar fascia and the course of the cluneal nerves into the superficial fascial layer

Fig. 9.2 Typical instrumentation using the original Belanger technique

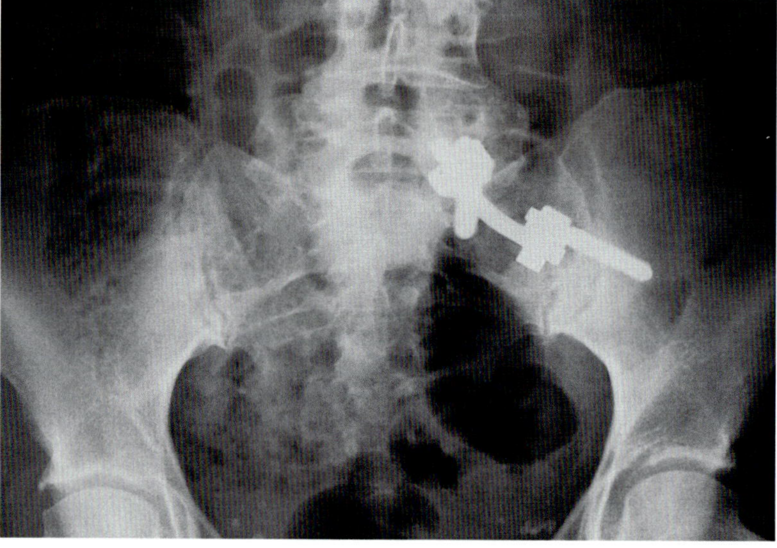

cortical layers of the ilium, a rod was placed between screws, compression was applied, and a tight fascial closure was done. The results from using this approach and technique in four patients were successful and the midline incision healed well, being in a low stress line, with cosmetically good results (Figs. 9.2 and 9.3).

Along with the posterior midline approach, the other firsts for SIJ fusion with this technique included using the S1 pedicle for fixation and the placing of a screw between the inner and outer cortical walls in the cephalad portion of the posterior ilium. This technique has gone through several evolutionary changes at the Borgess

Fig. 9.3 Ten-year follow-up showing incision and operated side post-original Belanger technique

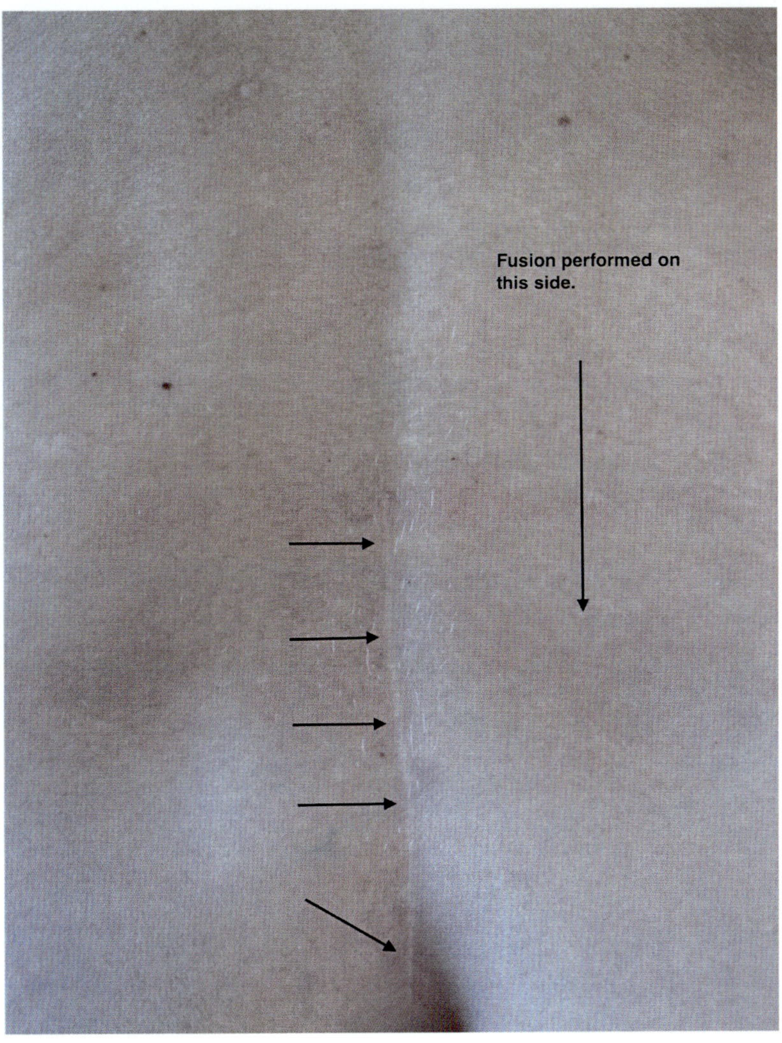

Brain and Spine Institute (BBSI) since that time, which have centered on preventing muscle injury and enhancing fixation.

Relative Indications and Contraindications

This approach should be considered secondary to any of the accepted minimally invasive procedures such as the lateral minimally invasive procedure discussed in Chap. 8. There are some conditions and situations that might make this method the most attractive option to the surgeon:

- If a repair of a previous lumbar fusion or extension of a lumbar fusion is required at the same setting as the SIJ fusion.
- When pathology that is thought to be both extra-articular and intra-articular.
- The patient is morbidly obese.
- Immediate full weight bearing is desired postsurgery.
- There is significant osteoporosis present in the sacrum.
- There is insufficient bone present dorsal to the gluteal ridge of the ilium.
- A failed lateral or posterior lateral minimally invasive fusion needs to be salvaged and current instrumentation cannot be removed.

There are no specific contraindications for this procedure once the decision has been made to go ahead with a SIJ fusion. If any of the other approaches discussed in this book can be used, then this procedure is possible to do.

As mentioned earlier, if a minimally invasive procedure can be done with a high likelihood of success, then that procedure should take preference to this muscle sparing yet more extensive procedure.

Posterior Midline Approach: Step by Step

Step 1: Positioning

The patient is placed in the prone position taking the same standard precautions as for a lumbar fusion surgery and allowing the abdomen to hang free (Fig. 9.4).

Step 2: Incision

The incision is made from approximately the lower border of the L3 spinous process and continues caudad to the S1–S2 level (Fig. 9.5).

Step 3: Identification and Separation of the Fascial Layers

The longitudinal dissection is carried down to the spinous processes of L3, L4, L5, and S1 without exposing bone and leaving the fascial layer intact

and well defined. Approximately 3–4 mm lateral to the midline at the level of the L3 spinous process, the fascia is incised longitudinally about

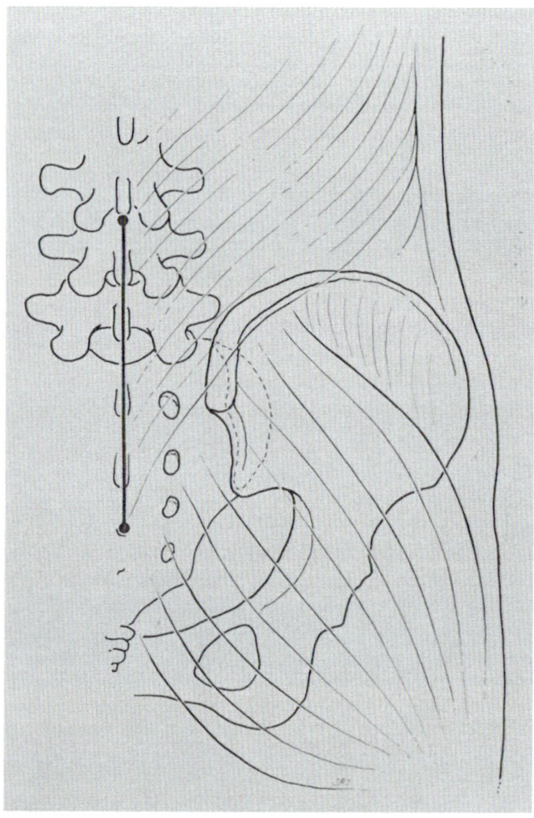

Fig. 9.5 Posterior midline incision from just below L3 to mid-sacrum

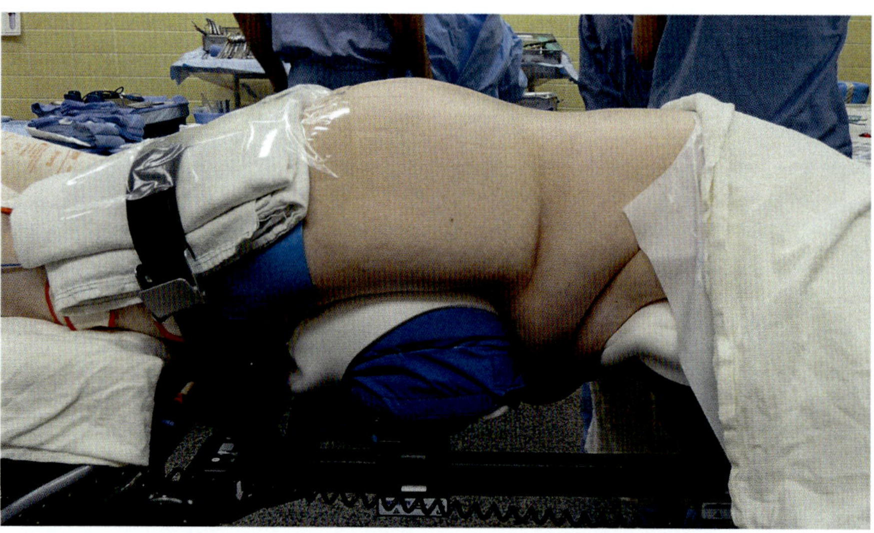

Fig. 9.4 Typical prone position as used for posterior lumbar fusions with the abdomen hanging free

3 cm, and the deep part of the two fascial layers is identified. This deep layer is not incised or violated. There is frequently a small layer of adipose tissue lying between the superficial and deep layers of fascia. The two layers are always distinctly separate and well defined at this level. Help in identification is that the superficial layer of fascia has a transverse or oblique pattern and the deep a longitudinal pattern. The dissection then continues in a caudad direction, approximately 3–4 mm lateral to the midline, and the superficial fascial layer is bluntly lifted off the deep fascial layer laterally the length of the incision. It should be noted that the two layers tend to blend somewhat as the dissection is carried caudally possibly necessitating some assistance with the Bovie or the scalpel for separation. Toward the caudal part of the dissection, bleeding might occur from what appears to be one or two small holes in the deep fascia each containing a perforating vein. To stop this bleeding, place the tip of the Bovie into the small hole, without making the hole bigger, and Bovie. If this is unsuccessful, place a figure of eight absorbable stitch closing the hole. With this fascial splitting dissection, the deep fascia attaches laterally to the medial border of the ilium. The lateral aspect of the superficial fascia attaches to the gluteal aponeurosis lateral to the ilium. This provides a clean blunt dissection, which exposes the PSIS and approximately 8–10 cm of the dorsal iliac wing. The cluneal nerves are in the reflected superficial fascial layer, which they access from the intrapelvic space to come over the iliac wing approximately 8–12 cm cephalad of the PSIS and subsequently spread out over the buttock. It is important to avoid transecting them where they cross the ilium (Fig. 9.6).

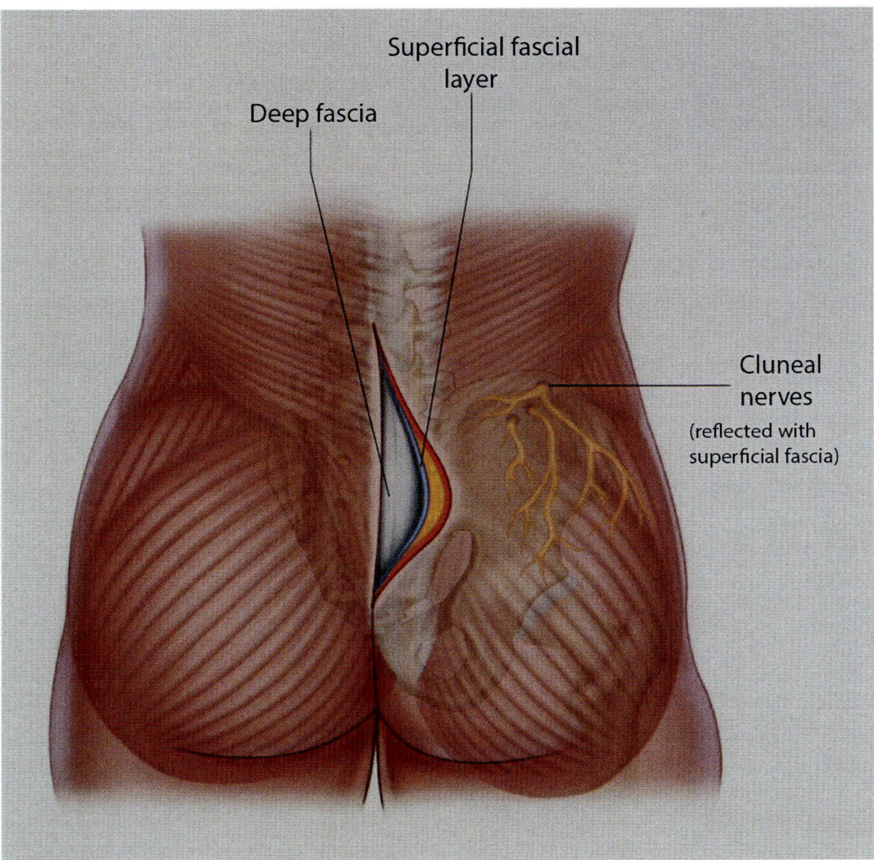

Fig. 9.6 Elevating the superficial fascial layer, which is an extension of the latissimus dorsi muscle and the cephalad portion of the gluteal muscles and contains the cluneal nerves

Step 4: Exposure of the PSIS

The dorsal iliac wing is incised with the Bovie along the entire length of exposure starting just caudal to the PSIS and ending approximately 8 cm cephalad along the iliac ridge. Subperiosteal dissection then progresses laterally to the gluteal line or ridge, and the medial dissection progresses to the dorsal sacrum. There may be bleeding along the medial edge which is stopped using the bipolar as the dorsal foramina of the sacrum are just medial to this (Fig. 9.7).

Step 5: Removal of Bone and Posterior Ligaments

The posterior transverse iliosacral and interosseous ligaments are then removed using a rongeur, which may necessitate the bipolar for control of bleeding. It is important to have all bleeding under control before proceeding. It is important to understand that the dorsal aspect of the sacrum in this location has very thin cortical bone. The proper direction for the removal of the ligaments is an anterior–lateral direction staying under the medial edge of the ilium. If the surgeon proceeds straight anterior here, he/she risks entering the dorsal body of the sacrum and creating a false passage that is in fact medial to the joint line. The PSIS is then removed the length of the exposure down to the gluteal line laterally and the sacrum medially. Bone wax is used for any persistent cancellous bleeding (Fig. 9.8).

Step 6: Placing Cage or Bone Dowel into Longitudinal Axis of the Joint

It is at the caudal end of this exposure where the ilium and the sacrum come closest together, and there is the least amount of dorsal ligament mass. This location is also straight dorsal to the apex and caudal portion of the true SIJ with the

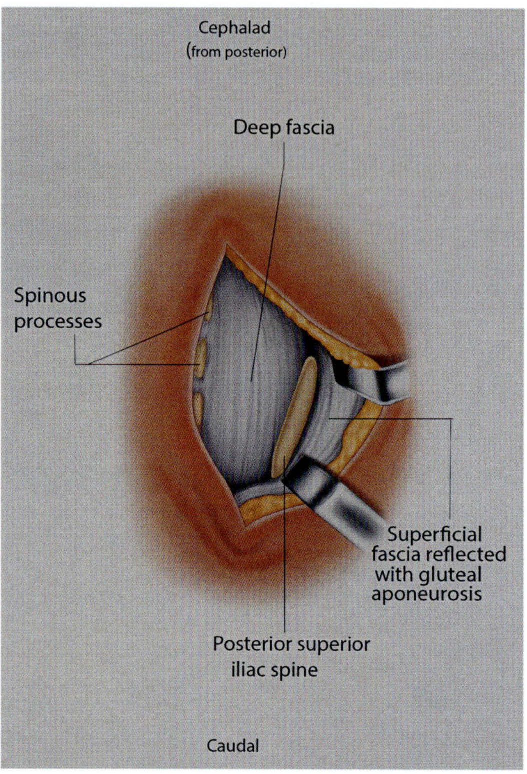

Fig. 9.7 Exposure between the superficial and deep fascial layers and exposure of the posterior superior iliac crest

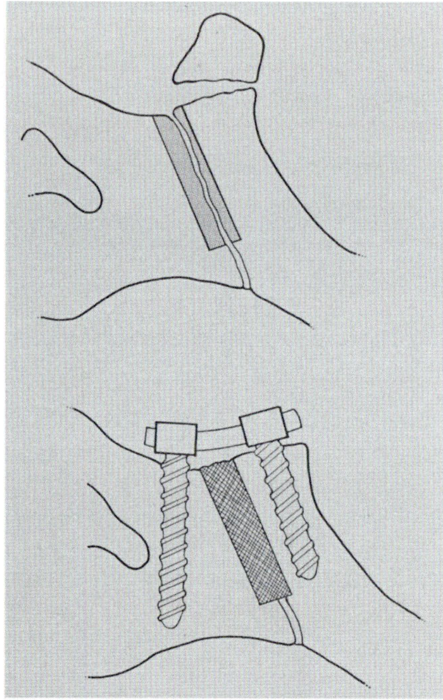

Fig. 9.8 Axial view of the operative area showing the PSIS being removed, the SIJ being cavitated, and bone grafting of the SIJ using the bone from the PSIS

longitudinal plane of the joint being almost perpendicular to the floor. It is here that the cage or bone dowel is placed. Image is brought in to visualize this caudal portion of the joint, and subsequently any of the remaining PSIS overlying this joint line is removed. A burr hole is made down into the joint line, a probe is placed, the image verifies that it is in the joint line, the probe is removed, and the burr is inserted again and so on back and forth until a depth of no more than 3 cm has been achieved. The average depth before entering the pelvis at this level can be 3–5 cm. The goal is not to come closer than 1 cm from entering the pelvis. This is where reviewing the preoperative CT scan and looking at the axial slice corresponding to this location can provide the surgeon with the exact number of centimeters that are available for this dissection in a given patient. The hole is then widened to a diameter less than the implant. Tapping is then done if necessary when using a bone dowel. The cage or bone dowel is then packed with iliac bone graft or bone-enhancing material and then screwed down into the provided space at least 1 cm deeper than the bone surface. The implant is then pulled on with a Kocher or similar instrument to assure rigid or very stable fixation (Figs. 9.9 and 9.10).

Step 7: Placing S1 Pedicle Screw

Having previously removed the posterior iliosacral ligaments at the cephalad portion of the dissection, we now have the ability to retract the paraspinous musculature medially and place a marker on our entrance point into the S1 pedicle. The hole for the pedicle screw is then made using image and a drill or awl depending on the surgeon's preference. The pedicle screw of choice is then inserted. We have used a multiaxial screw here. The actual placing of a pedicle screw is beyond the scope of this book and should be part of the inherent knowledge of the surgeon performing this procedure.

Step 8: Placing Iliac Screw

The placing of the iliac screw in this procedure is different than that used with long lumbosacral instrumentation to add further stability for the lumbosacral fusion. This screw is placed between the inner and outer iliac cortical layers but with a more cephalad starting point. This starting point is essentially in or close to the same axial plane as the S1 pedicle. At a point in the exposed

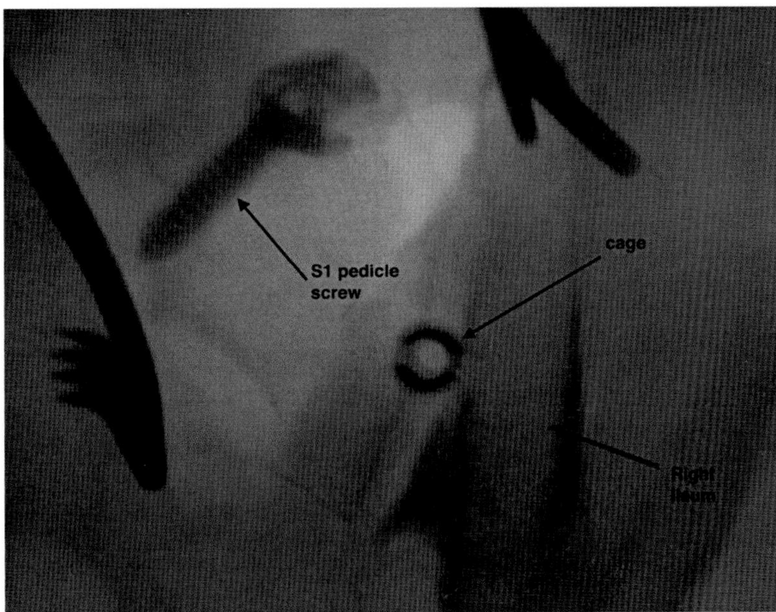

Fig. 9.9 Intraoperative AP image of the cage and the S1 pedicle screw in place

cancellous ilium in the cephalad one third of the exposure, a hole is made with the burr, and a ¼ in. drill is used to drill to a depth of 2 cm proceeding in a slightly lateral and slightly cephalad direction and staying between the outer and inner cortical layers, which are relatively close together in this location. A straight probe is then inserted into the hole and pushed through the remaining cancellous bone until it reaches the laterally curving medial cortical wall. This depth is measured and then tapped. A pedicle screw of choice, again we use a multiaxial screw, is placed. It is then pulled on to be sure it is rigidly stable. If this screw has any movement or sense of not being rigid and solidly stable, it should be replaced with a larger-diameter screw. It is important that this screw head is well seated into the cancellous bone, which, with the previous removal of the iliac bone to the level of the gluteal ridge laterally and the sacrum medially, allows for appropriate recessing of the screw head for complete fascial closure over it. Occasionally, the ventral tip of the screw penetrates the medial cortical wall of the ilium. This places the tip within the iliacus muscle. There have been no complications in long-term follow-ups when this has occurred, but the absolute outcome of this situation is yet to be determined and currently should be considered with caution (Figs. 9.11 and 9.12).

Step 9: Bone Grafting, Placing Rod, and Compression

The bulk of the bone grafting will occur posterior and caudal to the already placed cage or bone dowel. First, it is important to decorticate the

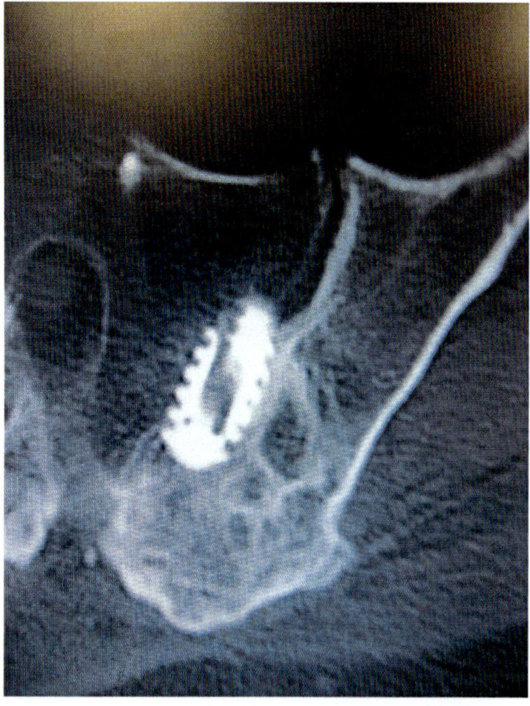

Fig. 9.10 Axial CT scan showing cage in position 1-year postsurgery with solid fusion

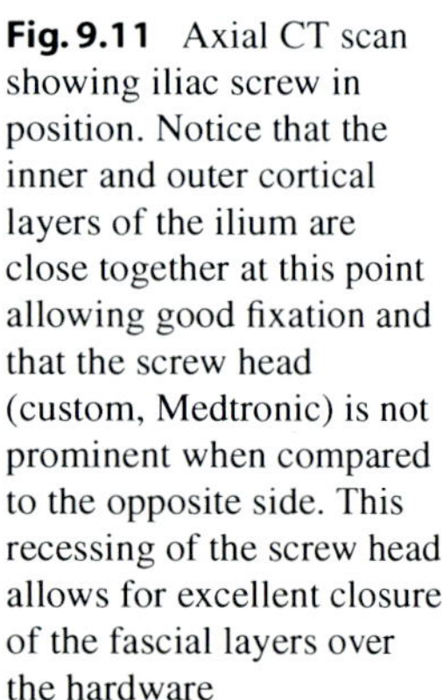

Fig. 9.11 Axial CT scan showing iliac screw in position. Notice that the inner and outer cortical layers of the ilium are close together at this point allowing good fixation and that the screw head (custom, Medtronic) is not prominent when compared to the opposite side. This recessing of the screw head allows for excellent closure of the fascial layers over the hardware

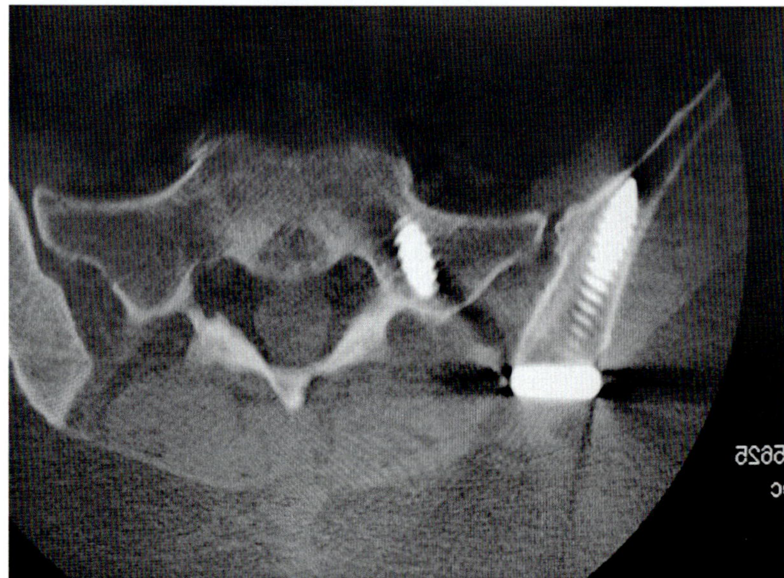

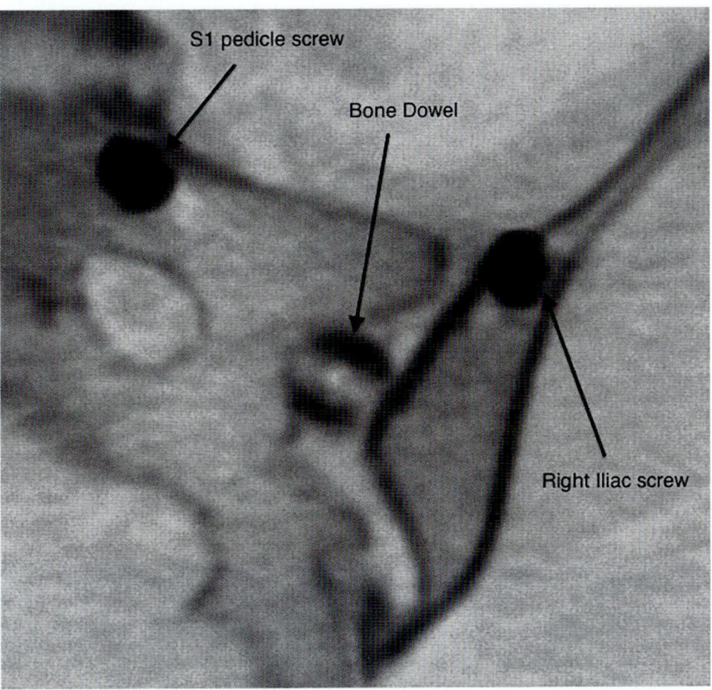

Fig. 9.12 Coronal CT scan showing positions of a bone dowel, the S1 pedicle screw, and the iliac screw. Note how that the iliac screw and the S1 screw are in approximately the same axial plane

bone on the dorsal sacrum at this level, which might involve removal of more ligamentous-type soft tissue on the sacral side. It is here that a non-union is most likely to develop. Iliac bone graft is used, which was harvested earlier in the procedure. A rod is then placed between the screw heads, and before tightening the setscrews, compression between screws is done. The setscrews are then tightened or broken off, depending on the system, and the instrumentation is complete. Using a large instrument or pliers, the construct is pulled on to assure it is rigid (Fig. 9.13).

Step 10: Tight Closure and Drain

This step is equally important to any that have preceded it. The approach, done correctly, helped to create medial and lateral to the ilium fascial layers that can be brought together for a tight interrupted closure over the bone graft and the instrumentation. When suturing, try to get a larger bite of tissue laterally with each interrupted stitch, and pull on it to be sure it is secure and does not easily pull out. Due to the removal of the entire PSIS, the instrumentation is subsequently recessed enough for complete coverage by the fascial layers.

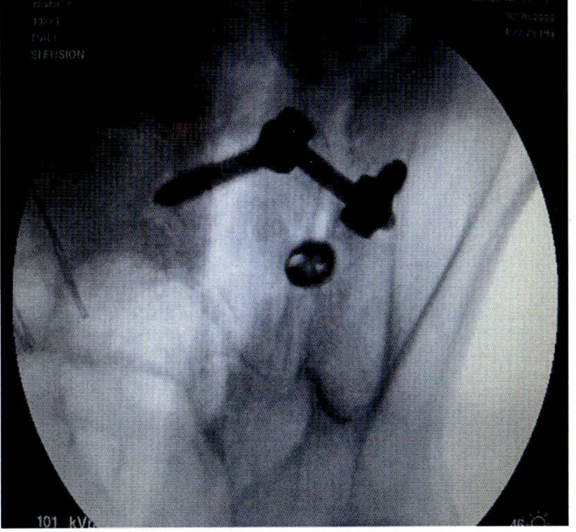

Fig. 9.13 Final AP image with the hardware in place

When done appropriately, this essentially reconstructs the previous medial and lateral attachments that existed before removing the PSIS. This helps with postoperative rehabilitation and is also the best protection for preventing the iliac screw head from being prominent and subsequently painful. A drain then is inserted deep to the fascial closure, as there will be drainage occurring during the first 24 h from this site (Fig. 9.14).

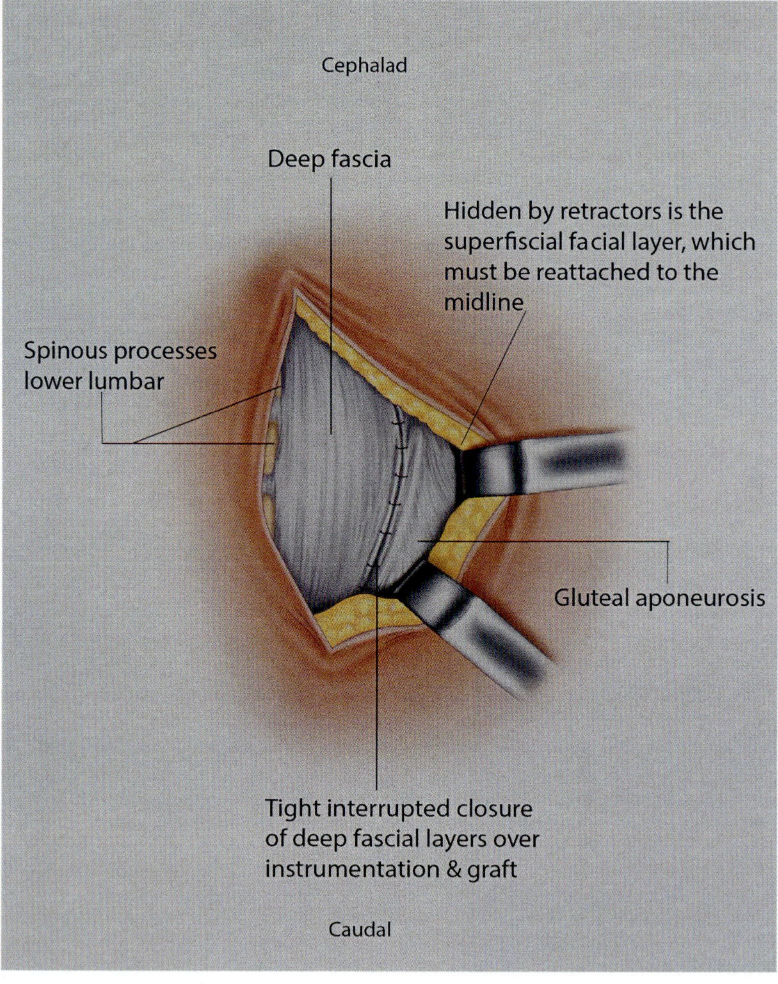

Step 11: Postoperative Management

Patients are kept at bed rest overnight with a Foley catheter and a drain. The following day, the catheter and drain are removed and the patient is mobilized. Full weight bearing as tolerated is allowed at this time. A sacral belt is used whenever up and is applied and removed in the standing position. It is removed for showers. A walker is substituted for the sacral belt in morbidly obese patients. If a lumbosacral fusion occurred with this procedure, the bracing is dictated by that procedure according to the standard protocols of the surgeon. Bracing is continued for 12 weeks during which the primary activity is walking with no excessive bending, twisting, or lifting activities. We allow patients to lift up to 15 lb during this period. After the initial 6 weeks, water therapy is allowed followed by formal physical therapy at 12 weeks postsurgery. Plain X-rays of the sacrum are taken at 6 weeks to assure no movement of the instrumentation, and a CT scan is performed at 3 months looking for any hardware loosening and to assure that the bone graft is healing well. When the patient is released from physical therapy, usually around

18 weeks postsurgery, they are allowed to return to work. If only the SIJ(s) was fused, there are no restrictions placed on activity unless symptoms persist. If a lumbosacral fusion was performed at the same time, then the restrictions would result from that fusion according to the standard protocol of the surgeon. Plain X-rays are taken at 18 weeks and 6 months. If at any time there is concern, a CT scan is performed to determine cause and further treatment.

Outcomes for the Posterior Midline Approach

Belanger in 2001 [1] presented long-term outcomes in four patients utilizing this procedure without the implementation of a cage or bone dowel. Also there were no bone graft-enhancing agents used. He reported successful results in all four patients; however, two required removal of the iliac screw due to point tenderness, after which those symptoms completely resolved. BBSI is currently in the process of submitting its review of 66 patients having had this procedure over a 5-year period with an average follow-up of 4 years. The results of that study will be summarized in the following paragraphs (Table 9.1).

Table 9.1 Preoperative data for all responding study patients

# of patients	66
Age	52.6 (31–76)
Sex	18 males, 48 females
BMI	29.2 (16.3–48.2)
Diabetes	9 %
Heart disease	41 %
Pulmonary disease	15 %
Obesity	42 %
Smoker	15 %
Disabled	36 %
Retired	20 %
Unemployed or workman's comp	20 %
Previous lumbosacral fusion	65 %
Time in conservative treatment	46.8 months (3.9 years)
Preoperative pain levels	All patients had pain levels of 7–10/10 at the time surgery was discussed

Procedural Data

Seventy-five individual SIJ fusions were performed consisting of 60 unilateral fusions and 15 bilateral fusions. This fusion procedure was combined with a lumbosacral fusion when both areas met appropriate criteria for fusion according to existing standards for the lumbosacral spine and as set forth in this book for the SIJ. Nine patients having had a unilateral SIJ fusion returned, during the study period, to have the contralateral side fused.

Off-Label Uses of Products

The FDA does not approve the use of the cage (Custom, Medtronic) and its placement into the longitudinal axis of the SIJ. The use of bone morphogenic protein (Infuse, Medtronic) is not approved by the FDA for use in this fashion. The use of these items in this procedure is "off label."

Complications and Reoperations

A complication occurred in 15 % of patients. There were no deaths, neurovascular complications, or infections. Complications had no correlation with the performing of a bilateral SIJ fusion or performing an accompanying lumbosacral fusion. All complications were temporary and self-limiting except for two patients with a nonunion of their fusion and one patient with point tenderness over the iliac screw head. All three required reoperation with long-term successful results. In the case of the painful iliac screw head, reoperation consisted only of iliac screw removal, as the fusion was solid (Table 9.2).

Table 9.2 All complications occurring in study group

Complications	Occurrence #
Confusion	1
Pulmonary embolism	1
Urinary tract infection	1
Nonunion	2[a]
Postoperative anemia	2
Hemorrhagic esophagitis	1
Painful iliac screw head	1[a]
Totals	10/66 (15 %)

[a]Required second surgery (3/66, 5 %)

Satisfaction and Function Statistics

Satisfaction results were in the 80 % range for all patients in terms of their long-term result, being willing to have it again for the same result and being willing to recommend the procedure to another. Two subgroups in our retrospective follow-up database for this procedure had the best overall results. The first group consisted of all those having bilateral SIJ fusions and the second group consisted of all those having either one or both SIJs fused in conjunction with either a lumbosacral fusion repair or extension. In each group, there was a significant decrease in pain scores (visual analog scale) and satisfaction scores greater than 85 %. Both groups are discussed further later in this chapter. Follow-up function in these patients as a whole is difficult to assess considering that the average patient going into the process of having a SIJ fusion at our institution had been in conservative treatment for 4 years, was in a pain clinic, was on chronic narcotics, and was not working or disabled (Chap. 7). Our findings were that, despite lower pain scores and high degrees of satisfaction, the variables of narcotic use and disability remained essentially the same. There was, however, a significant decrease in those requiring a pain clinic (Table 9.3).

Table 9.3 Operative and follow-up data on all patients in study group

# Patients	66
Avg age (years)	52
# Surgeries	75
# Unilateral/bilateral	60/15
# Returning for opp. side	9
Duration/surg (min)	187
Blood loss/surg (ml)	573
Complications/surgery	10/75 (13 %)
Follow-up (months)	50
Disabled	45 %
Retired	22 %
Working	25 %
Others (WC, auto, legal, etc.)	8 %
Pain level	5.0/10
Satisfied with procedure	83 %
Would do again for same result	80 %
Would recommend to another	77 %
Avg. sat score	80 %

What Is the Effect of Performing This Procedure Bilaterally?

Performing bilateral SIJ fusions at the same setting has been a routine at our institution for over a decade not only with this procedure but with posterior lateral minimally invasive procedures as well. In reviewing our retrospective long-term follow-up data using the posterior midline approach, we had 15 patients who underwent bilateral SIJ fusions over a 5-year period. At an average follow-up of 2.5 years for this group, the pain levels had dropped 2.4 points and the patient satisfaction rates averaged 87 %. This is our experience using one type of posterior approach for SIJ fusion, and it will be necessary for other institutions using this or other procedures to ultimately prove the validity of these results. We have not performed bilateral fusions using the lateral minimally invasive techniques, as they require limited weight bearing for several weeks in the postoperative period.

What Is the Effect of Performing This Procedure Concurrently with a Lumbosacral Fusion?

Many patients having a dysfunctional SIJ requiring surgery will also have lumbosacral pathology requiring a fusion. Our experience at BBSI is that 65 % of patients presenting for a SIJ fusion will have had a previous lumbosacral fusion. Frequently, the lumbosacral fusion needs repair or further disabling symptoms have developed in the cephalad segments adjacent to the lumbosacral fusion that an extension of that fusion is needed. It has been the philosophy at BBSI that when both areas are found to have pathology that warrants fusion, both are performed at the same setting. When reviewing our long-term results, we have found no correlation with satisfaction rates, complications, and the performing of a lumbosacral fusion at the same setting as the SIJ fusion. In patients with the specific diagnosis of dysfunctional SIJ(s) and in need of a lumbosacral fusion repair or extension, if both were done at the same setting, the 4-year follow-up decrease in pain levels using the VAS was statistically significant ($p=0.02192$, "paired 't'-test") with patient satisfaction rates averaging 85 %. A technical point to be made here is that when both the SIJ and the lumbosacral spine are fused at the same setting through a posterior midline incision, the rod used to cross the SIJ and connect the spinal pedicle screw with the iliac screw is passed under (anterior to) the paraspinal muscle belly (Fig. 9.15). This allows for the entire rod and screw fixation device to be deep to muscle and fascia limiting instrumentation problems postoperatively.

When the situation of having a patient with both the SIJ and the lumbosacral spine meeting the criteria for fusion presents itself to the surgeon, the posterior midline approach allows for both areas to be operated on successfully through the one incision. The impact on the patient is no greater than performing a lumbosacral fusion with an IBG. Further study is needed to validate these current assumptions (Fig. 9.16).

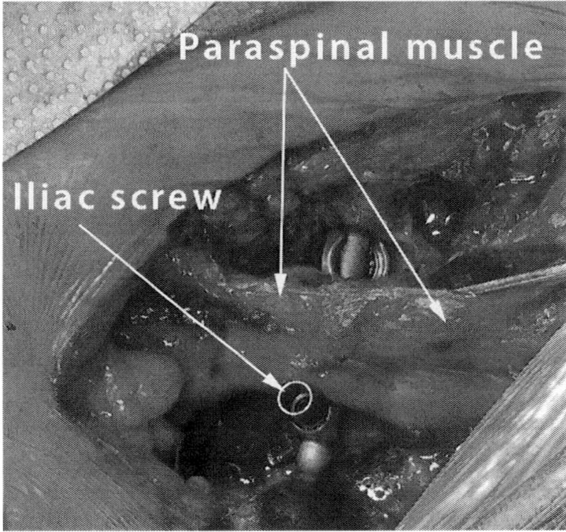

Fig. 9.15 Intraoperative photo showing the placement of the rod crossing the posterior aspect of the SIJ and anterior to the paraspinous muscle belly. This patient was also undergoing a revision of a failed lumbosacral fusion, thus the generous midline exposure

What Type of Patient Is Most Likely to Benefit from This Procedure?

- When a lumbosacral fusion needs to be repaired or extended in conjunction with the SIJ(s) fusion.
- When bilateral SIJ fusions are required.

What Type of Patient Is Least Likely to Benefit from This Procedure?

- When the patient has not had previous lumbar or SIJ surgery and both areas meet all criteria for fusion surgery. These patients had an approximately 70 % long-term success in our experience. Reasons for this are currently unknown.

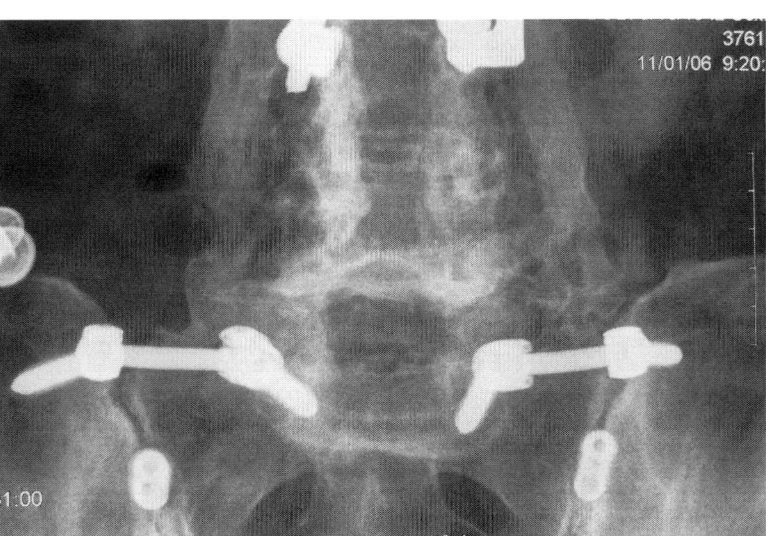

Fig. 9.16 AP X-ray showing a posterior midline approach bilateral sacroiliac joint fusion coupled with a cephalad extension of a lumbosacral fusion

Salvage Surgery for a Failed Posterior Midline Approach as Described in This Chapter

The two reasons for salvage surgery following a posterior midline approach to fuse the SIJ(s) as described in this chapter are a painful hardware situation consisting of point tenderness over the head of the iliac screw and a painful nonunion most likely accompanied by loose hardware. When the iliac screw is painful and needs to be removed, we recommend opening the posterior midline incision; approaching the surgical area between fascial layers, as described in the posterior midline approach technique; and then making a small incision in the fascia to cut the rod and remove the iliac screw followed by secure fascial repair. The rest of the hardware is left as the fusion has already been determined to be solid. If it is not solid, that then becomes the primary reason for revision as described above. For the second reason, there are a variety of methods to attempt to achieve a solid fusion. One method is to remove the screws and rod and add a second and possibly a third cage into the longitudinal joint line. Usually, if the screws are loose, it has not been fruitful to replace them, especially in the iliac wing. It is possible to use the lateral approach with a screw in device that could be maneuvered between the existing sagittal instrumentation to secure the joint in a different plane. At our institution, adding more cages or bone dowels into the longitudinal axis of the joint has resulted in fusion, decreasing pain, and improved patient satisfaction (Fig. 9.17).

Chapter Summary

This procedure is relatively new to the literature making its debut in 2001. It is the first SIJ fusion procedure to utilize the posterior midline fascial splitting approach and S1 pedicle screw fixation. This procedure also introduces a novel way to place a cancellous screw between cortical layers of the ilium for fixation. This surgical technique

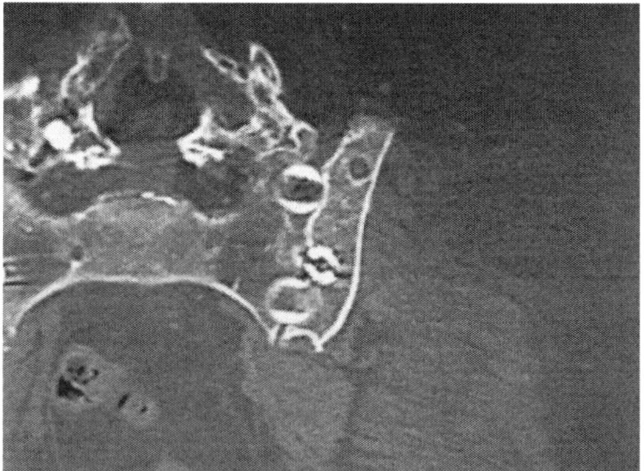

Fig. 9.17 Coronal CT scan showing a 6-month follow-up of a salvage procedure for a failed posterior midline sacroiliac joint fusion using two bone dowels (Medtronic) with BMP (Infuse, Medtronic) placed using the Stryker Virtual Navigation System (Infuse is not FDA approved for this purpose and in this case it was used "off label")

is a safe procedure for the patient, and a relatively straightforward one for the spine surgeon, who has experience with pedicle screw fixation, to perform. It has been proven to have a high fusion rate, low morbidity, and a low reoperation rate. Although many patients in our experience still have issues with disability and with their previously acquired narcotic addictions, the patient satisfaction rates averaging 4 years after surgery are very high. Recommendations have been suggested for the type of patient who might benefit the most from this procedure as well as in what circumstances it should be used with caution. This is the first textbook description of this procedure, and it reflects the results from one major institution that has been devoted to the diagnosis and treatment of the dysfunctional SIJ for over two decades. The reader should understand that this procedure is not fully understood at this point in time, and more information needs to be generated, not only from BBSI but also from other institutions as well to fully understand exactly what the patient and the surgeon can expect from it. It should be reiterated at this time that if a minimally invasive procedure can accomplish all the surgical goals for a patient, that procedure should take precedence over this more extensive posterior midline approach.

References

1. Belanger TA, Dall BE. Sacroiliac arthrodesis using posterior midline fascial splitting approach and pedicle instrumentation: a new technique. J Spinal Disord. 2001;14(2):118–24.
2. Hutchinson M, Dall BE. Midline fascial splitting approach to the iliac crest for bone graft: a new approach. Spine. 1994;19:62–6.

Bruce E. Dall

Introduction

This chapter will discuss the unique nature of this approach and fixation that allow it to be minimally invasive and yet highly effective in achieving surgical goals. Its etiology as an Investigational Review Board (IRB) hospital study will be discussed as well as limitations based on the lack of current FDA approval for implanting instrumentation in the longitudinal axis of the sacroiliac joint (SIJ). The indications, contraindications, and specific technical challenges to this procedure will be discussed as well as relative outcomes. Lastly, the method of salvaging this procedure in the event of failure will be discussed as well as using this approach for SIJ aspiration and biopsy in the event of suspected joint infection or other pathologic process.

Etiology of Procedure and Literature Review

The first paper in the literature explaining this unique approach was by Wise in 2008 [1]. This procedure utilizes two threaded cages, each with bone or bone-enhancing elements packed inside, placed via a posterior lateral minimally invasive approach into the longitudinal axis of the SIJ. The procedure concept and design were based on the need for a minimally invasive technique that would not go through muscle, avoid neurovascular structures, meet minimal hardware requirements for joint stabilization, allow for a very solid fusion, and permit immediate full weight bearing with minimal bracing postsurgery. This procedure was first performed and studied under an IRB in 2004, after which it became a useful addition to our surgical armamentarium for SIJ fusion. The procedure's main limitation is that placing a cage into the longitudinal axis of the SIJ line is not FDA approved for this purpose. Unlike the direct lateral approaches with predicates preexisting the FDA and allowing for approval via the 510(k) process, this approach has no such predicates. Bone morphogenic protein (BMP) (Infuse, Medtronic), which is used inside the cages, is also not FDA approved for this use. Surgeons using this method and approach must declare that what they are doing is "off label." As a result of needing pre-market approval for this procedure to be FDA approved,

B.E. Dall, M.D. (✉)
Neurosurgery of Kalamazoo, Borgess Brain
and Spine Institute, 1541 Gull Road, Kalamazoo,
MI 49048, USA

Orthopedic Spine Division, Western Michigan
University Medical School, Kalamazoo, MI, USA
e-mail: dall.bruce@yahoo.com

B.E. Dall et al. (eds.), *Surgery for the Painful, Dysfunctional Sacroiliac Joint*,
DOI 10.1007/978-3-319-10726-4_10, © Springer International Publishing Switzerland 2015

industry is less willing to bear the expense of bringing this procedure to market.

Indications and Contraindications for Procedure

The absolute indications for this procedure can only be estimated secondary to following approximately 40 patients having had this procedure either unilaterally or bilaterally at the same sitting and followed long term. The circumstances where this procedure was used successfully include:

- Single or bilateral joint involvement
- Gross or morbid obesity
- When full weight bearing postsurgery is required
- As an adjunct to a lumbosacral fusion at same setting

  Absolute contraindications for this procedure would include:

- Significant osteoporosis
- When there is a damaged or missing portion of the posterior superior iliac spine (PSIS)
- When intraoperative imaging cannot give a clear anterior posterior (AP) image
- When this procedure has failed to achieve fusion
- Gross joint instability
- Lack of stable anterior or posterior SIJ ligament structures
- Unusual anatomy making landmarks unclear

Posterior Lateral into the Longitudinal Axis of the Joint: Minimally Invasive Approach, Step by Step

Step 1: Preoperative Preparation

In order for this procedure to proceed quickly and smoothly in the operating room, significant work must be done prior to ensure complete cage containment. Since, in the absence of a navigation system, which will not be discussed here, the surgeon only has real-time fluoroscopic image to rely on, he/she must know ahead of time where

the cephalad and caudal margins of the SIJ "safe zone" are. The safe zone is defined as, when viewing the SIJ in the coronal plane, that portion of the SIJ having adequate bone on the iliac and sacral sides of the joint to support a full insertion of the cage. A preoperative CT scan is obtained of the entire pelvis. From this the axial cuts are evaluated looking for the most cephalad and most caudal slices that would allow full cage containment. These two views also allow the surgeon to know exactly the distance from the most palpable bone of the dorsal ilium to the anterior aspect of the sacrum in each of the axial slices (Figs. 10.1 and 10.2).

Utilizing CT scanner software, these margins are printed out as horizontal lines on an AP scout radiograph of the pelvis, appearing as the surgeon would visualize it with fluoroscopy in surgery. The space between the lines represents the "safe zone" (Fig. 10.3).

Now the surgeon has knowledge of the safest space to place cages from posterior into the longitudinal axis of the SIJ in both the coronal and axial planes. There is no useful imaging that will assist the surgeon with this approach in the lateral plane, as the SIJ cannot be reliably imaged laterally. If any of the preoperative preparation images cannot be obtained, this technique should be abandoned in favor of another procedure.

Step 2: Positioning

The patient is placed in the prone position taking the same standard precautions as for a lumbar fusion surgery and allowing the abdomen to hang free (see Fig. 9.4). Image is then brought in and an AP view of the involved SIJ is obtained to assure good visibility. This can usually be accomplished even in the most obese patient, as there is actually less soft tissue muscle and bony obstruction in this plane than in the lateral plane. The image is then moved live approximately 10–25° cephalad and, in the axial plane, posterior medial and anterolateral, until the best overall image of the joint is obtained. This becomes the angle of insertion for the cages and provides the last necessary angular information for the surgeon before beginning the operation.

Fig. 10.1 Preoperative axial CT showing the cephalad-most margin for total cage containment. Also shown is the measurement from the tip of the PSIS to the anterior aspect of the sacroiliac joint bilaterally. Stopping 1 cm short of that distance is considered a safe depth for drilling, in surgery, to avoid entering the pelvic cavity

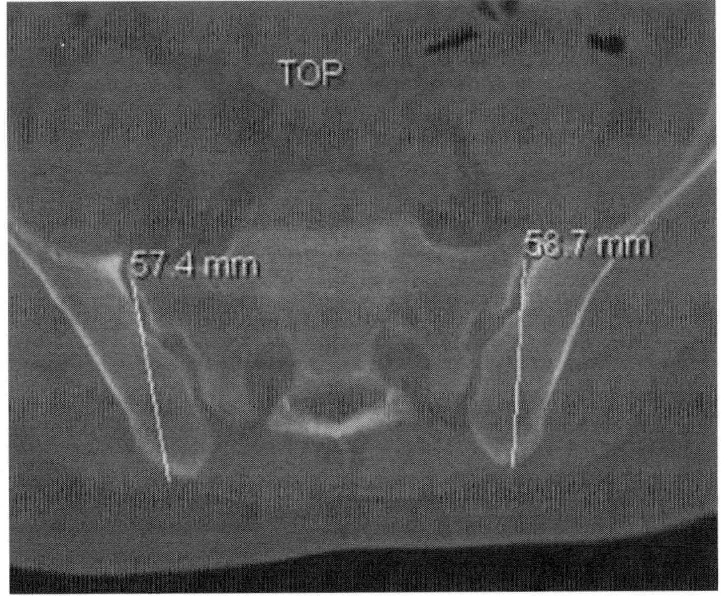

Fig. 10.2 Preoperative axial CT showing the caudal-most margin for total cage containment. Note that the measurement from the tip of the PSIS to the safe anterior aspect of the sacroiliac joint is shorter in this axial plane than in the previous more cephalad section

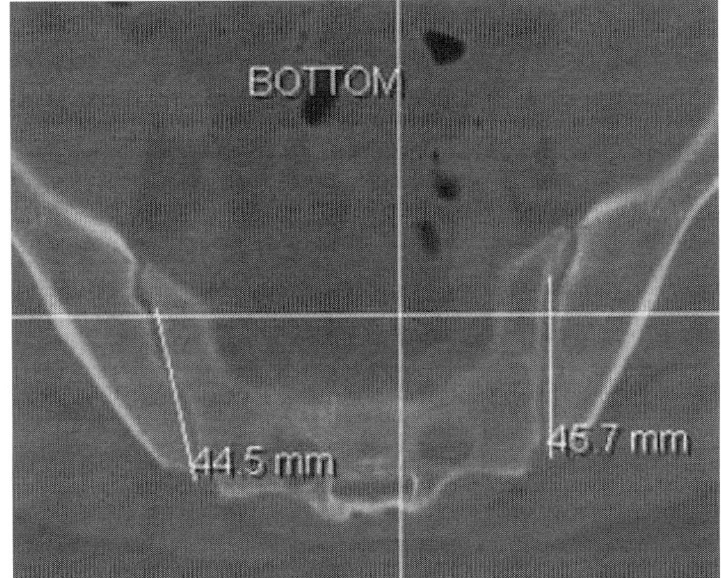

Step 3: Incision

The most prominent tip of the PSIS is palpated, and a 1–2 in., depending on the size of the patient, vertical incision is made. This dissection is carried down to the bone. In an obese patient, the PSIS tip might not be felt externally and may need to be visualized with image after which the incision and blunt finger dissection are needed to physically feel the PSIS (Fig. 10.4).

Step 4: Preparing the Space for the Cage

With the image remaining in position, a ¼ in. drill bit is then tapped into the bone of the PSIS with a mallet just far enough to hold it upright. Image is used to verify that the bit is in the lower 1/3 of the safe zone and aimed straight into the joint following the same angles as the imaging (Fig. 10.5).

Fig. 10.3 Preoperative coronal image generated by the CT scan as a scout film showing the upper and lower margins of the "safe zone" for placing two cages, as defined in this chapter, with total longitudinal cage containment based on the data in Figs. 10.1 and 10.2

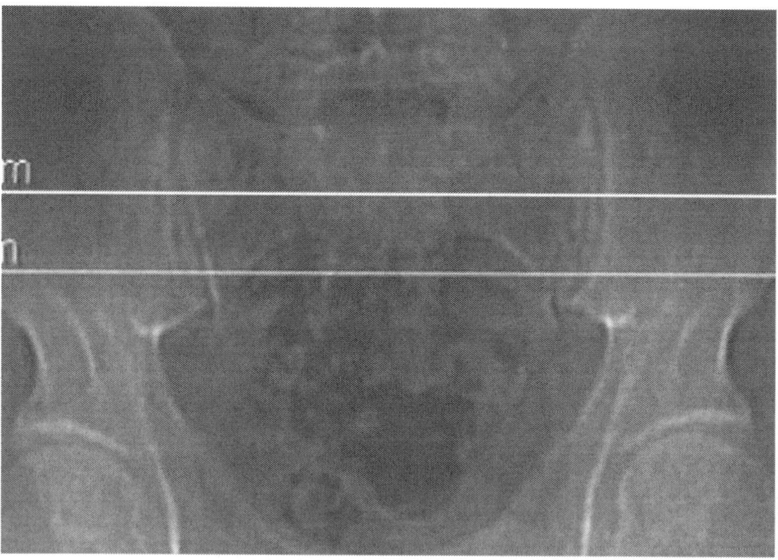

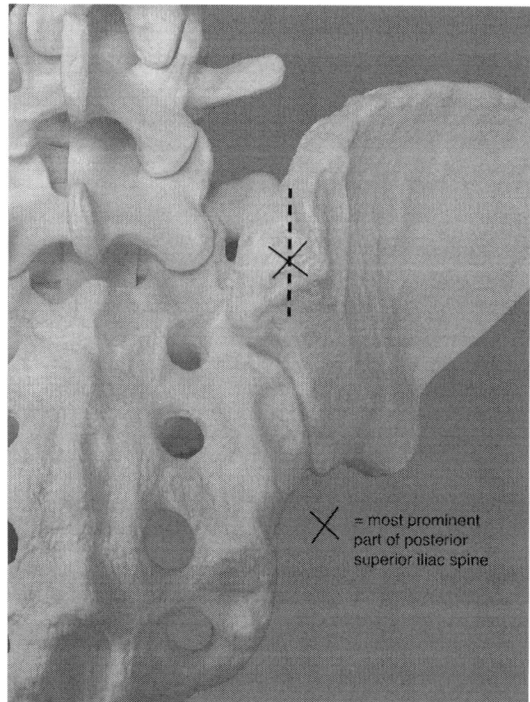

Fig. 10.4 The vertical incision is in line with and just cephalad and caudal to the PSIS

The drill is then advanced through the PSIS and into the joint, frequently verifying with image that it is staying in the joint line. Once the depth, predetermined by preoperative CT scan, is reached, the drill is removed and a K-wire is placed, blunt end first, into the hole. The surgeon verifies with this that there is bone at the hole's depth. After creating the channel for the inverted K-wire, the surgeon will have a good understanding as to the density of the subchondral bone. It is with this knowledge that he/she decides whether an awl can be used to make the channel larger or whether a power drill will be needed. A cannulated awl or drill bit is then placed over the K-wire, approximately 2 mm less in width than the cage that will be placed, and the hole is made larger to the same depth as the K-wire. This is when a lateral image becomes important. All that needs to be seen is the position of the tip of the blunt end of the K-wire. If, when using the awl or the drill to widen the channel, the tip of the K-wire moves, further drilling is stopped. The K-wire is removed and the hole is palpated to be sure that bone still remains at the base of the hole and no soft tissue is palpable.

Caution! If after measuring the channel appears to be deep enough for total cage containment to include some subsidence of it at the dorsal surface, the procedure can continue. If not the decision to make the hole deeper using a "freehand" technique while watching the lateral image is an option, but only in the hands of a very technically capable and experienced surgeon keeping

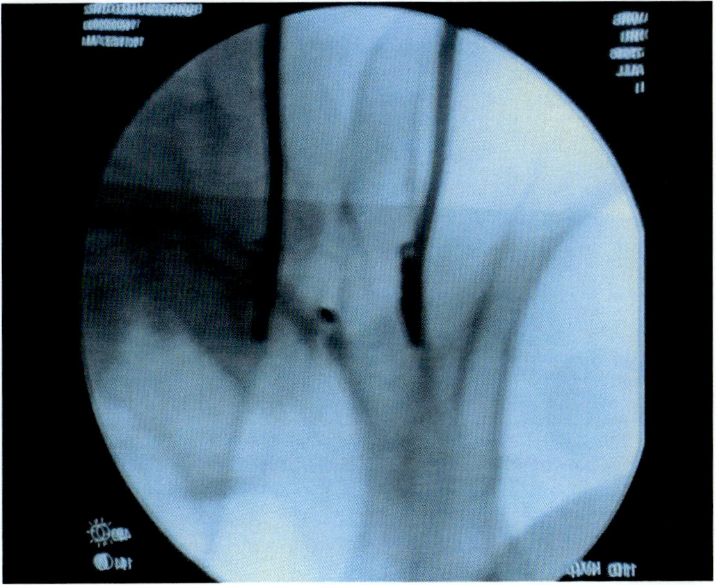

Fig. 10.5 Intraoperative AP image showing the drill bit aimed at the sacroiliac joint

in mind that plunging through the anterior SIJ into the pelvis is potentially "life threatening"! We are not recommending that option here and our advice is that if there is any hesitation or concern on the part of the surgeon, another method to fuse the SIJ should be entertained.

All hardware is then removed and the hole is palpated to insure that bone is present both deep and all around the created canal. It is also visualized on image to assure that the created hole is inside the center of the joint line. We use a 9 mm-diameter awl or drill bit for an 11 mm-diameter cage placed at an average depth of 4.5–5.5 cm depending on the preoperative studies.

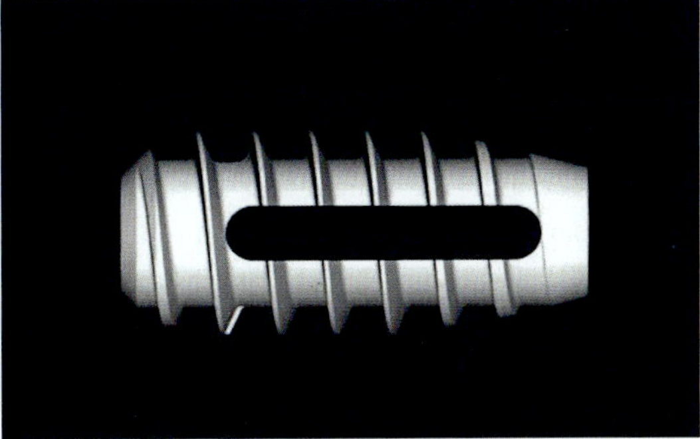

Fig. 10.6 The cage (Medtronic, Custom) is cylindrical, threaded, and hollow and measures 25 mm in length and 11 mm in diameter

Step 5: Insertion of Cage

At our institution, the cages used in our study were custom (Medtronic) and filled with BMP (Infuse, Medtronic). With the hole properly prepared, the cage is then inserted to a depth of tightening by two fingers. It is then visualized on image in both the AP and lateral planes. A clamp is then placed on the dorsal aspect of the cage, and vigorous pulling is done to verify that the cage is indeed very stable. If it moves, then a larger cage must be inserted. The success of the cage placement is based on the concept of distracting the joint against the opposing tension forces of the intact anterior and posterior SIJ ligaments. If these structures are severely compromised, other methods for SIJ fusion should be considered (Figs. 10.6 and 10.7).

Step 6: Insertion of Second Cage

The lowest cage was placed first as the landmarks and the qualities of bone are best in this location. Once the first cage is placed successfully, the

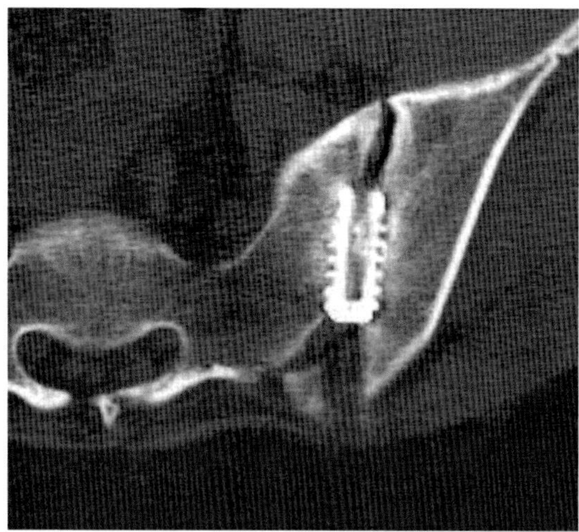

Fig. 10.7 Axial CT showing the path of the cage through the tip of the PSIS and then into the longitudinal axis of the sacroiliac joint

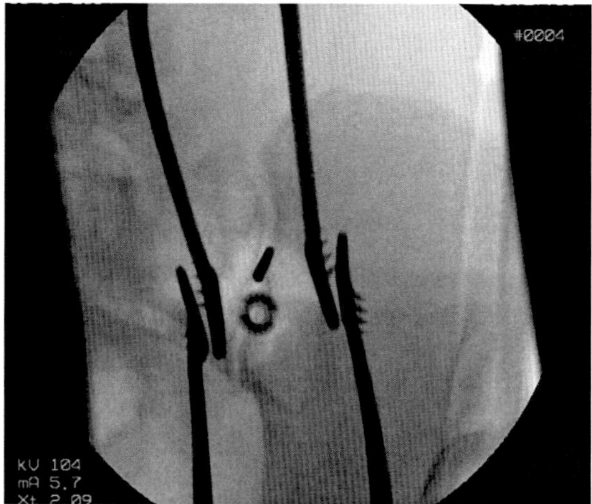

Fig. 10.8 Intraoperative AP image showing the first cage in place and the drill bit accessing the path for the second cage

second cage placement goes fairly quickly. Steps 4 and 5 are repeated with placement aimed at putting this cage just cephalad to the first cage. It should be noted that the depth of drilling for the cephalad cage may be slightly deeper than the caudal cage. This was defined with the preoperative CT scan (Figs. 10.1 and 10.2). Once the cage is placed, a clamp is used to verify the stability of this one as well. Again, if either cage is loose, they must be replaced with something larger in diameter (Figs. 10.8–10.10).

Caution! If a cage cannot be placed, that is, rigidly stable when tested, this procedure will not work in the long run, and other options for further instrumenting the SIJ should be considered. This would be considered a very rare situation.

Step 7: Closure

The deepest tissues, consisting only of fascial and subcutaneous tissues, which have been minimally violated, are closed with heavy absorbable suture followed with routine closure after that. These incisions have routinely healed well with very good cosmetics.

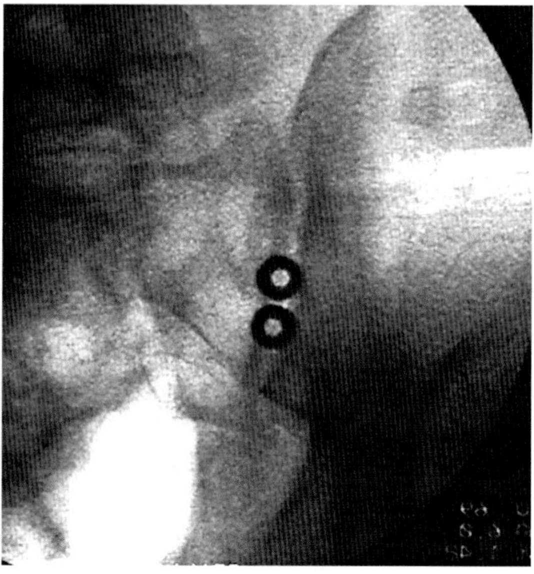

Fig. 10.9 Intraoperative AP image showing both cages in place within the longitudinal axis of the sacroiliac joint

Step 8: Postoperative Management

This procedure has been performed as an outpatient with equal results to the IRB study, in which the patients were kept overnight. Patients are allowed to immediately weight bear and use a sacral belt whenever up for 12 weeks. In the case

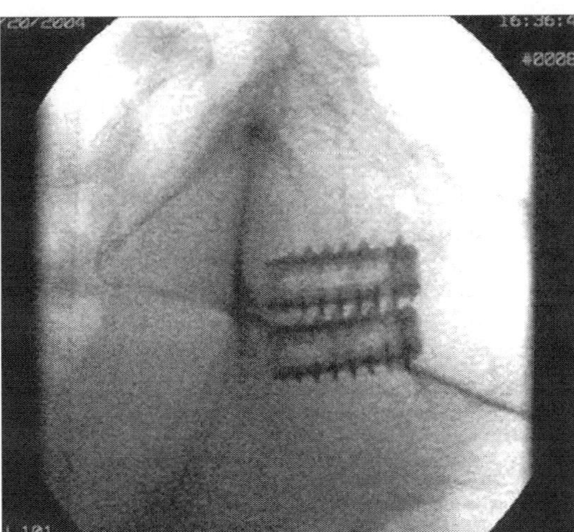

Fig. 10.10 Intraoperative lateral image showing both cages in place. Note how the lower cage appears anterior to the midline of the sacrum demonstrating that the joint line extends farther into the pelvis lateral to the midline. This also demonstrates the inability of the lateral image to assist in proper cage placement

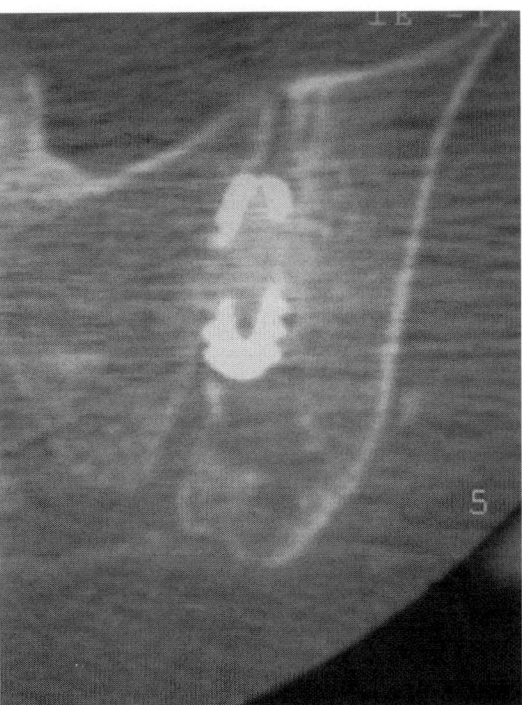

Fig. 10.11 One-year postoperative axial CT scan showing bone fusion of the sacroiliac joint occurring directly through the cage

of the very obese patient, a walker is substituted and used whenever up for 12 weeks. No lifting more than 15# is allowed for 12 weeks, and the main exercise is walking using a shorter stride. After this 12-week period, therapy is begun to fully strengthen the patient, and they are allowed to return to work without restrictions at 18 weeks. Restrictions are only applied if the patient still has residual pain or there are other issues occurring requiring the restrictions (e.g., associated lumbar fusion). X-rays are taken at 6 and 18 weeks postsurgery with a CT scan being performed at the 12-week mark (Fig. 10.11). If at any time there is concern about the status of the cage or fusion, a CT scan is performed with treatment as needed.

Procedural Data

This procedure was performed as part of an IRB protocol on 13 consecutive patients during the course of 1 year. Of these, six had bilateral SIJ fusions performed. There were more females and the average age was 53. The average BMI was 31. Blood loss averaged less than 100 cc in all cases, and the average length of stay was 1.7 days, with a mean follow-up of 2.4 years.

Off-Label Use of Products

The FDA does not approve either the cage (custom, Medtronic) or the BMP (Infuse, Medtronic) for this use. These were used "off-label" in these patients.

Complications and Reoperations

Two of the 19 joints (11 %) developed a nonunion of the fusion. One patient was converted to a posterior midline fusion as described in Chap. 9, leaving the original cage in place, with ultimate success. The other patient was not revised, as they were not symptomatic and happy with their result. There were no infections, neurovascular complications, or lasting morbidity.

Satisfaction, Pain, and Functional Statistics

Satisfaction for the procedure was 79 % at long-term follow-up with those patients stating they would do the procedure again for the same result. Using the VAS (0–10), the average drop in back pain levels averaged 4.9 ($p = <0.001$), and for leg pain, it was 2.4 ($p = <0.013$). Dyspareunia dropped by an average 2.4 ($p = <0.0028$). No data on functional activities pre- or postsurgery was gathered.

What Is the Effect of Performing This Procedure Bilaterally?

This was not statistically evaluated, although the three patients who were not satisfied with the procedure long term did not have bilateral fusions. Information as to whether a bilateral fusion verses spacing the procedures is not available at this time (Fig. 10.12).

What Is the Effect of Performing This Procedure with a Lumbosacral Fusion?

It can be performed with a lumbosacral fusion, but we have no current data to recommend for or against performing this combination.

Salvage Surgery for a Failed Posterior Lateral into the Longitudinal Axis of the Joint Minimally Invasive Approach Procedure

The most assured method for salvaging this surgery in our hands has been to perform a posterior midline surgery as described in Chap. 9, leaving the current cages in place and not inserting more. We have one instance of removing both cages, which had become loose, and reinserting larger cages with an overall excellent result in a moderately obese patient.

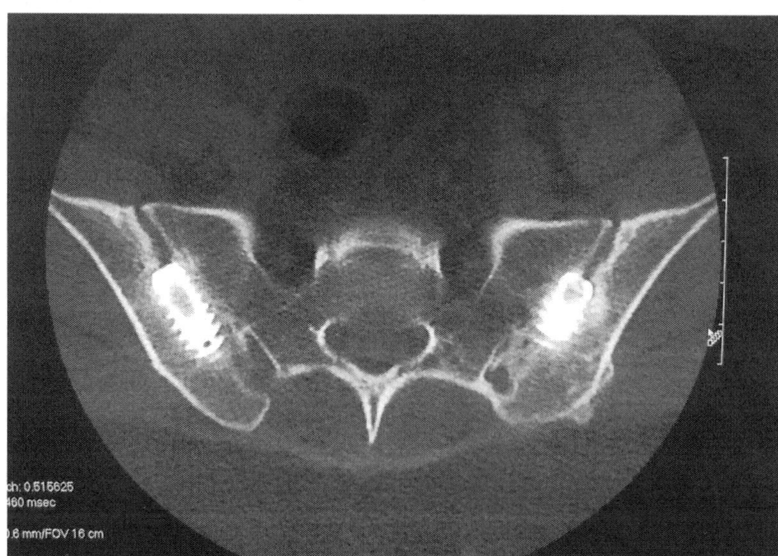

Fig. 10.12 Long-term follow-up axial CT scan showing bilateral sacroiliac joint fusions using this technique

Method for Using This Approach for Aspiration and Biopsy

Although this book's primary function is not to discuss infection or other acute processes that may affect the SIJ, this particular approach offers a simple mechanism for aspiration and/or biopsy of the joint should the situation occur. The following discussion will provide the technical details for performing this procedure; however, it is up to the individual surgeon to decide under what circumstances to use it.

Procedure

Steps 1, 2, 3, and 4 are followed in an identical fashion as described in the preceding discussion for this approach. At this point, any of the bone or debris residing in the cannulated drill is cultured and sent for histology, each based on the surgeon's preferences. With the passage now established into the joint, further swabbing, curetting, or other is performed to acquire further fluid or tissue specimen for analysis. A permanent image should be obtained in various planes to verify the position of a probe in the joint. Closure is accomplished, if appropriate, depending on potential drainage, as discussed in the preceding step 7. The surgeon, based on the potential diagnosis of the patient, determines further decisions on treatment and patient function (Figs. 10.13, 10.14, 10.15, and 10.16).

Our experience with this technique is limited and should be used by the experienced surgeon understanding that each patient with his or her associated pathology is unique and results may vary. This is meant to be considered as an option for aspiration and biopsy of the SIJ understanding that several other options, with no given standard, exist for the surgeon's consideration.

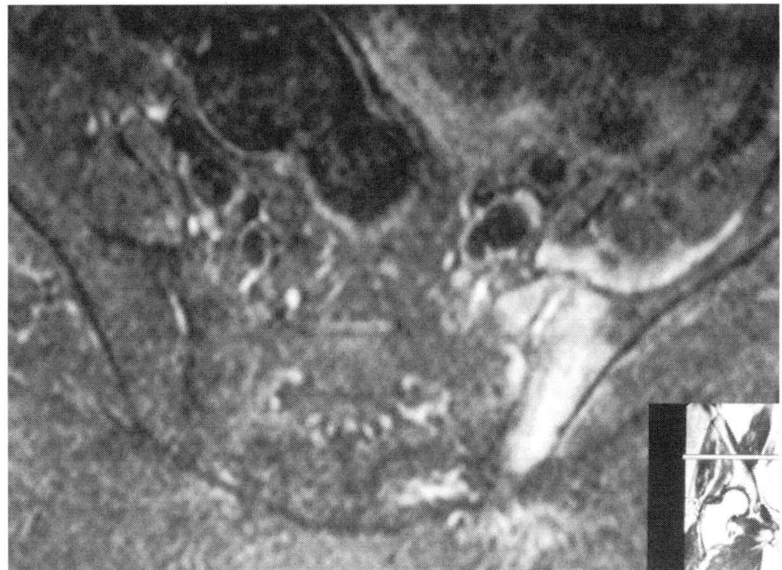

Fig. 10.13 Axial T2 STIR MRI showing hyperintensity of the area surrounding the sacroiliac joint

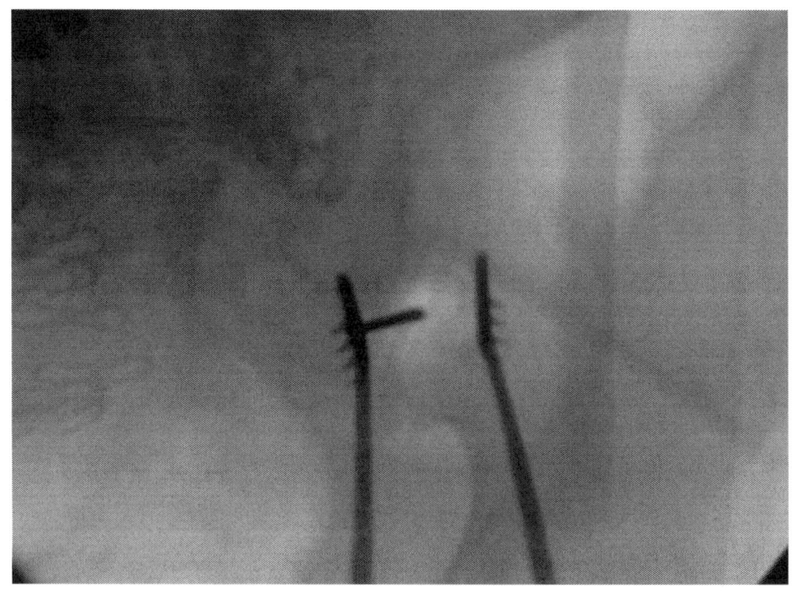

Fig. 10.14 Intraoperative AP image showing probe inside the sacroiliac joint

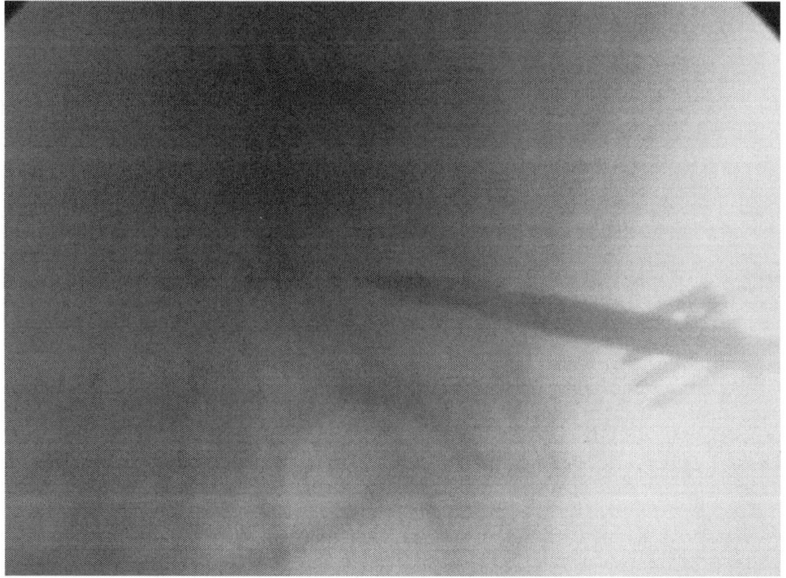

Fig. 10.15 Intraoperative lateral image showing cannulated drill inside the sacroiliac joint

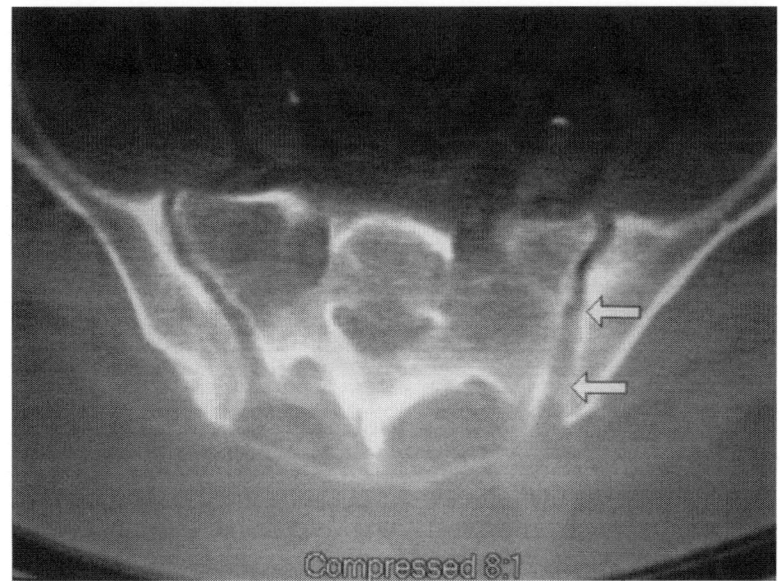

Fig. 10.16 Six-month follow-up axial CT scan showing the previous path created into the sacroiliac joint using this approach with possible auto-fusion beginning to occur. The patient was asymptomatic at the time this image was obtained

Chapter Summary

There is minimal data available for the insertion of cages, bone dowels, or other into the longitudinal axis of the SIJ. Our work is unique and was initially performed under the auspices of an IRB to insure patient safety and appropriate follow-up with subsequent publication in a peer review journal [1]. This surgery requires detailed preoperative steps, which are paramount to successful placement of the cages. The approach used, starting at the tip of the PSIS, allows for the surgeon to have a secure landmark from which to proceed through the rest of the procedure. The ability to operate on obese patients with immediate weight bearing and minimal bracing with a procedure that takes a short period of time make this an attractive first procedure to perform when a more complicated procedure may not be deemed desirable or appropriate. This surgery needs to be trialed in prospective multicenter studies to completely understand its exact indications, contraindications, and long-term results. The main clinical limitation to this procedure at this time is the need for it to go through "pre-market approval" to be approved for use by the FDA. This approach can also be used to access the SIJ for other purposes like acute infection, and as with its use for performing a minimally invasive fusion, should be considered as a new procedure with limited and incomplete experience and one of many options in existence with no current standard model to follow.

Reference

1. Wise CL, Dall BE. Minimally invasive sacroiliac joint arthrodesis: outcomes of a new technique. J Spinal Disord Tech. 2008;21:579–84.

Michael R. Moore

Introduction

The open posterior lateral, or transiliac, approach to the sacroiliac joint (SIJ) is considered by many to be the standard open approach for either arthrodesis or drainage of septic sacroiliitis. This chapter will describe the historical background and development of the transiliac approach and will review results and complications observed utilizing this technique.

Historical Background

Smith-Petersen provided the first description of the transiliac approach to the SIJ in 1921 [1]. He suggested that anterior and superior approaches were impractical because of the difficulty in reaching the joint by those approaches and opined that an earlier approach described by Painter which involved reflecting a large flap of bone from the posterior Ilium was too extensive [2]. Smith-Petersen's operation involved a long curved incision overlying the posterior portion of the iliac crest, continuing across the posterior superior iliac spine (PSIS) and curving laterally following the fibers of the gluteus maximus muscle for an additional 4 in. (Fig. 11.1a).

The gluteal musculature was detached and subperiosteal dissection carried out until the posterior and lateral portions of the ilium were exposed (Fig. 11.1b).

The anatomic projection of the articular portion of the SIJ on the ilium was visualized using the sciatic notch and the "medial gluteal line", what anatomists refer to as the anterior gluteal line [3], as landmarks. A rectangular "window" was then cut through the ilium through which the articular surface of the sacral side of the joint was visualized. Cartilage and subchondral bone was removed from the sacral side of the joint as well as from the removed block of bone. The block was then countersunk across the defect, which allowed for opposition of cancellous surfaces with the bone block spanning the joint. In his original publication Smith-Petersen made passing reference to seven cases of sacroiliac tuberculosis and three cases of "relaxation" of the joint that had undergone the procedure with successful results though, as was common at the time, no specific data were reported. In the same year Gaenslen reported on a transiliac approach in which a similar window was made after reflecting a partial thickness flap of bone from the posterior ilium (Fig. 11.2) [4].

A triangular window was then made into the synovial portion of the joint through the exposed cancellous surface of the ilium. Decortication of

M.R. Moore, M.D. (⊠)
Department of Surgery, University of North Dakota Medical School, Bismarck, ND, USA

The Bone & Joint Center,
310 N 9th St, Bismarck, ND, 58501, USA
e-mail: mmoore@bone-joint.com

B.E. Dall et al. (eds.), *Surgery for the Painful, Dysfunctional Sacroiliac Joint*,
DOI 10.1007/978-3-319-10726-4_11, © Springer International Publishing Switzerland 2015

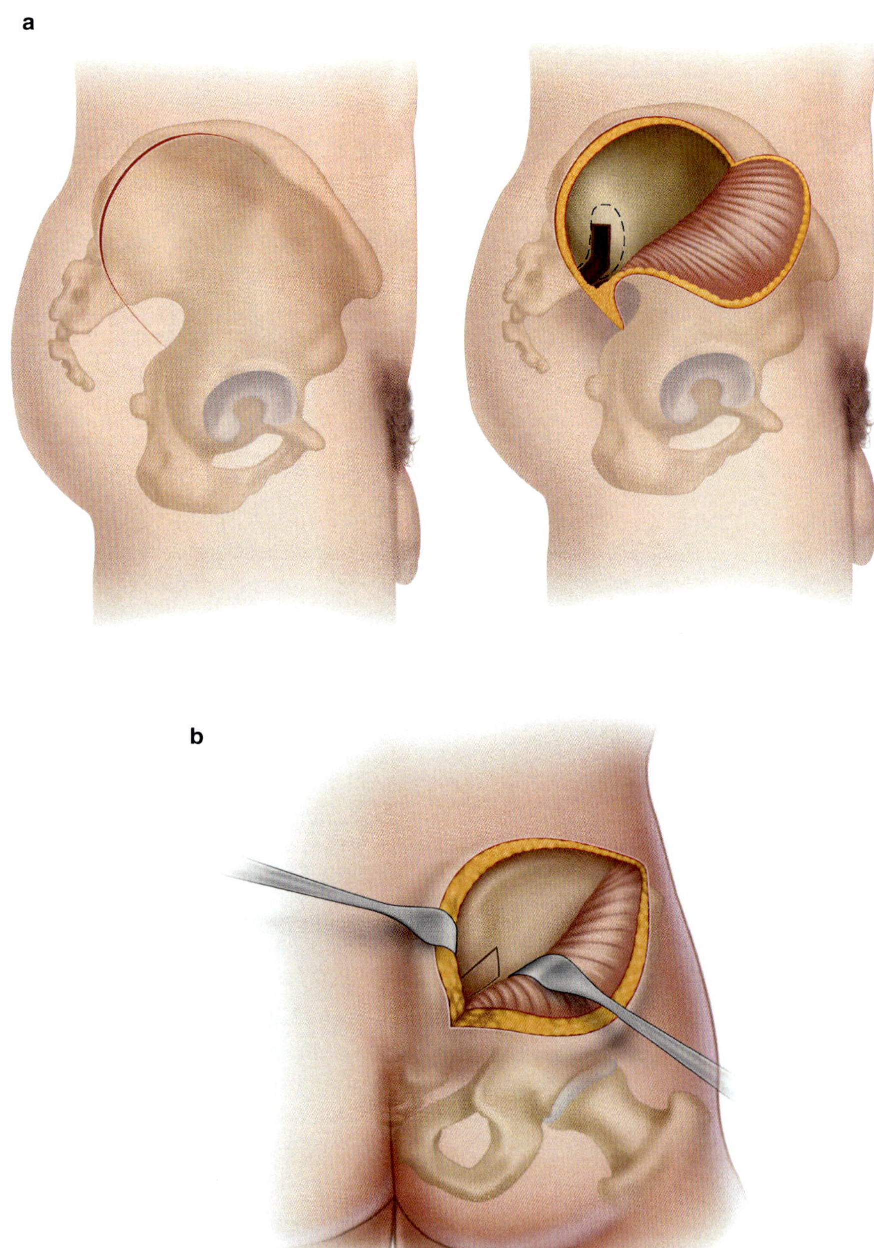

Fig. 11.1 Smith-Petersen transiliac approach for sacroiliac arthrodesis. (**a**) Incision and window in original description. (**b**) Exposure of lateral ilium and subse-quent modification of transiliac bone window into synovial portion of sacroiliac joint

the sacral side of the joint was carried out and local bone graft was placed. The reflected flap of bone and attached musculature were approximated back to the crest using sutures. Blood loss was not reported, but it could be expected that with the exposure of a large area of cancellous bone, blood loss would be higher than with the Smith-Petersen technique.

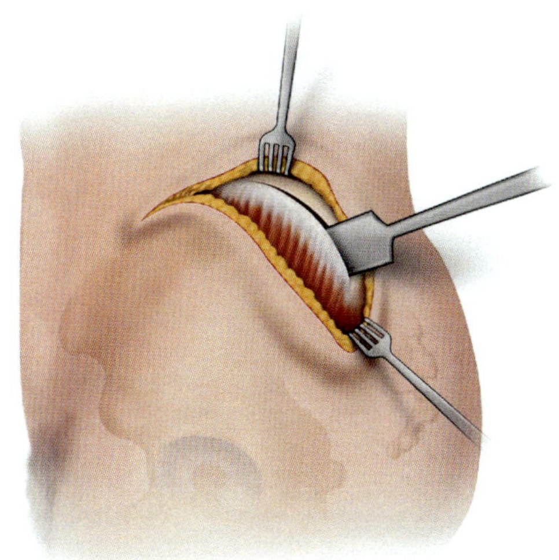

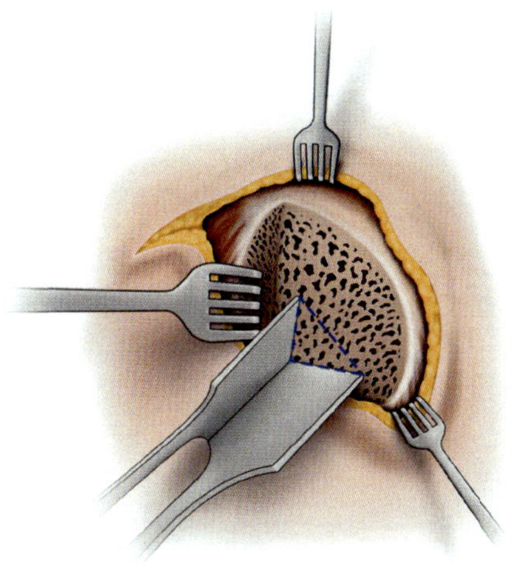

Fig. 11.2 Gaenslen's transiliac approach for sacroiliac arthrodesis. The outer table of the ilium is osteotomized and a flap reflected with attached gluteal musculature. A triangular window is made to access the sacroiliac joint. After decortication and grafting, the flap was reapproximated with sutures

Smith-Petersen later reported on end results of his technique for patients with tuberculosis of the SIJ [5] and patients with non-tuberculous disorders of the SIJ [6]. Twelve of thirteen (12/13 = 92 %) of patients operated on for tuberculosis had complete resolution of pain following surgery and eight of thirteen (8/13 = 69 %) returned to their prior occupation. It was noted, however, that four patients eventually died from tuberculosis, three from distant involvement due to meningitis or peritonitis and one from a secondary infection and abscess who left the hospital against advice and died 3 months after surgery. In patients with non-tubercular arthritis of the SIJ, 23/26 (88 %) had complete relief of pain. In a follow-up report on his technique, Gaenslen reported on nine patients undergoing surgery either for tuberculosis of the SIJ or sacroiliac "strain" [7]. One patient was considered a failure on the basis of a probable incorrect diagnosis. One patient developed a severe deep infection but ultimately had a good result.

Harris reported on a series of 67 consecutive cases of sacroiliac disease treated with arthrodesis using a transiliac approach similar to that described by Smith-Petersen [8]. He reported 68 % had excellent results, 18 % partially improved, and 3 % had no relief and 1 patient died. Nine percent were lost to follow-up.

Bloom should be credited with the first attempt to perform a minimally invasive sacroiliac arthrodesis [9]. He described a much smaller straight-line incision based on landmarks relating to a line drawn from the (PSIS) to the anterior superior iliac spine (ASIS) (Fig. 11.3a).

A perpendicular to this line was drawn inferior to a point 1.5 in. anterior to the PSIS along the first line. A point ½ inch from the original line along the perpendicular was selected as the center of a 3-in. incision that was made in the direction of the gluteus maximus muscle fibers. Blunt dissection was utilized to separate muscle fibers and palpate the ilium and the sciatic notch (Fig. 11.3b).

The central point of this incision overlies the synovial portion of the SIJ. A Steinman pin was then driven across the joint perpendicular to the surface of the ilium. A 1.25 in. diameter hole saw (Fig. 11.3c) was then used to cut a cylindrical core of bone through the ilium and across the joint into the sacrum.

The plug was removed, the opposing cartilage surfaces were excised, and the plug was then reinserted and countersunk providing a cancellous plug spanning the joint (Fig. 11.3d).

Per Bloom, the operation could be accomplished bilaterally in "...fifteen to twenty-five

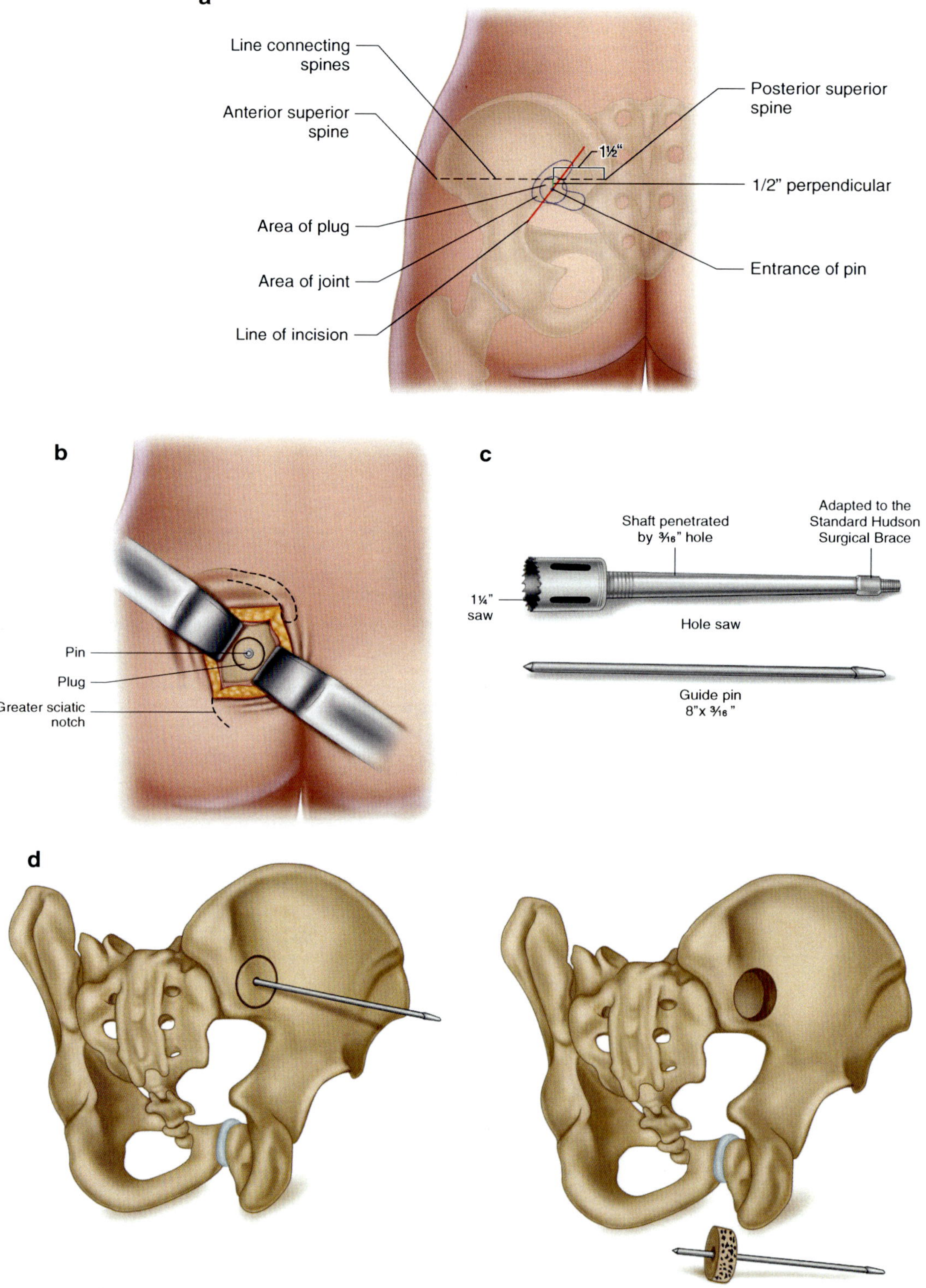

Fig. 11.3 Bloom's description of novel technique for sacroiliac arthrodesis with minimal soft tissue disruption. (**a**) Landmarks and planning for incision. (**b**) Exposed outer surface of ilium and planned bone plug cut. (**c**) "Hole saw" used for removal of bone plug accessing the sacroiliac joint. (**d**) Cadaver pelvis showing location of graft [9]

minutes, including closure of skin, without any undo haste." Bloom noted that patients felt well the day following surgery and did not require pain medication. He allowed them to be mobilized early in contrast to other postoperative regimens at the time that prescribed plaster beds and spica casts for up to 5 months [10]. He allowed them to "sit up as soon as they desire" and to be without restrictions in 14 days.

Unfortunately, Bloom only reported on the procedure in four patients and never published any further information on his technique. In the same year, Key also reported on a variation of the Smith-Petersen technique intended to reduce the exposure and soft tissue trauma [11]. Key described a straight-line incision parallel to the fibers of the gluteus maximus just below the PSIS. Blunt dissection was used to separate the gluteus maximus from the gluteus medius, and the ilium was exposed. The standard Smith-Petersen window was then made with much less exposure than in the original description. The author described having used the procedure in eight patients with good results, but, as was common at the time, no specific data were given.

There is a marked absence of mention of sacroiliac arthrodesis in general in the literature for most of the next 50 years. Hodgson reported on 11 cases of pyogenic SIJ infection, which were drained by a Smith-Petersen transiliac approach with 100 % satisfactory results but did not describe the surgical procedure as an arthrodesis per se [12]. Waisbrod et al. [13] reported on arthrodesis of the SIJ for chronic low back pain in 1987 with a very limited description of their technique. It is clear from CT scans included in the article, however, that they used a direct posterior open approach rather than a transiliac approach. Moore first reported on results from a modified Smith-Petersen approach using a smaller incision and incorporating internal fixation in 1992 [14]. Thirteen patients were presented in his initial report who had been diagnosed by CT scan or fluoroscopically guided injections and who had failed conservative treatment. All 13 patients underwent fusion by a modified Smith-Petersen approach with internal fixation. Results were reported as excellent in ten patients, fair in one, and poor in two patients. The only complication

reported was a pseudarthrosis in two patients. Subsequent reports by the same author [15–21] using the same transiliac approach documented favorable results with few approach-related complications. In the final review of 120 operations in 110 patients, there was one superficial wound infection, one incidence of over-penetration of a fixation screw causing temporary neuritic pain requiring screw removal, and one case where an intraoperative fracture into the sciatic notch occurred when creating the bone window using an osteotome. The fracture was fixed with a single screw during the index procedure without subsequent morbidity. A symptomatic pseudarthrosis rate of 8.9 % (10/110 cases) was reported, seven of which were reoperated with five going on to radiographic union and a good clinical result. Eight of ten patients with pseudarthrosis were smokers. In patients with isolated sacroiliac pathology, 90 % were classified as clinical successes. Operative time averaged 1 h and 15 min and blood loss averaged 200 cc.

Kurica reported on 32 patients who underwent open sacroiliac arthrodesis by a modified Smith-Petersen transiliac approach without instrumentation and reported a fusion rate of 94 % (30/32) but did not detail clinical results [22]. Giannikas et al. reported on five patients operated on using two Cloward-type grafts placed across the SIJ without any associated instrumentation [23]. Four of five operated patients reported complete relief of symptoms at a mean follow-up of 29 months (range 25–41 months) with one patient reporting partial improvement. Residual symptoms in the fifth patient were ascribed to coexistent lumbar osteoarthropathy.

Buchowski et al. [24] reported on functional and radiographic outcomes of 20 patients who had undergone sacroiliac arthrodesis using a modified Smith-Petersen technique with screw and plate fixation. Solid arthrodesis was found in 17/20 patients (85 %) though only plain radiographic criteria were used. Only 15/20 (75 %) of patients completed preoperative and postoperative SF-36 forms, but of those completing forms, significant improvements were seen in physical functioning, role physical, bodily pain, vitality, social functioning, role emotional, and pain indices. Complications included pseudarthrosis

(15 %), deep wound infection (10 %), and painful hardware (5 %).

One frequently cited but seldom critiqued report is the article by Schutz and Grob that describes poor outcomes from sacroiliac arthrodesis [25]. This article stands in distinction from virtually every other article on sacroiliac arthrodesis in that satisfactory results are generally reported in the literature and this article reports negative results in the experience at a single center using a novel technique. Critics of sacroiliac arthrodesis often cite this reference as being evidence that SIJ arthrodesis has been associated with poor outcomes [26, 27]. Examination of the study, however, reveals multiple factors that limit any generalization of their observed results to the subject of sacroiliac arthrodesis.

The authors reported on 17 patients thought to have SIJ-mediated pain who underwent surgical treatment, though diagnostic criteria varied from image-guided diagnostic injection to positive bone scans to pain relief from a trial of external fixation. By their own report, only 30 % of the patients were considered to have "definite" indications for a sacroiliac fusion. Additionally, 10/17 (59 %) had an average of 2.7 prior surgeries on the lumbar spine and/or SIJs. Of the group of patients who had prior surgery, only two patients reported significant improvement from prior surgical interventions with the remainder reporting limited, transient, or no improvement. As the absence of a symptom-free interval following prior surgery is well known to be correlated with an unsatisfactory outcome from a subsequent surgical intervention [28], the study group was likely predisposed to negative outcomes regardless of the intervention. The authors instrumented and fused both SIJs routinely utilizing a technique that involved bilateral exposure of both lateral and medial surfaces of the ilium, direct decortication of (presumably) the articular portion of the joint, and compression instrumentation that spanned both ilia and included screws placed through the ilium into the sacral ala (Fig. 11.4)

They do not cite a rationale or literature support for routinely fusing both joints, nor do they indicate if any of the patients in the series were experiencing bilateral pain. Operative time was 121.3 min and mean blood loss was 794 cc

Clinical results were reported as satisfactory in 3/17 (18 %) and unsatisfactory in the remaining 14 patients (82 %). They reported their nonunion rate however to be between 41 % (definite nonunion and instability) and possibly 65 % (including those with questionable union). Furthermore, there was a statistically significant association between nonunion and poor clinical result. These data would seem to lead to a conclusion that this

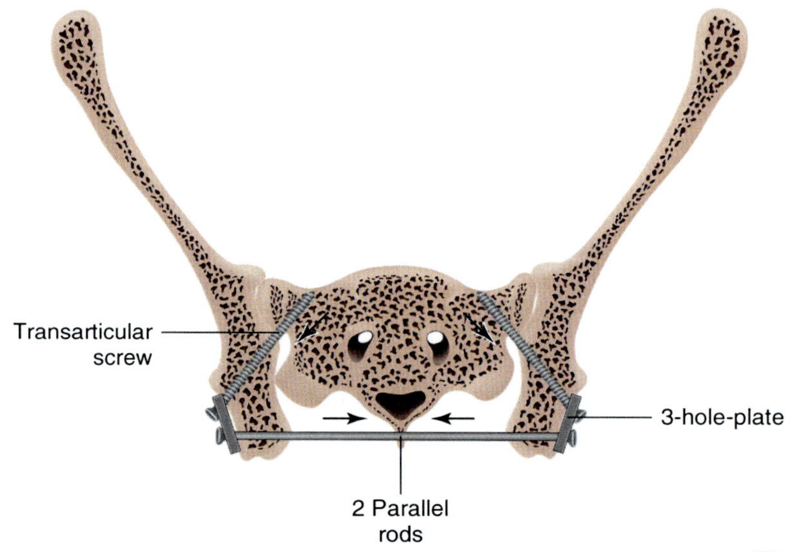

Fig. 11.4 Drawing from Schutz and Grobs article showing technique of novel bilateral sacroiliac arthrodesis and fixation spanning both ilia. Extensive bilateral exposure is necessary involving access to both lateral and medical aspects of ilium for posterior decortication of joint and lateral placement of plate and screws. Posterior sacroiliac ligaments were removed inferiorly

particular technique was not effective in achieving the surgical goal. The reported blood loss of 794 cc exceeds that of other reports by nearly a factor of 4, which, even allowing for the fact that bilateral fusions were done, suggests that the technique utilized in this study is associated with greater tissue damage than other techniques [15, 17]. Based on a critical review of the article, the poor results were likely due to variable patient selection criteria, a high percentage of failed low back surgery patients, and a surgical technique that resulted in a very high rate of nonunions. The frequent use of this study as a reference purporting to documenting poor results from sacroiliac fusion represents a lack of familiarity with the details of the report.

Indications for Open Transiliac Approach

The indications for the open posterior lateral or transiliac approach for sacroiliac arthrodesis are the same as indications for sacroiliac arthrodesis in general. Pain arising from the SIJ, which is causing significant disability that has been recalcitrant to conservative measures, represents an indication. Recently developed minimally invasive approaches for sacroiliac fusion are arguably preferable to open approaches because of decreased blood loss, reduced operative times, and shorter hospitalization times [29]. Factors that might mitigate toward an open approach include aberrant anatomy, the need to carry out extensive bone grafting, or the need to disassemble existing instrumentation (see Figs. 11.5, 11.6a, b, and 11.9).

Relative Advantages and Disadvantages of Transiliac Approach vs. Other Open Approaches

The open posterior lateral or transiliac approach has the advantage over the open posterior approach in that the entire posterior ligamentous complex is avoided. Advocates argue that sacrificing any portion of the posterior ligamentous complex increases instability and might in theory increase the rate of pseudarthrosis and/or long-term pain because of scarring in the area of densely innervated ligaments. Clinical reports of direct open posterior approaches, however, have not shown this to be the case [30, 31].

Precise localization of the synovial portion of the SIJ and its projection onto the outer table of the ilium has been cited by some authors as being problematic for planning the transiliac window [32]. As early as 1935 Gellman suggested an acoustic technique for solving this problem [33].

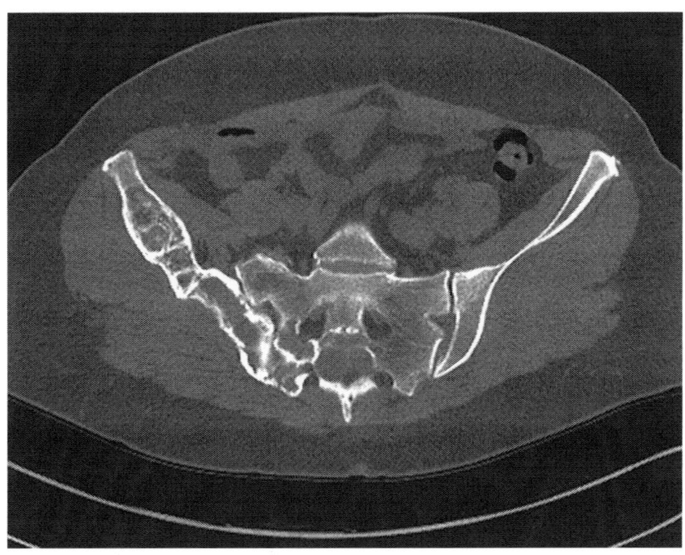

Fig. 11.5 Patient with fibrous dysplasia affecting innominate bone and sacrum and ipsilateral sacroiliac pain confirmed by injection. Minimally invasive approach relatively contraindicated because of the lack of bone to anchor into on either side of joint. Open in situ fusion with extensive bone grafting would be likely recommendation if patient elected surgery. Patient at this time is not interested in surgical treatment

Fig. 11.6 Patient with history of major pelvic trauma requiring internal fixation. This patient had persistent pain in left sacroiliac joint. Open posterior lateral approach is likely the best option because of the need to remove retained implants. (**a**) Plain film. (**b**) CT scan showing implants in position making transiliac minimally invasive technique difficult. Note persistent widening of contralateral joint. Patient's predominant symptoms were left sided

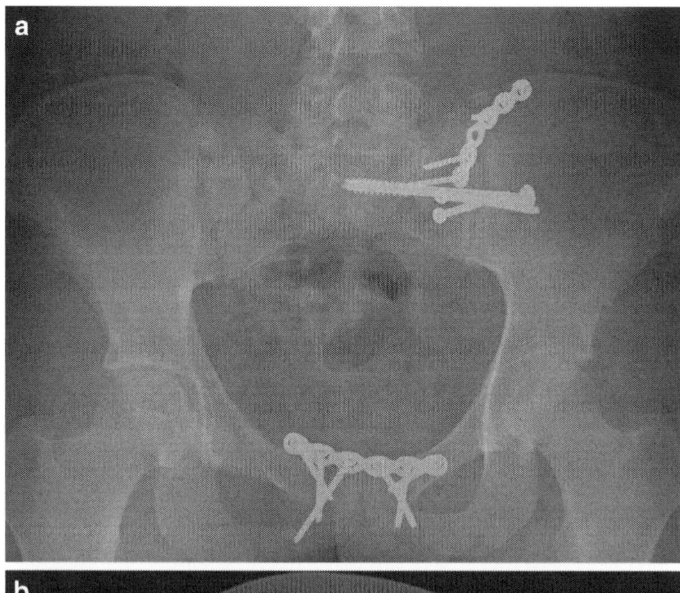

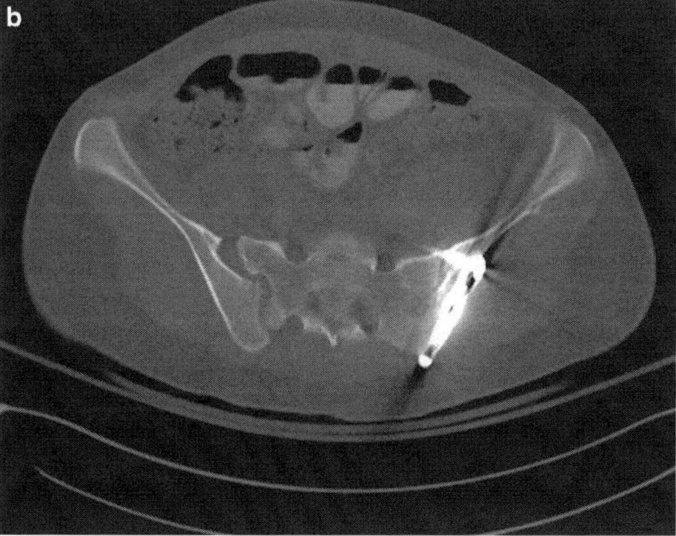

He recommended percussion of the ilium over the exposed area with the handle of an osteotome. Gellman claimed that percussion allowed identification of the superior, inferior, posterior, and anterior borders of the joint. Use of a modern image intensifier also allows more precise localization of landmarks. Preoperative CT imaging provides precise delineation of anatomic variations and the ability to measure distances from easily identified landmarks such as the PSIS and sciatic notch, which make appropriate placement of the transiliac window a manageable problem. If surgical navigation is available, very little difficulty is experienced in localizing the joint.

Description of Technique of Open Posterior Lateral (Transiliac) Approach to the SIJ

The following is the author's preferred technique based on experience in 235 cases. The patient is placed supine on chest rolls on a radiolucent table after induction of general anesthesia and placement of a Foley catheter. No bowel preparation is necessary. Prior to draping, the image intensifier is used to check AP, inlet, outlet, oblique, and inlet-oblique and outlet-oblique views. The lateral view may be checked but is generally not necessary intraoperatively. A CT scan of the pelvis with 3-D, sagittal, and coronal reconstructions is obtained preoperatively in every case. Several measurements are made on the preoperative CT scan that are useful intraoperatively (see Fig. 11.7).

The distance from the PSIS to the most anterior extent of the joint is noted as well as the thickness of the Ilium at the level of the planned transiliac window. After sterile preparation and draping, a curvilinear incision is made centered on the PSIS (Fig. 11.8a).

The length of the incision varies with the size of the patient but a 4–5 in. incision is usually sufficient. Dissection is taken through subcutaneous tissue with electrocautery until the fascial attachments to the iliac crest are identified. Subperiosteal dissection of the outer surface of the ilium is carried out beginning at the PSIS. Dissection is continued anteriorly for the premeasured distance noted on the preoperative CT scan and inferiorly until the margin of the sciatic notch can be palpated. Some fibers of the gluteus maximus must usually be divided inferiorly to expose the ilium at the inferior portion of the SIJ. A Taylor retractor is placed and may be held in place with sterile roller gauze looped around the handle of the retractor and dropped down to the foot of the surgeon who then can maintain retraction with both

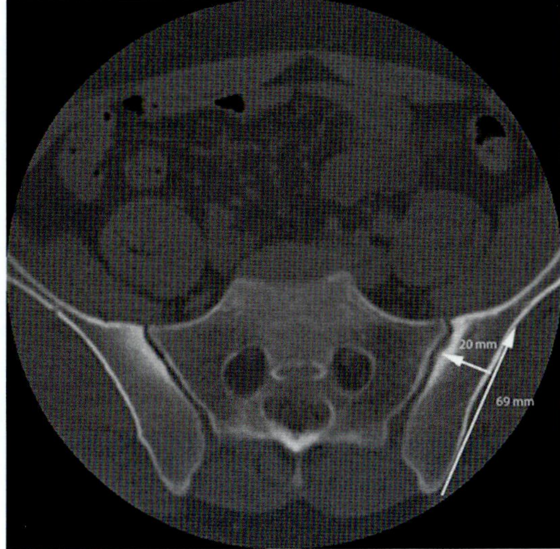

Fig. 11.7 Preoperative CT for planning open transiliac approach. The distance from the PSIS to the most anterior portion of the joint is measured and used to plan both screw placement and placement of transiliac bone window. The thickness of the ilium is noted to allow guidance in anticipating depth of transiliac window

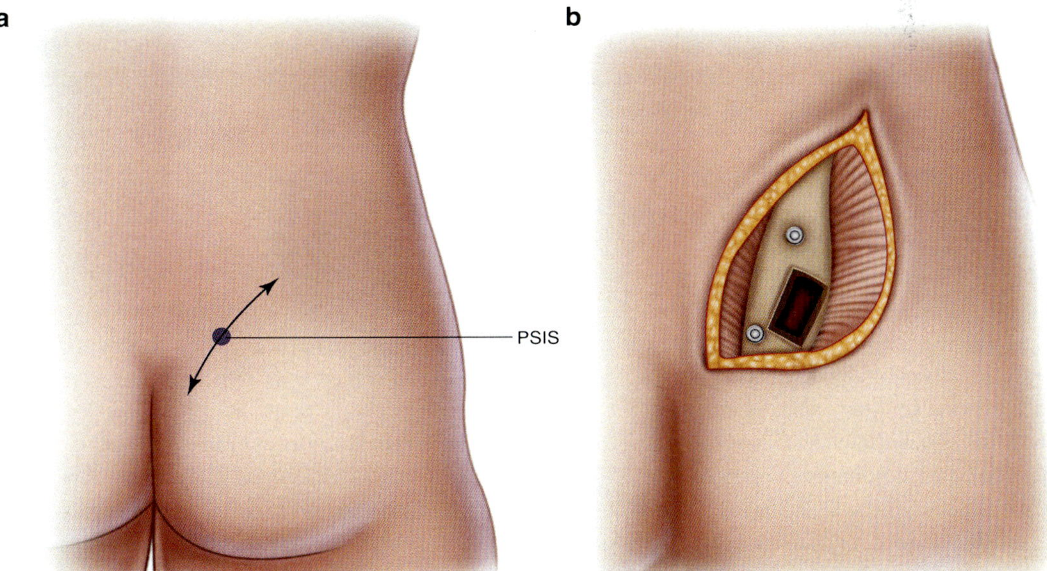

Fig. 11.8 Author's preferred technique for open posterior lateral (transiliac) approach for sacroiliac arthrodesis. (**a**) Incision made based on fluoroscopic identification of PSIS. (**b**) Exposure of outer table of ilium showing completed bone window with fixation screws in place caudally and inferiorly

of his and his assistant's hands free. A cerebellar or Weitlaner retractor is often helpful in the caudal portion of the wound.

Cancellous screws are then placed across the joint in superior and inferior positions. The position and trajectory can be planned with reference to the PSIS based on the preoperative CT scan. AO large fragment non-cannulated screws are used. The image intensifier can be used to check position and trajectory. Care is taken while drilling to assure that only three cortical surfaces are penetrated. If only three cortical surfaces are penetrated as the joint is crossed, the drill cannot be in the pelvis or in a sacral foramen. Penetration of a cortical surface is usually very easily discriminated. The drill is withdrawn and a depth gauge is used to assess the appropriate length of screw. AP, inlet, outlet, and oblique image intensifier views can verify satisfactory position. The outer cortex is tapped and 6.5 mm cancellous screws with short threads are placed with washers. The superior screw is usually approximately 50–55 mm, and the inferior screw, which is placed across the most inferior portion of the joint, is usually 20–25 mm in length. The length of screws can be anticipated based upon the preoperative CT scan.

The transiliac window will lie between and anterior to the two screws. The cortex of the ilium is entered using a Midas Rex K-1 bit. A rectangular window is created and then completed with straight and curved osteotomes. The thickness of the ilium and the geometry of the interior iliac surface are variable and can be anticipated based upon the preoperative CT scan. The ilium at its thickest portion may be 15–20 mm or greater in thickness. A distinct change in tone of the sound the mallet makes when contacting the osteotome can be identified when the osteotome has reached the subchondral bone on the iliac side of the joint. Once this is penetrated the osteotome is removed and curved osteotomes are used to work around the window until it can be removed en bloc from the wound. If this is done correctly, the removed block of bone should have the appearance of hyaline cartilage overlying the subchondral bone on the medial surface, and hyaline cartilage on the sacral side of the joint should be visible through

the window. A headlight is imperative for this portion of the operation. Cartilage and subchondral bone is removed from the bone plug and it is set aside. The sacral side of the joint is decorticated through the window with a combination of osteotomes and curettes. Angled curettes are used to decorticate the margins of the synovial portion of the joint from within the window. Care must be taken to avoid penetration into the pelvis and sacral foramina.

Additional bone graft may be harvested from the PSIS and packed into the marginal decorticated area within the joint. The bone plug is then impacted across the joint and countersunk to produce opposing cancellous surfaces spanning the joint (Fig. 11.8b).

The divided fascial attachments are approximated with 1-0 Vicryl, and a drain is placed in the subcutaneous space. Subcutaneous closure is with 0 Vicryl and the skin is closed with staples or sutures as preferred. A dressing is applied and the patient is taken to the recovery room.

The patient is mobilized on the evening of surgery. Discharge is anticipated at 24–48 h. Touchdown weight bearing is maintained for 6–8 weeks. A brief period of physical therapy (3–6 weeks) is often necessary to normalize gait. Gluteal strengthening and avoidance of the tendency to walk with an externally rotated hip usually constitute the focus of the postoperative physical therapy.

Results

A retrospective review of 110 patients with recalcitrant sacroiliac pain demonstrated an average operative time of 75 min and average blood loss of 200 cc. In the subgroup with no prior spine surgery and no coexistent spinal pathology, successful outcomes were seen in 90 % (53/59). Of the six patients considered to be failures in this group, four had pseudarthrosis. All four patients underwent reoperation and three went on to successful clinical and radiographic outcomes. The fourth patient remained a clinical failure and had evidence of persistent pseudarthrosis. In patients with coexistent spinal pathology or prior surgery, outcomes were more difficult to categorize as residual pain from other interventions or coexistent spinal pathology confounded evaluation of the success of the sacroiliac intervention. Forty-three of 51 patients (84 %), however, stated they felt improved after the sacroiliac fusion [18].

Complications

A known pseudarthrosis rate of 9.1 % (10/110) was observed, although only patients with recurrent or persistent symptoms underwent CT imaging to detect nonunion. Eight of the ten patients with pseudarthrosis were smokers. Seven reoperations for repair of pseudarthrosis were undertaken, and five patients went on to radiographic union and clinical success. Two patients had persistent nonunions and were clinical failures. There was one superficial wound infection, which responded to local care and oral antibiotics. Early in the series a fixation screw was purposely placed through the inner cortex of the sacrum to improve purchase, and this resulted in radicular pain and required removal. The radicular pain resolved immediately and there were no long-term sequela. There was one intraoperative fracture of the ilium into the sciatic notch during creation of the transiliac window. This was repaired with a single AO large fragment screw, and the patient went on to heal without further complication.

Posterior Lateral Open Approach vs. Minimally Invasive Approaches

A literature is emerging with regard to minimally invasive approaches to arthrodesis of the SIJ [29, 34–36]. Based upon these early data, it appears that similar or improved results can be achieved by minimally invasive approaches, though no randomized comparisons are available. The minimally invasive approaches have the advantages of lower blood loss, less tissue damage, reduced postoperative pain, and potentially quicker recovery of function. Intuitively, it would seem that if patient selection is done carefully, a minimally invasive approach should be a superior alternative to open posterior lateral or transiliac approaches for sacroiliac arthrodesis. Exceptions might include cases where an open approach is required to remove existing implants or when bone graft harvest has left insufficient bone for either healing or implant capture on the iliac side of the joint. Another relative indication might be when dysmorphic anatomy and/or prior surgery makes some minimally invasive approaches particularly difficult (Fig. 11.9).

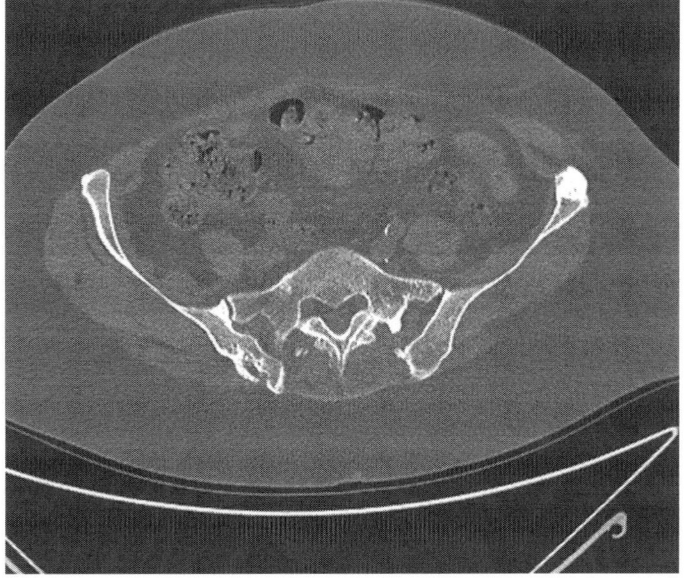

Fig. 11.9 Patient with small pelvis, prior lumbar surgery, ipsilateral bone graft harvest, and dysmorphic sacrum with right-sided sacroiliac pain recalcitrant to conservative treatment. Minimally invasive approach with transiliac implants thought not to be practical because of anatomic considerations and limited space for placing implants with adequate bony contact. Patient was treated with open in situ transiliac arthrodesis with excellent clinical result at 12 months

As noted previously, if extensive bone grafting is required because of tumor or dysplastic condition, current minimally invasive techniques probably cannot be utilized.

Conclusions

Since its original description in 1921, the transiliac approach to the SIJ has been the most frequently reported open technique for accessing the joint for incision and drainage or for arthrodesis. The vast majority of reported cases document satisfactory results and low complication rates. The most frequently reported complication is pseudarthrosis. It remains a viable technique when minimally invasive techniques are difficult or impossible because of anatomic considerations, prior surgery, dysplastic conditions, and the presence of implants, which requires an open approach for removal, or when extensive bone grafting is required. Recent reports of a variety of minimally invasive techniques suggest that the open transiliac approach should be reserved for those cases in which a minimally invasive approach is not possible or practical.

References

1. Smith-Petersen MN. Arthrodesis of the sacroiliac joint. A new method of approach. J Bone Joint Surg. 1921;3(8):400–5.
2. Painter CF. Excision of the os innominatum. Arthrodesis of the sacroiliac synchondrosis. Boston Med Surg J. 1908; Aug 13, p 207.
3. Warwick R, Williams PL. Gray's anatomy 35th British edition. Philadelphia, PA: WB Saunders Co; 1973. p. 345–6.
4. Gaenslen FJ. Sacroiliac joint arthrodesis by bone splitting technique. Wis Med J. 1921;20:20–2.
5. Smith-Petersen MN, Rogers WA. Arthrodesis for tuberculosis of the sacroiliac joint. JAMA. 1926;86(1):26–30.
6. Smith Petersen MN, Rogers WA. End-result study of arthrodesis of the sacroiliac joint for arthritis-traumatic and non-traumatic. J Bone Joint Surg. 1926;8:118–36.
7. Gaenslen FJ. Sacroiliac arthrodesis: indications, author's technic and end-results. JAMA. 1927;89(24):2031–5.
8. Harris CT. Operative treatment of sacroiliac disease. Analysis of cases and end-results. J Bone Joint Surg. 1933;15:651–60.
9. Bloom FA. Sacroiliac fusion. J Bone Joint Surg. 1937;19:704–8.
10. Verrall PJ. A bone graft for sacro-iliac fixation. J Bone Joint Surg. 1926;8:491–3.
11. Key JA. A straight line incision for arthrodesis or drainage of the sacroiliac joint. J Bone Joint Surg. 1937;19(1):117–20.
12. Hodgson BF. Pyogenic sacroiliac joint infection. Clin Orthop Relat Res. 1989;246:146–9.
13. Waisbrod H, Krainick JU, Gerbershagen HU. Sacroiliac arthrodesis for chronic lower back pain. Arch Orthop Trauma Surg. 1987;106:238–40.
14. Moore MR. Diagnosis and surgical treatment of chronic sacroiliac arthropathy. Presented at the 1992 North American Spine Society Annual Meeting, Boston, MA, July 10, 1992. Orthop Trans 1992. 1994;18(1):255.
15. Moore MR. Diagnosis and surgical treatment of chronic painful sacroiliac dysfunction. Presented at the second interdisciplinary world congress on low back pain, the integrated function of the lumbar spine and sacroiliac joint, San Diego, California, November, 1995.
16. Moore MR. Surgical treatment of chronic painful sacroiliac joint dysfunction. In: Vleeming A, Mooney V, Dorman T, Snijders C, Stoeckart R, editors. Movement, stability, and low back pain. New York: Churchill Livingstone; 1997. p. 563–72.
17. Moore MR. Outcomes of surgical treatment of chronic painful sacroiliac joint dysfunction. In: Vleeming A, Mooney V, Tilscher H, Dorman T, Snijders C, editors. 3rd Interdisciplinary World Congress on Low Back and Pelvic Pain, 19–21 Nov, 1998, Vienna, Austria, ECO Rotterdam, pp 218–226.
18. Moore MR. Surgical treatment of chronic painful sacroiliac joint arthropathy. Poster presentation, 13th annual meeting of the North American Spine Society, San Francisco, 28–31 Oct 1998.
19. Moore MR, Chaussee KP. Surgical treatment of sacroiliac joint pain. Presented at the first world congress 2000 on minimally invasive spinal medicine and surgery, Las Vegas, 7–10 Dec 2000.
20. Moore MR, Chaussee KP. Sacroiliac arthrodesis for chronic sacroiliac pain. Poster, 8th international meeting on advanced spine techniques (IMAST). Paradise Island, Bahamas, 12–14 Jul 2001.
21. Moore MR. Surgery for sacroiliac joint syndrome, chapter 117. In: Slipman CW, Derby R, Simeone FA, Mayer TG, editors. Interventional spine: an algorithmic approach. Philadelphia, PA: Saunders; 2008. p. 1269–75.
22. Kurica KB. A prospective study of sacroiliac joint arthrodesis with one to six year follow-up. In Vleeming A, Mooney V, Dorman T, Snijders C, editors. 2nd Interdisciplinary world congress on low back pain: the integrated function of the lumbar spine and sacroiliac joints, San Diego, CA, 9–11 Nov 1995, ECO, Rotterdam; 1995.
23. Giannikas KA, Khan AM, Karski MT, Maxwell HA. Sacroiliac joint fusion for chronic pain: a simple

technique avoiding use of metalwork. Eur Spine J. 2004;13(3):253–6.

24. Buchowski JM, Kebaish KM, Sinkov V, Cohen DB, Sieber AN, Kostuik JP. Functional and radiographic outcome of sacroiliac arthrodesis for the disorders of the sacroiliac joint. Spine J. 2005;5:520–8.

25. Schutz U, Grob D. Poor outcome following bilateral sacroiliac joint fusion for degenerative sacroiliac joint syndrome. Acta Orthop Belg. 2006;72:296–308.

26. Schaffrey CI, Smith JS. Neurosurg Focus. 2013;35(Suppl):1 (Editorial).

27. Kitchel SH, Lieberman I, Mroz T. Curve/outercurve: Is SIJ fusion effective for SIJ pain? SpineLine. 2007;14(4):14–9.

28. Finnegan WJ, Fenlin JM, Marvel JP, Nardini RJ, Rothman RH. Results of surgical intervention in the symptomatic, multiply operated low back patient: analysis of 67 cases followed for three to seven years. J Bone Joint Surg. 1979;61:1077–82.

29. Smith AG, Capobianco R, Cher D, Rudolf L, Sachs D, Gundanna M, Kleiner J, Mody MG, Shamie AN. Open versus minimally invasive sacroiliac joint fusion: a multi-center comparison of perioperative measures and clinical outcomes. Ann Surg Innov Res. 2013; 7:14.

30. Keating J, Sims V, Avilar M. Sacroiliac fusion is a chronic low back pain population. In: 2nd interdisciplinary world congress on low back pain. The integrated function of the lumbar spine and sacroiliac joints, San Diego, CA: ECO, 1995; pp 261–365

31. Belanger TA, Dall BE. Sacroiliac arthrodesis using a posterior midline fascial splitting approach and pedicle screw instrumentation: a new technique. J Spinal Disord. 2001;14:118–24.

32. Stark JG, Fuentes JA, Fuentes TI, Idemmili C. The history of sacroiliac arthrodesis: a critical review and introduction of a new technique. Curr Orthop Pract. 2011;22(6):545–57.

33. Gellman M. A suggestion for a more accurate localization of the sacroiliac joint. J Bone Joint Surg. 1935;17(1):235.

34. Wise CL, Dall BE. Minimally invasive sacroiliac arthrodesis: outcomes of a new technique. J Spinal Disord Tech. 2008;21(8):579–84.

35. Sachs D, Capobianco R. One year successful outcomes for novel sacroiliac joint arthrodesis system. Ann Surg Innov Res. 2012;6(1):13.

36. Rudolf L. Sacroiliac joint arthrodesis with titanium implants: report of the first 50 patients and outcomes. Open Orthop J. 2012;6(1):495–502.

Posterior Inferior Approach, Minimally Invasive

E. Jeffrey Donner

Introduction

The authors of previous chapters have identified the anatomy, biomechanics, and the potential for the sacroiliac joint (SI joint or SIJ) to cause pain severe enough for the patient and surgeon to consider surgical options after conservative measures have failed to control their disabling pain. I will defer the details to those authors and their references and primarily report on my personal experience of surgically treating hundreds of painful SI joints over the past 25 years as well as my personal medical history of having traumatic SIJ pain diagnosed and treated nonoperatively at age 18 by Dr. John Royal Moore who was the Chief of Orthopedic Surgery at Temple University Hospital and Shriners Hospital in Philadelphia, PA. I also have the insight to differentiating between other confounding pain generators by way of a 40-year history of chronic L5-S1 discogenic pain diagnosed primarily by discography 20 years ago and requiring spinal injections and two subsequent discectomies. To add to my experience, I have had bilateral arthroscopic reconstructive hip surgeries

E.J. Donner, M.D. (✉)
Colorado Spine Institute, 5285 McWhinney
Boulevard, Suite 145, Loveland, CO 80538, USA

University of Colorado Health, Medical Center
of the Rockies, 2500 Rocky Mountain Avenue,
Loveland, CO 80538, USA
e-mail: ejdonner@gmail.com

5 years ago for chronic symptoms associated with femoroacetabular impingement (FAI).

Pain and the SIJ

As previously discussed, pain localized in the buttock area can be caused by maladies of the hip joint, such as FAI, piriformis syndrome, and degenerative joint disease, but more commonly by pathology of lumbar and sacral spinal structures which primarily includes the intervertebral discs, facet joints, and nerve roots, as well as the more recently recognized painful conditions of the SIJ [1–5].

It is the author's opinion, and consistent with Dreyfuss, Lippitt, and others, that the etiology of a painful or dysfunctional SIJ can be divided into two main categories. The first category is due to a damaged or degenerated extra-articular ligamentous complex, which includes the commonly described sacroiliac sprain strain. The second category is caused by the damaged or degenerative articular cartilage of the synovial portion of the joint [1, 6–8]. Periarticular and intra-articular injections and radiofrequency ablation are reasonable treatment options for chronic SIJ pain that fails to improve with a combination of rest, physical therapy, and oral nonsteroidal anti-inflammatory drugs [9–11]. In the author's opinion, when nonoperative treatment fails and the SI ligaments are determined to be the main source of the pain, it is intuitive to only stabilize the joint

B.E. Dall et al. (eds.), *Surgery for the Painful, Dysfunctional Sacroiliac Joint*,
DOI 10.1007/978-3-319-10726-4_12, © Springer International Publishing Switzerland 2015

without fusion using screws or rods across the joint. If the articular surface of the joint is the source of the pain, then removal of the painful articular surface followed by bone grafting and placing stabilization/fixation devices is advised which should also address the pain caused by the damaged ligamentous complex and subsequent unstable SI joint. This concept is analogous to other orthopedic procedures used to treat recalcitrant joint pain and based on accepted orthopedic principles [12].

Surgical Techniques for Fusing the SIJ

The two primary surgical options for treating SIJ pain are with an open procedure or with a minimally invasive surgical (MIS) technique. Both options involve either stabilization of the SIJ with a variety of screw designs with or without ongrowth surface coatings, titanium rods with a plasma spray on-growth surface, or stabilization with screws combined with an SI joint fusion (SIF) by a variety of methods through the same lateral approach.

Open Procedures

The open procedure can be performed through the standard surgical routes to the SIJ which include the direct posterior, lateral, or anterior approaches which allows reasonable but often limited access to a portion of the intra-articular and/or extra-articular SI joint.

The classic Smith-Petersen technique, first described in the early 1900s, requires a fairly large incision and reflection of the gluteus muscle attachments with subperiosteal stripping of the lateral ilium followed by excision of a large block of the lateral ilium, removal of the articular cartilage, and reapplication of the resulting bone block into the joint. Later techniques added multiple screws or a plate and screws for fixation [13]. The open anterior approach requires a similar amount of muscle disruption and plate and screw fixation after cartilage removal, but only a

small portion of anterior SIJ is accessible for bone grafting. There is also an additional reported risk of injuring the L4 and L5 nerve roots located in close proximity to the SIJ where anterior plate fixation is performed [14–16].

The direct posterior open approach once again requires extensive muscle dissection, removal of a large portion of the PSIS, which fortunately has the advantage of allowing direct visualization of the entire SIJ including the extra- and intra-articular surfaces while providing a large quantity of autogenous bone graft and surface area for performing a fusion. The added advantage of this technique includes the extensive removal of the articular portion of the SIJ which based on orthopedic principles is a significant source of the patient's pain similar to what is accepted to be the cause of pain in other degenerative joints commonly treated by orthopedic surgeons [12]. Percutaneous fixation of the joint with transsacroiliac screws or a S1 pedicle screw/iliac screw/connecting rod fixation is subsequently added to stabilize the joint until fusion occurs (Figs. 12.1, 12.2, 12.3, and 12.4).

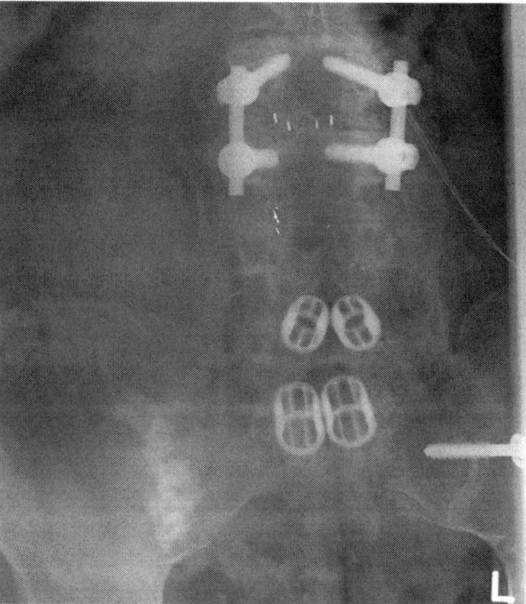

Fig. 12.1 An AP view of the *left* and *right* SI joints (SIJs) after fusion using a direct posterior approach and fixation with trans-SIJ screws. Note that the *right* SIJ screw was removed after successful fusion due to soft tissue irritation (permission to use photo by E. Jeffrey Donner)

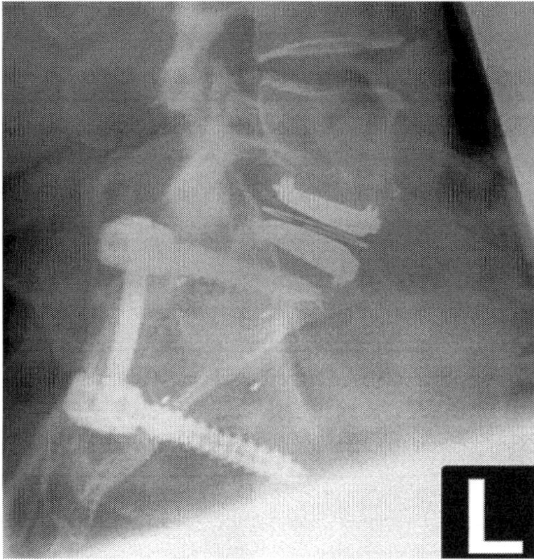

Fig. 12.2 An AP view of PEEK Intervertebral Body Fusion Devices (IBFDs) in the SIJ and fixation with S1 and iliac pedicle screws joined by a rod (permission to use photo by E. Jeffrey Donner)

Fig. 12.3 A lateral view of PEEK IBFDs in the SIJ and fixation with S1 and iliac pedicle screws joined by a rod in the same patient from Fig. 12.2 (permission to use photo by E. Jeffrey Donner)

In 1996 Donner and Browne [17] reported on a 3-year retrospective follow-up study on 18 patients (25 SIFs) who had undergone an SIF with a posterior approach with the addition of internal fixation (Fig. 12.1). There were 11 unilateral fusions and seven bilateral fusions. The average duration of symptoms was 3.25 years. There was a minimum 1-year follow-up with an average follow-up of 20 months. The indications for surgical treatment were chronic disabling SIJ pain, which failed to improve with nonoperative treatment. The pain was localized to the SIJ using CT-guided or fluoroscopic-guided SIJ injections with an anesthetic and steroid solution. Discography and facet injections were often utilized to rule out possible lumbar pathology, and if they were significant pain generators, they were also treated simultaneously. Fourteen out of the 18 patients improved from the procedure. The average overall symptom improvement is 89 % for unilateral SIJ fusions (range: 75–100 %) and 79 % for bilateral SIFs (range: 50–100 %). The average leg pain improvement was 86 %. The purpose of the study was to evaluate the efficacy of posterior SIJ fusion for chronic intractable SIJ-related pain syndrome. Long-term follow-up on this study group has demonstrated durability of this procedure.

Minimally Invasive Surgical (MIS) Techniques

The most commonly utilized MIS techniques involved performing a percutaneous lateral approach and placing fixation screws across the SIJ without a fusion (as popularized by Lippitt in the 1990s) is similar to the method used for pelvic trauma, with the belief the primary cause of the patient's pain was due to excessive instability of the joint [8]. Additional products have been introduced into the market, and these techniques primarily incorporate stabilization of the joint with a variety of screws with the addition of bone grafting techniques from the same lateral approach. All of these techniques may have their perceived advantages, but some of the disadvantages based on the author's experience primarily include a limited ability to visualize and assure adequate removal of the articular cartilage as well as sufficient decortication of the subchondral bone which is often very dense on the iliac surface. Both of these limitations may limit the ability to obtain a reliable boney fusion. This

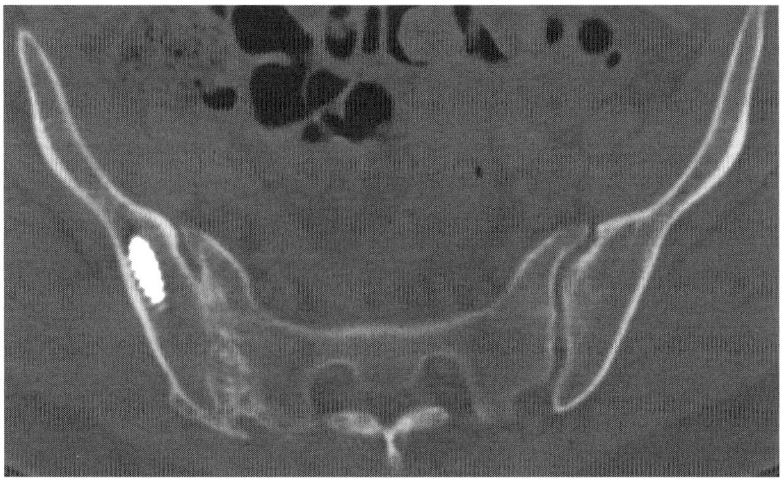

Fig. 12.4 PEEK IBFDs in the SIJ and fixation with S1 and iliac pedicle screws joined by a rod (permission to use photo by E. Jeffrey Donner)

issue is emphasized by Dr. Christopher Shaffrey in a 2013 editorial regarding SIJ stabilization wherein he states: "concern with this implant [fusion rods] is whether the porous plasma spray coating on the implant actually results in bone growth across the SIJ or only serves as a stabilizer. If true fusion does not result, deterioration in the clinical result could occur over time" [18]. Furthermore, the majority of the MIS techniques are performed with a fluoroscopic-guided lateral approach which on the surface appears minimally invasive when visualizing the 2–3 cm incision, but in reality there is a significant amount of deep tissue disruption when making multiple passes with a variety of instruments in multiple locations through the gluteus muscles and in close proximity to their accompanying neurovascular bundles.

Author's Experience with Minimally Invasive SIJ Fusions

Having performed the majority of these open procedures and MIS techniques, the author prefers performing a less invasive procedure. This procedure accomplishes the principle mission of thoroughly removing the painful cartilage, decorticating the subchondral bone, and obtaining a boney fusion of the SIJ. This is performed by directly accessing the articular portion of the joint through a posterior inferior access "window" in the plane of the SIJ with a minimally invasive approach located above the sciatic notch and below the PSIS (Figs. 12.5, 12.6, and 12.7).

Advantageously, this approach allows conversion of an MIS technique to a mini-open technique where direct visualization of the joint surfaces is possible if the surgeon so desires or to an open procedure if the situation necessitates greater visualization and access to the joint, ligaments, or surrounding neurovascular elements.

It is also the author's opinion, based on orthopedic principles and analogous to other pathologic orthopedic joint conditions, that the main pain generator from a dysfunctional or degenerative SI joint is related to disruption, injury, or degeneration of the articular surface of the joint and not gross instability. Based on this hypothesis, the surgeon's attention should be directed toward removal of the painful degenerative cartilage followed by fusion and fixation. This is typical of the approach and orthopedic logic applied to most other degenerative joints where a joint replacement is not available or not the best-proven option [12, 19].

The unique anatomy of the SIJ is well described in Chap. 3 by Dr. Michael Rahl. Basically, the joint has been classified as both diarthrodial, based on satisfying the criteria of having a hyaline articular surface, surrounding capsule and synovium, and supporting ligaments,

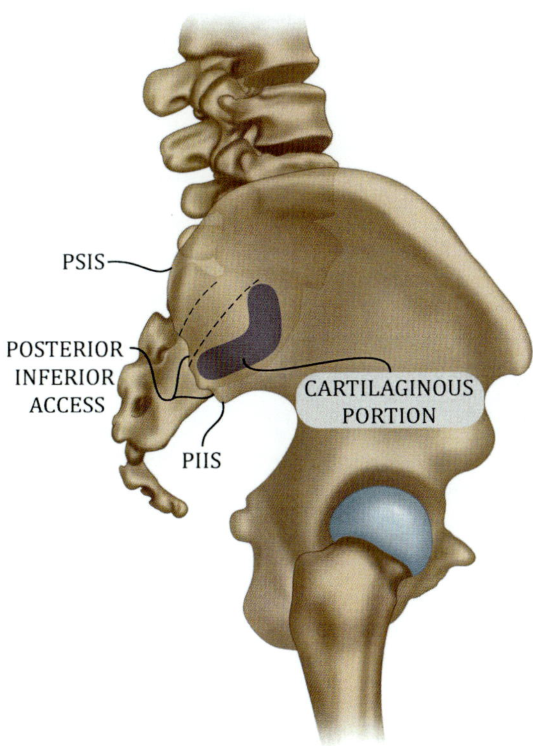

Fig. 12.5 Shows a lateral view illustrating the posterior inferior access region (permission to use photo by Springer illustration (permission to use duplicate image in book by G Sartorius))

and more specifically as amphiarthrodial since there is very limited motion of the joint [20]. The motion itself is described as nutation where there is a sliding, rotational movement of the joint between the articular surfaces which has many matching undulations constrained by strong ligaments. Another unique characteristic of this vertically oriented joint is its keystone type configuration, where the wedge-shaped sacrum is situated in the middle of the arch created by the ilia of the pelvis [1]. A majority of the body weight is transmitted through each SIJ when on a single leg stance, and therefore, the movement of the joint within this unique interlocking and constrained anatomy is critical to understanding the pathologic degenerative process and clinical symptoms. These same anatomic features and movements help create high contact stresses which may lead to early degeneration and pain especially if there is trauma or a malalignment of

the sacroiliac undulations which can occur with SIJ traumatic injuries such as with motor vehicle accidents or through normal activities such as lifting and jumping. Cartilage injury in other joints has been demonstrated to induce chondrocyte apoptosis [21–23]. Even a small amount of malalignment may markedly increase the contact stresses across the SI joint surfaces, analogous to malalignment of the ankle joint where the stress per unit area increases as the total contact area decreases. The malalignment of the matching undulations may lead to a decrease in normal contact area similar to what has been identified with even 1 mm of talar displacement in the ankle mortise, which leads to a 42 % reduction in the contact area between the tibia and talus [24]. According to the author's experience, patients will often describe severe pain with the sensation that the joint is "out of place" when a malalignment occurs. And when realigned, either spontaneously or with the assistance of a manipulation by a chiropractor or physical therapist, these patients describe the feeling as though the joint "pops back into place" often followed by relief of the pain. The long-term sequela of malalignment of the SIJ is analogous to what is observed when an ankle fracture dislocation is not anatomically aligned during ORIF and early degeneration of the joint and pain develops [12].

Obesity is another major risk factor which adds significant loads and stresses to weight-bearing joints, further increasing the chance of degeneration, pain, and dysfunction [25, 26]. In addition to this, more patients are undergoing longer instrumented fusions in the lumbar spine which typically end at the sacrum which creates a large lever arm and markedly increased stresses across the SIJ elucidated by multiple clinicians through radiographic surveys as well as biomechanical analysis [4, 5, 27, 28].

The author has extensive experience fusing hundreds of SI joints through a direct open posterior procedure over the course of 20 years and rarely visualized movement of the SI joint with mechanical testing. Some joint motion was observed after removal of the PSIS and posterior interosseous ligaments (ISL). Further removal of the joint surfaces led to mechanical instability, but

Fig. 12.6 Shows a posterior view illustrating the posterior inferior access region (permission to use illustration by Christopher Donner)

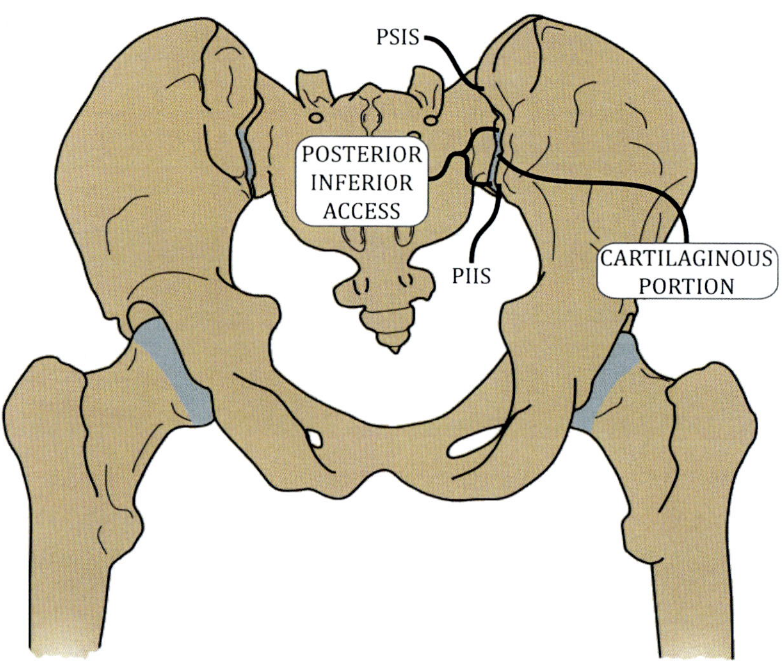

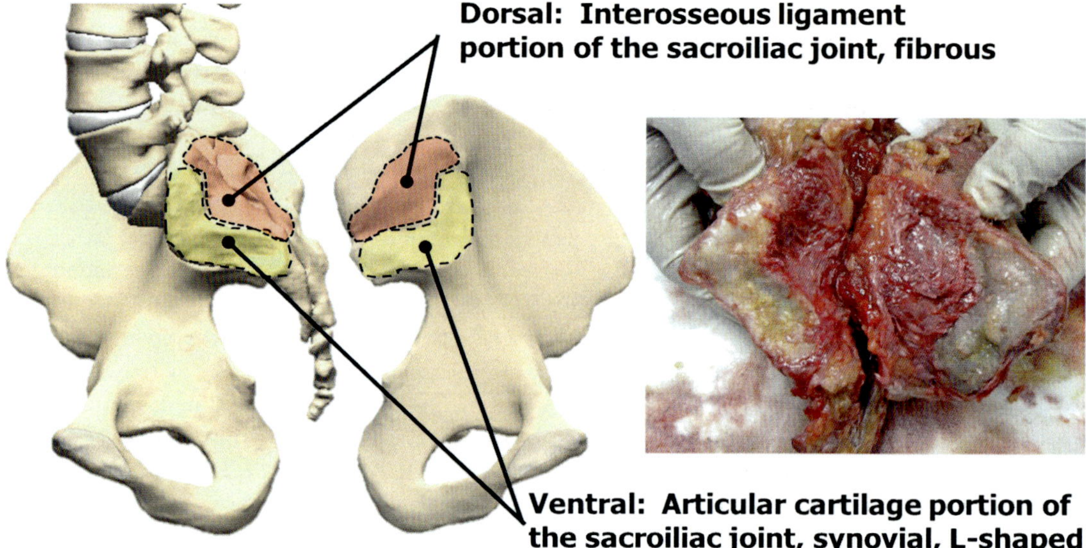

Fig. 12.7 Drawings and photo illustrating the cartilaginous portion of the SIJ. Courtesy and copyright of ZYGA TECHNOLOGY, Inc. (permission to use photo by Zyga Technology, Inc.)

stability was restored by impacting bone graft with off-label intervertebral interbody cages into the joint space followed by sacroiliac screw fixation across the joint. The surgical technique involves removing as much of the joint surfaces as possible, similar to the orthopedic concepts used for joint fusions such as the subtalar joint, in order to eliminate the painful abnormal articular cartilage but also in order to obtain a large fusion surface area for long-term stability and pain relief [12].

The above-described approaches disrupt significant dorsal ligaments, and therefore, it is prudent to utilize a technique which preserves the integrity of the ligamentous complex in order to enhance stability for obtaining a fusion. The vast ISL is the strongest of the SIJ-supporting ligaments providing for major multidirectional structural stability. Not only is the ISL the strongest SIJ-supporting ligament, but it also has the most extensive bony origin and overall volume of all SIJ ligaments [20, 29].

A surgical technique, which significantly disrupts the ISL, may lead to further joint instability than techniques, which attempt to spare or minimally disrupt it. This may be one of the reasons for Dr. Smith-Petersen's findings of when "[a] wedge [is] driven in between the posterior crest of the ilium and the dorsum of the sacrum [it] would tend to spread the joint and consequently would not render the local condition in the joint as favorable for bony ankylosis as an operation that aims to eradicate the joint. I have seen three cases in which the wedge operation was performed. The results were far from satisfactory [30]." Perhaps his unsatisfactory results were due to a gross violation of the ISL which may have consequently compromised the stability of the joint and therefore the ability of the joint to fuse; or, rather, as Dr. Smith-Petersen implies, the failure to resolve the patient's condition may lie with the increased distance the fusion must overcome given the distraction of the joint or the fact that the joint surfaces were insufficiently prepared.

As evidenced by a 2013 study conducted by Dr. Stefan Endres in Germany on 19 patients who had prior multilevel lumbar or lumbosacral fusion procedures, the patients' VAS scores improved 30 % from an 8.5 pre-op to a 6 at an average 13.2-month follow-up following an extra-articular distraction interference arthrodesis of the SIJ with an average length of stay of 7.3 days while obtaining a fusion rate of 79 % [31]. While this represents an improvement in the patients' condition, the author's experience with techniques which specifically address the articular surfaces of the SI joint and provide adequate fixation yields a much greater amount of pain relief with significantly shorter duration of hospitalization.

Over time, it was recognized this procedure could be performed less invasively through a small incision below the PSIS and above the sciatic notch while not removing the PSIS and interosseous ligaments. Following cartilage removal from this limited exposure, local autogenous bone graft may still be obtained from the "noncontact" portion of the inferior PSIS (the posterior inferior overhang of the PSIS), which may then be packed into the decorticated joint along with a variety of sized interbody spacers. The technique is further augmented with trans-sacroiliac screw fixation under fluoroscopic guidance with neural monitoring. The author was able to identify the advantages of this technique by witnessing quicker recovery and less pain than the traditional more extensive open posterior approach previously described. The remainder of this chapter will be dedicated to describing the steps of this specific minimally invasive technique and the important anatomy and technical issues which need to be recognized in order to achieve the best fusion and clinical result while avoiding complications.

Posterior Inferior Fusion-Minimally Invasive Surgical (PIF-MIS) Technique of the SIJ

Figures 12.5, 12.6, and 12.7 illustrate the relevant anatomy for the surgical approach to the posterior inferior articular access to the caudal end of

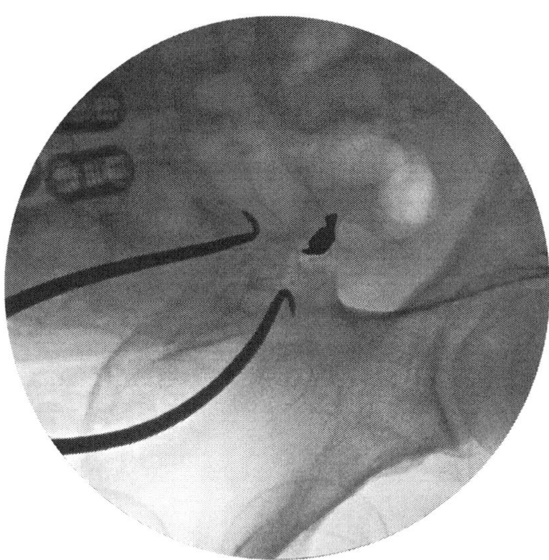

Fig. 12.8 An AP view illustrating the step of finding the posterior inferior access region with a probe placed between the joint surfaces (permission to use photo by E. Jeffrey Donner)

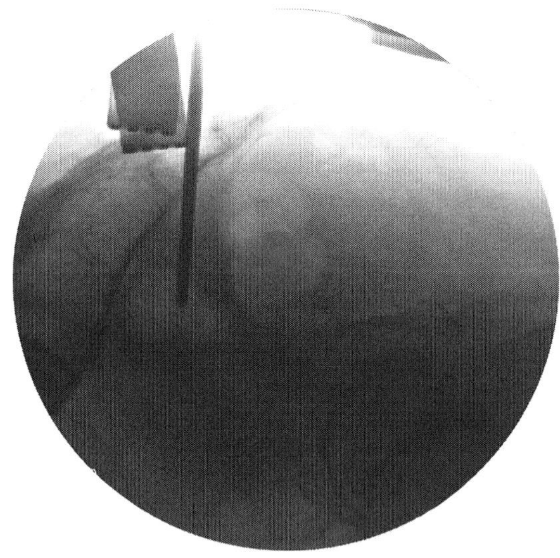

Fig. 12.9 A lateral view illustrating the step of advancing a probe anteriorly through the caudal portion of the cartilaginous portion of the SIJ via a posterior inferior access region (permission to use photo by E. Jeffrey Donner)

the "boot-shaped" articular cartilage portion of the joint which also allows access to the cephalad arm of the joint and subtotal removal of the articular surfaces across the deepest point of the extra-articular recess. The surgical approach utilizes the standard prone position on the translucent operating room table to allow intraoperative fluoroscopy. After the patient is prepped and draped in the usual aseptic manner and a sterile covered C-arm is positioned in the AP plane, the inferior portion of the joint is identified above the sciatic notch and a metallic instrument is placed on the skin over this anatomic landmark just inferior to the PSIS. A lateral view is then obtained with the sciatic notches and hip joints overlapped to obtain a true lateral image, and the direction of the probe is aligned parallel to the caudal articular arm of the joint, and the C-arm image is adjusted so that the probe is perpendicular to the floor (Fig. 12.8).

After anesthetizing the skin and soft tissues with anesthetic, a small incision, approximately 2–4 cm, is made over this anatomic landmark, and the proximal fibers of the gluteus maximus muscle near its insertion point are divided. A self-

retaining retractor is then placed. The articular portion of the joint is easily identified by using a Bovie tip to essentially "melt" the articular cartilage, which is often very narrow, degenerative, and likely covered by a dorsal spur, which may need to be resected using an instrument such as a Cobb elevator or Leksell rongeur.

Once the joint has been clearly defined with the Bovie, a blunt gearshift-type pedicle probe is then placed just above the sciatic notch and down the depth of the joint to create the initial access hole to identify the most inferior portion of the articular joint space. The gearshift is then removed, and a blunt-tipped "feeler" probe can be placed into the void in the cartilage made by the probe to confirm the access hole is not outside of the joint. A small straight curette is then used to remove the cartilage under direct visualization aided by lateral fluoroscopy. Aggressive removal of the cartilage is then performed using a combination of drill bits, typically performed manually, burs, rasps, and a variety of straight and angled curettes until the articular portion of the joint including the cephalad arm has been substantially removed down to bleeding bone (Figs. 12.9, 12.10 and 12.11).

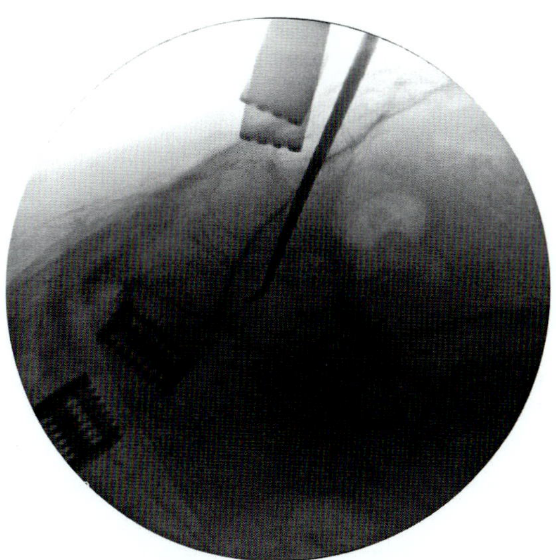

Fig. 12.10 A lateral view illustrating the step of advancing a curette anteriorly and cephalad between the joint surfaces of the SIJ via a posterior inferior access region (permission to use photo by E. Jeffrey Donner)

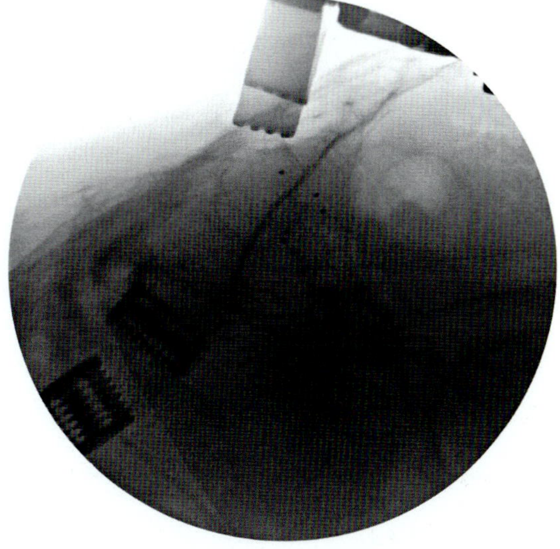

Fig. 12.12 A lateral view illustrating the final placement of titanium plasma-spray coated PEEK IBFDs between the joint surfaces of the SIJ within the caudal portion of the cartilaginous portion of the SIJ via a posterior inferior access region (permission to use photo by E. Jeffrey Donner)

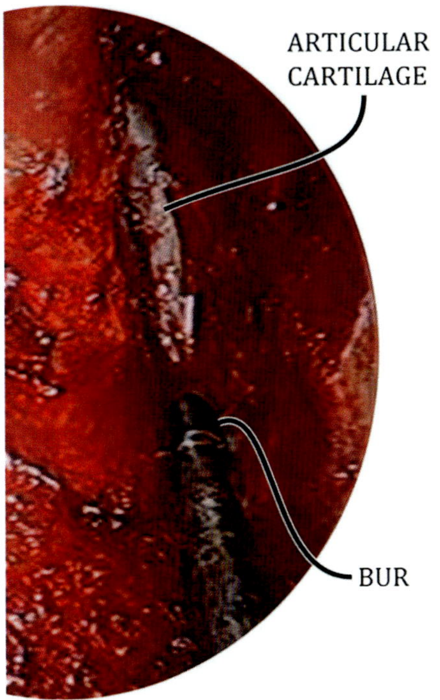

Fig. 12.11 A view down the plane of the SIJ illustrating the lustrous articular cartilage and a bur (permission to use photo by E. Jeffrey Donner)

Following cartilage removal, broaches matching the shape of the implant are employed and trial spacers for either cervical or lumbar interbody devices of a variety of compositions are used to size the spacers, which are filled with a combination of local autogenous bone graft from the posterior superior iliac spine and allograft paste and then impacted into the joint space. Additional bone graft paste is placed around the spacers to increase the fusion area. Fixation is then performed using AP, lateral, inlet, and outlet view fluoroscopic images in a standard fashion to aid in fixation. One or two additional screws are placed depending upon the clinical situation accounting for prior long fusions, obesity, and bone quality (Figs. 12.12 and 12.13).

The procedure is typically performed with neural monitoring, and trigger EMGs are performed after screw insertion to confirm the implants are not impinging any exiting nerve roots. Final images are obtained, following which the retractor is removed. The deep fascial layer is closed with interrupted #1 Vicryl suture. The subcutaneous tissue is closed with interrupted 2-0

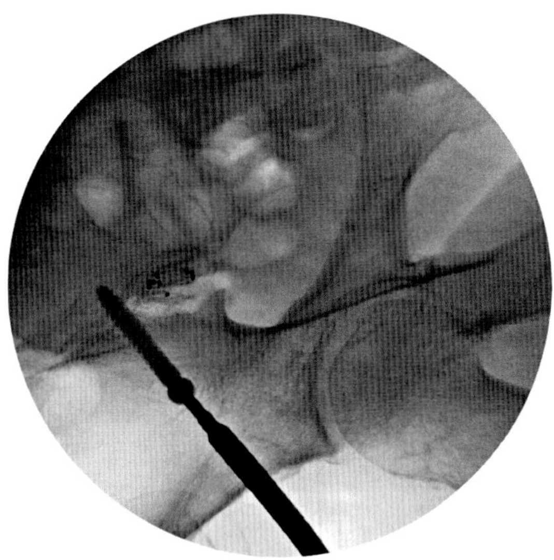

Fig. 12.13 An AP view illustrating the step of advancing a bone screw in a lateral to medial direction across the SIJ adjacent the titanium plasma-spray coated PEEK IBFDs (permission to use photo by E. Jeffrey Donner)

Vicryl, and the skin is closed with staples. Sterile dressings are then applied and the patient is awakened and transferred to the recovery room. The patient is then instructed on partial weight bearing of the operative side as tolerated, and patients are encouraged to avoid overstrain on the joint for at least 6 weeks postoperatively (Figs. 12.14 and 12.15).

The preliminary results from this technique have been very encouraging with substantially decreased operative time, blood loss, and pain following a PIF-MIS procedure versus the standard open posterior operation previously described. Noteworthy, the editor of Evidence-Based Spine-Care Journal who reviewed "Dual fibular allograft dowel technique for sacroiliac joint arthrodesis" by McGuire et al. confirmed the validity of this approach and technique: *"his [Dr. McGuire] technique is different as it does not attempt to cross the SIJ but rather provides an interference fit within the main excursion of the joint. This promises to be a safer and less complex undertaking than either crossing the SI joint or placing hardware through an anterior approach"* [32].

Case Study Examples

Case Study Example 1

64-year-old female with a 5-year history of left SIJ pain confirmed with independent SIJ fluoroscopic injections and surgically treated with the PIF-MIS technique utilizing ZIMMER SPINE's TRABECULAR METAL® tantalum cervical IBFDs. VAS improved from 7 to 0 and ODI 40 % to 2 % by 3 months post-op and was durable at 2 ½-year follow-up (Figs. 12.16, 12.17, and 12.18).

Case Study Example 2

38-year-old female with a 1-year history of right SIJ pain confirmed by independent fluoroscopic injections and surgically treated with the PIF-MIS technique utilizing ZIMMER SPINE's TRABECULAR METAL® tantalum cervical IBFDs. VAS improved from 8 to 2 and ODI from 32 % to 4 % by 3 months post-op and was durable at 2 ½-year follow-up (Figs. 12.19, 12.20, 12.21, 12.22, and 12.23).

Case Study Example 3

55-year-old female with a history of a L4-S1 fusion in 2000 and progressive SIJ determined pain effectively treated with an open posterior right SIF in 2009 and a temporarily effective IFUSE® of the left SIJ in 2010. A fluoroscopic left injection confirmed the recurrent pain was due to the SIJ; a successful PIF-MIS was performed in 2013. VAS improved from 8 to 2 and ODI improved from 40 % to 28 % at 14 months post-op (Fig. 12.24, 12.25, 12.26, 12.27, 12.28, and 12.29).

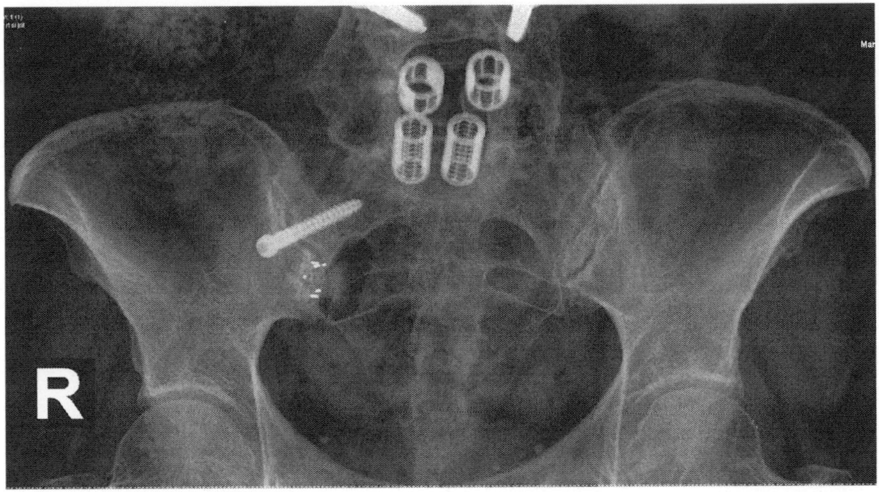

Fig. 12.14 An AP view illustrating the final placement of the bone screw across the SIJ and the titanium plasma-spray coated PEEK IBFDs between the joint surfaces of the SIJ (permission to use photo by E. Jeffrey Donner)

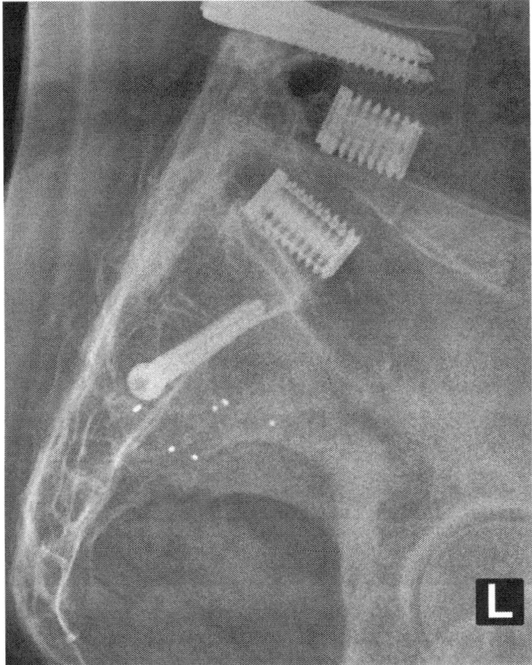

Fig. 12.15 A lateral view illustrating the final placement of the bone screw across the SIJ and the titanium plasma-spray coated PEEK IBFDs between the joint surfaces of the SIJ (permission to use photo by E. Jeffrey Donner)

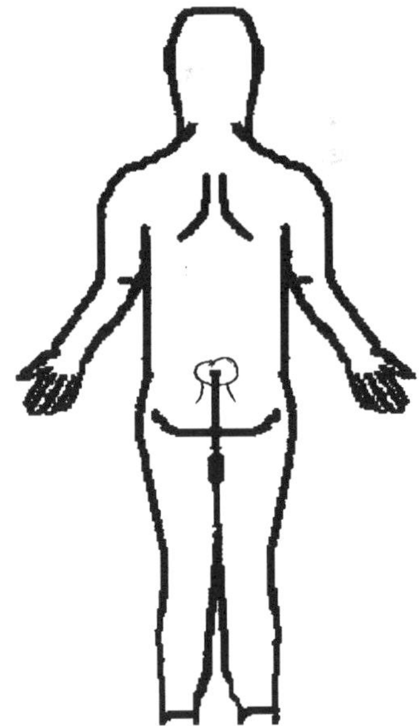

Fig. 12.16 Case Study Ex 1: Pre-op Pain Diagram (permission to use photo by E. Jeffrey Donner)

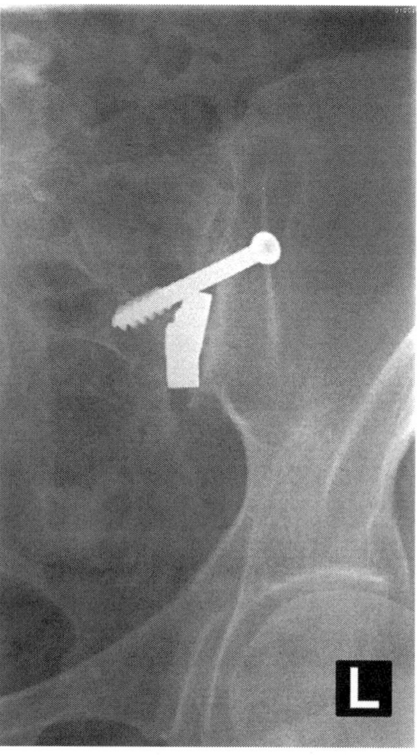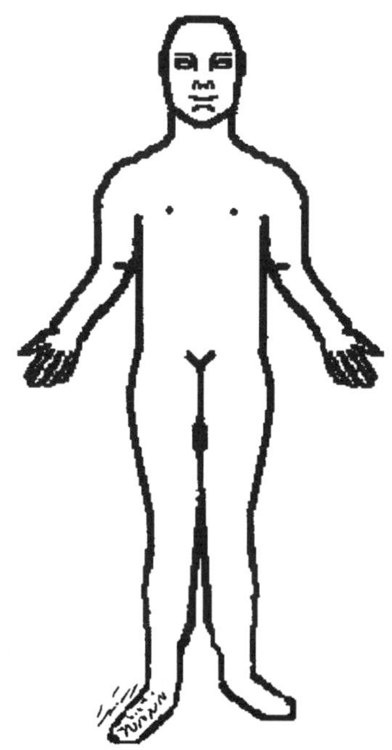

Fig. 12.17 Case Study Ex 1: Oblique view (permission to use photo by E. Jeffrey Donner)

Fig. 12.19 Case Study Ex 2: Pre-op Pain Diagram (permission to use photo by E. Jeffrey Donner)

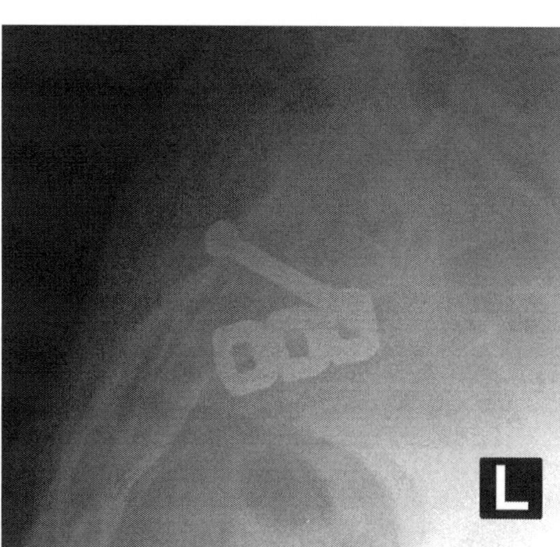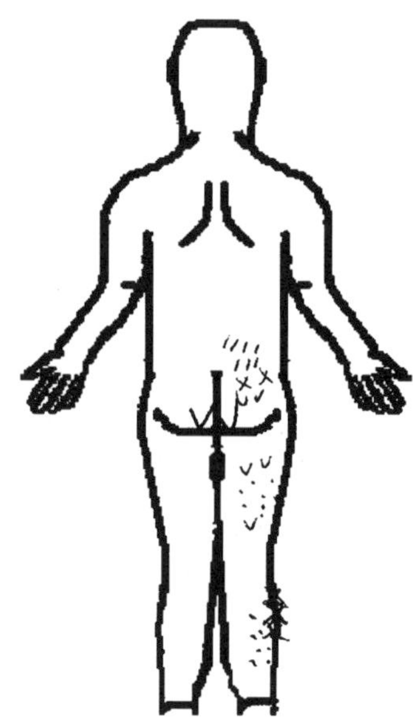

Fig. 12.18 Case Study Ex 1: Lateral view (permission to use photo by E. Jeffrey Donner)

Fig. 12.20 Case Study Ex 2: Pre-op Pain Diagram (permission to use photo by E. Jeffrey Donner)

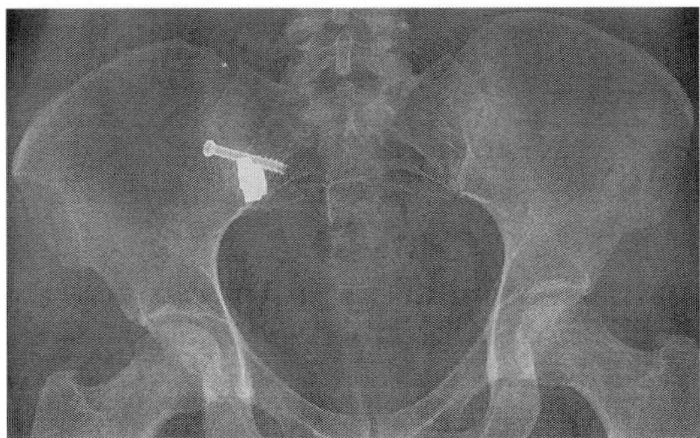

Fig. 12.21 Case Study Ex 2: AP view (permission to use photo by E. Jeffrey Donner)

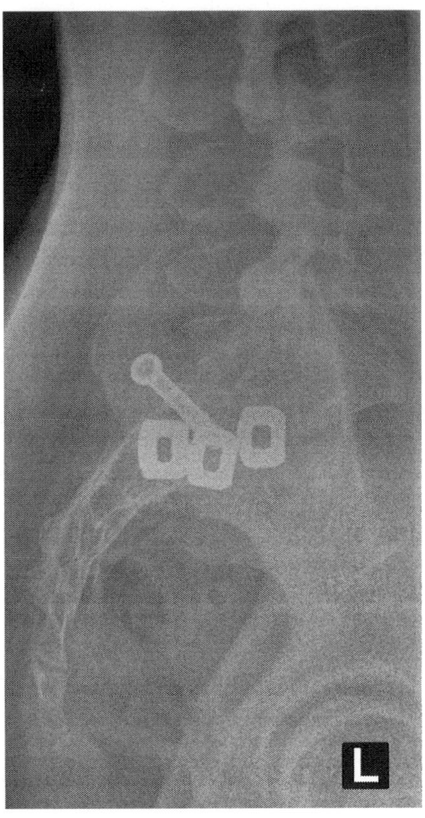

Fig. 12.23 Case Study Ex 2: Lateral view (permission to use photo by E. Jeffrey Donner)

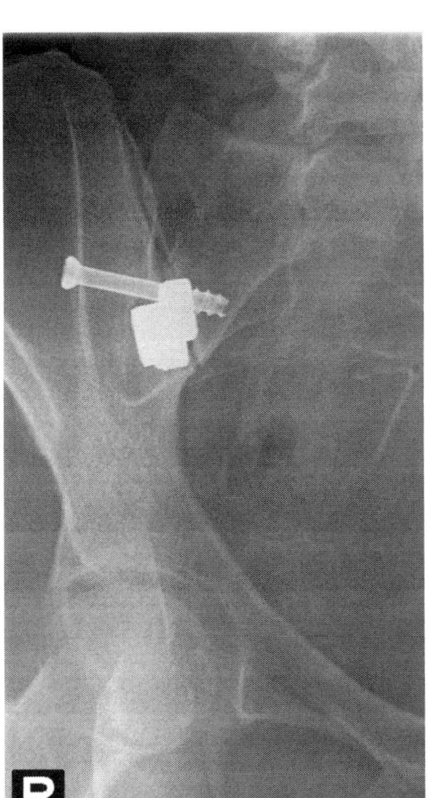

Fig. 12.22 Case Study Ex 2: Oblique view (permission to use photo by E. Jeffrey Donner)

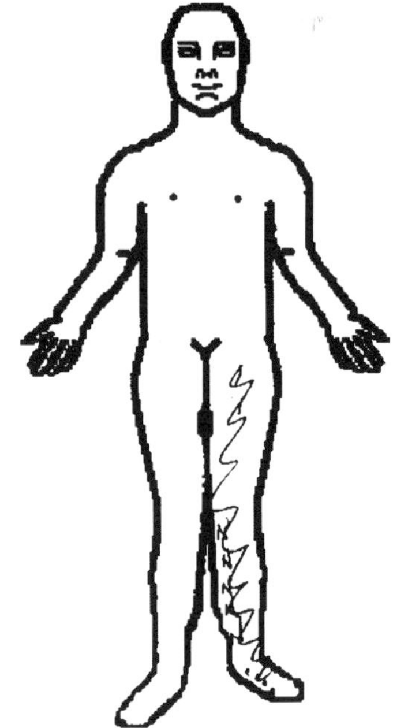

Fig. 12.24 Case Study Ex 3: Pre-op Pain Diagram (permission to use photo by E. Jeffrey Donner)

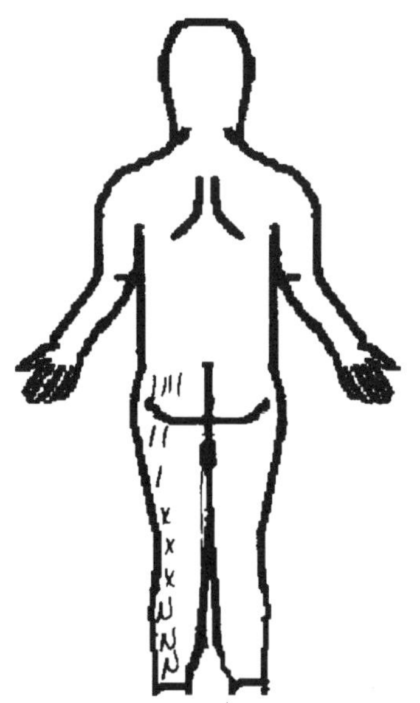

Fig. 12.25 Case Study Ex 3: Pre-op Pain Diagram (permission to use photo by E. Jeffrey Donner)

Conclusion

In conclusion, multiple approaches and techniques have been described and continue to be developed to address the painful SIJ. The safest, most reliable, and effective method has not yet been fully confirmed; however, it is reasonable to conclude that a method, which incorporates known and proven orthopedic principles, has the best opportunity for a successful and durable outcome. Presently, this unique minimally invasive posterior inferior fusion surgical technique is limited to using off-label spinal implants; however, in the near future we anticipate FDA clearance for a surgeon-friendly SIJ-specific implant system which incorporates structural features designed to enhance fixation and fusion of the SIJ.

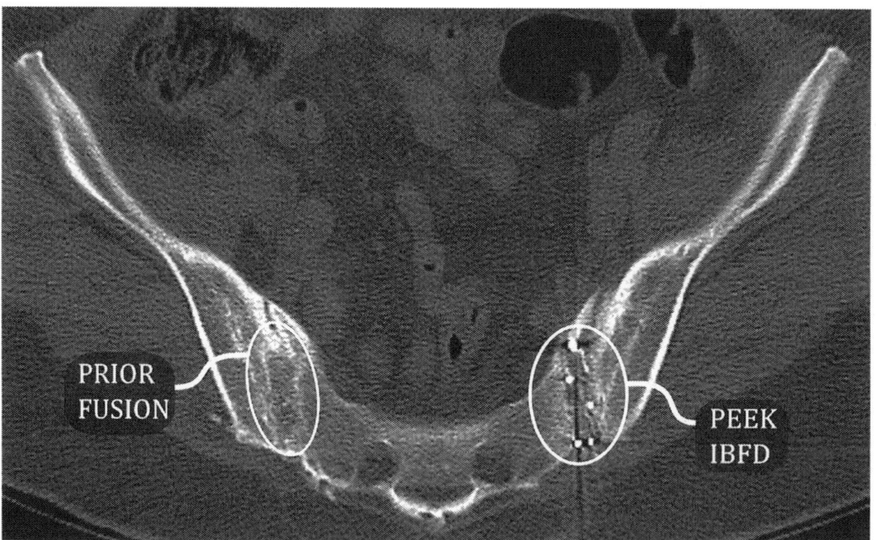

Fig. 12.26 Case Study Ex 3: CT transverse plane cuts illustrating the prior right SIJ open posterior fusion, prior left SIJ IFUSE®, and the most recent left SIJ PIF-MIS with titanium plasma-spray coated PEEK IBFDs (permission to use photo by E. Jeffrey Donner)

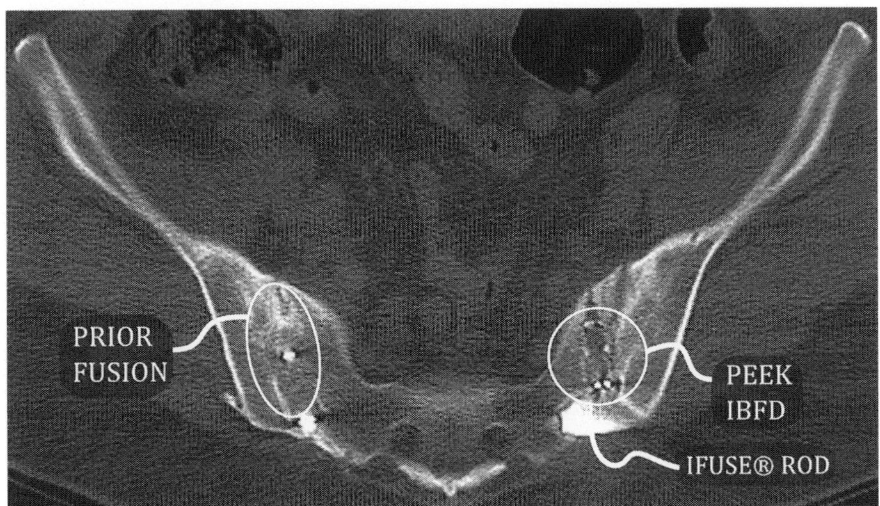

Fig. 12.27 Case Study Ex 3: CT transverse plane cuts illustrating the prior right SIJ open posterior fusion, prior left SIJ IFUSE®, and the most recent left SIJ PIF-MIS with titanium plasma-spray coated PEEK IBFDs (permission to use photo by E. Jeffrey Donner)

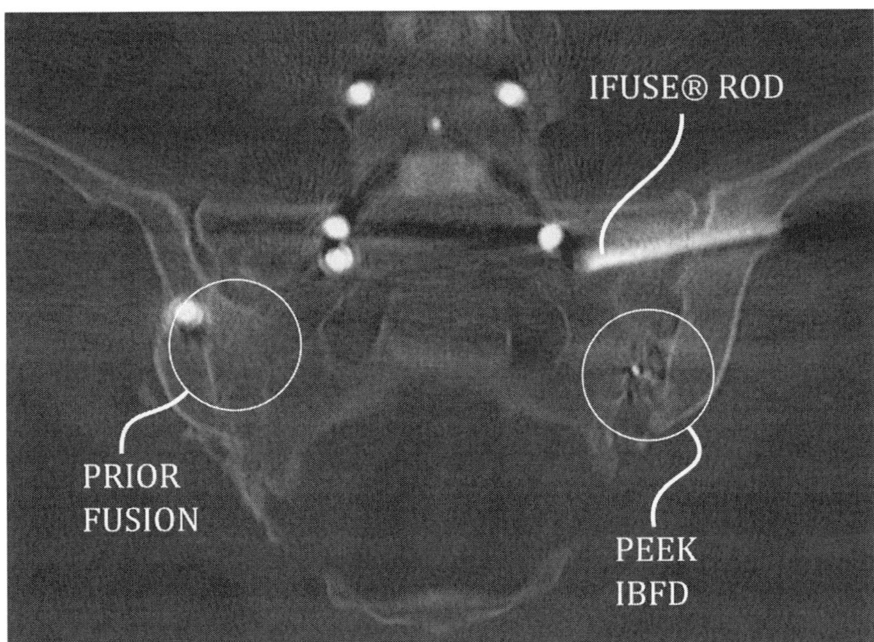

Fig. 12.28 Case Study Ex 3: CT coronal plane cut illustrating the prior right SIJ open posterior fusion, prior left SIJ IFUSE®, and the most recent left SIJ PIF-MIS with titanium plasma-spray coated PEEK IBFDs (permission to use photo by E. Jeffrey Donner)

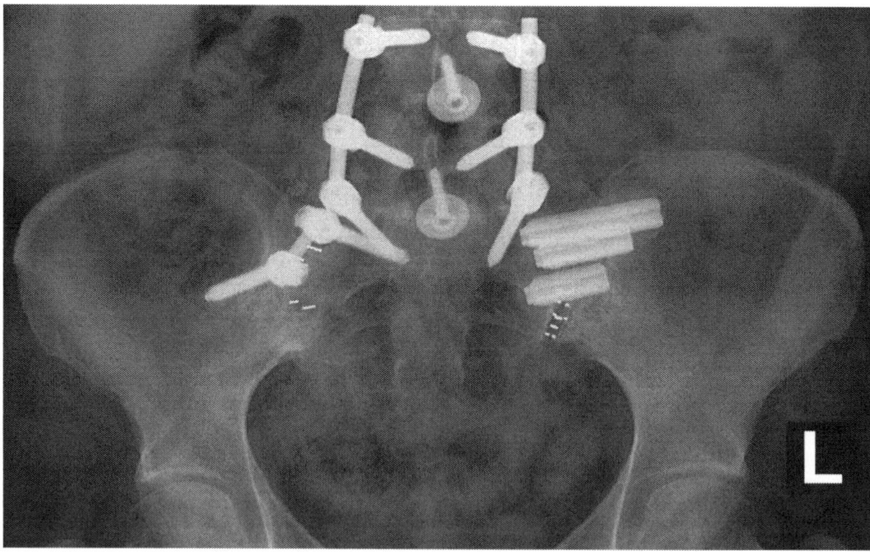

Fig. 12.29 Case Study Ex 3: AP view illustrating the prior right SIJ open posterior fusion, prior left SIJ IFUSE®, and the most recent left SIJ PIF-MIS with tita- nium plasma-spray coated PEEK IBFDs (permission to use photo by E. Jeffrey Donner)

References

1. Dreyfuss P, Dreyer SJ, Cole A, Mayo K. Sacroiliac joint pain. J Am Acad Orthop Surg. 2004;12(4):255–65.
2. Young S, Aprill C, Laslett M. Correlation of clinical examination characteristics with three sources of chronic low back pain. Spine J. 2003;3(6):460–5.
3. Schwarzer AC, Aprill CN, Bogduk N. The sacroiliac joint in chronic low back pain. Spine. 1995;20(1):31–7.
4. DePalma MJ, Ketchum JM, Saullo T. What is the source of chronic low back pain and does age play a role? Pain Med. 2011;12(2):224–33.
5. DePalma MJ, Ketchum JM, Saullo TR. Etiology of chronic low back pain in patients having undergone lumbar fusion. Pain Med. 2011;12(5):732–9.
6. Smith-Petersen MN, Rogers WA. End-result study of arthrodesis of the sacroiliac joint for arthritis—traumatic and non-traumatic. J Bone Joint Surg. 1926;8(1):118–36.
7. Vanelderen P, Szadek KM, Cohen SP, Witte J, Lataster A, Patijn J, et al. Sacroiliac joint pain. Pain Pract. 2010;10(5):470–8.
8. Lippitt AB. Percutaneous fixation of the sacroiliac joint. In: Vleeming A, editor. Movement, stability, and low back pain: the essential role of the pelvis. New York: Churchill Livingstone; 1997. p. 587–94.
9. Hansen H, Manchikanti L, Simopoulos TT, Christo PJ, Gupta S, Smith HS, et al. A systematic evaluation of the therapeutic effectiveness of sacroiliac joint interventions. Pain Physician. 2012;15(3):E247–78.
10. Ho KY, Hadi MA, Pasutharnchat K, Tan KH. Cooled radiofrequency denervation for treatment of sacroiliac joint pain: two-year results from 20 cases. J Pain Res. 2013;6:505–11.
11. Stelzer W, Aiglesberger M, Stelzer D, Stelzer V. Use of cooled radiofrequency lateral branch neurotomy for the treatment of sacroiliac joint-mediated low back pain: a large case series. Pain Med. 2013;14(1):29–35.
12. Crenshaw AH, Daugherty K, Campbell WC. Campbell's operative orthopaedics. St. Louis: Mosby Year Book; 1992.
13. Buchowski JM, Kebaish KM, Sinkov V, Cohen DB, Sieber AN, Kostuik JP. Functional and radiographic outcome of sacroiliac arthrodesis for the disorders of the sacroiliac joint. Spine J. 2005;5(5):520–8.
14. Ebraheim NA, Lu J, Biyani A, Yeasting RA. Anatomic considerations of an anterior approach to the sacroiliac joint. Am J Orthop (Belle Mead, NJ). 1996;25(10):697–700.
15. Alla SR, Roberts CS, Ojike NI. Vascular risk reduction during anterior surgical approach sacroiliac joint plating. Injury. 2013;44(2):175–7.
16. Atlihan D, Tekdemir I, Ateŝ Y, Elhan A. Anatomy of the anterior sacroiliac joint with reference to lumbosacral nerves. Clin Orthop Relat Res. 2000;376:236–41.
17. Donner EJ, Browne DJ. Sacroiliac joint fusion follow-up study. Presented, 11th annual meeting of the North American Spine Society, Vancouver, October 26, 1996.

18. Shaffrey CI, Smith JS. Editorial: Stabilization of the sacroiliac joint. Neurosurg Focus. 2013;35.
19. DeHeer PA, Catoire SM, Taulman J, Borer B. Ankle arthrodesis: a literature review. Clin Podiatr Med Surg. 2012;29(4):509–27.
20. Vleeming A, Schuenke MD, Masi AT, Carreiro JE, Danneels L, Willard FH. The sacroiliac joint: an overview of its anatomy, function and potential clinical implications. J Anat. 2012;221(6):537–67.
21. D'Lima DD, Hashimoto S, Chen PC, Colwell CWJ, Lotz MK. Human chondrocyte apoptosis in response to mechanical injury. Osteoarthritis Cartilage. 2001; 9(8):712–9.
22. D'Lima DD, Hashimoto S, Chen PC, Lotz MK, Colwell CWJ. Cartilage injury induces chondrocyte apoptosis. J Bone Joint Surg Am. 2001;83:19–21.
23. D'Lima DD, Hashimoto S, Chen PC, Lotz MK, Colwell CWJ. In vitro and in vivo models of cartilage injury. J Bone Joint Surg Am. 2001;83:22–4.
24. Ramsey PL, Hamilton W. Changes in tibiotalar area of contact caused by lateral talar shift. J Bone Joint Surg Am. 1976;58(3):356–7.
25. Berenbaum F, Sellam J. Obesity and osteoarthritis: what are the links? Joint Bone Spine. 2008;75(6):667–8.
26. Zhai G, Cicuttini F, Ding C, Scott F, Garnero P, Jones G. Correlates of knee pain in younger subjects. Clin Rheumatol. 2007;26(1):75–80.
27. Ha KY, Lee JS, Kim KW. Degeneration of sacroiliac joint after instrumented lumbar or lumbosacral fusion: a prospective cohort study over five-year follow-up. Spine. 2008;33(11):1192–8.
28. Ivanov AA, Kiapour A, Ebraheim NA, Goel V. Lumbar fusion leads to increases in angular motion and stress across sacroiliac joint: a finite element study. Spine. 2009;34(5):162–9.
29. Steinke H, Hammer N, Slowik V, Stadler J, Josten C, Böhme J, et al. Novel insights into the sacroiliac joint ligaments. Spine. 2010;35(3):257–63.
30. Smith-Petersen MN, Rogers WA. Arthrodesis for tuberculosis of the sacro-iliac joint: Study of the end-results. Jama. 1926;86(1):26–30.
31. Endres S, Ludwig E. Outcome of distraction interference arthrodesis of the sacroiliac joint for sacroiliac arthritis. Indian Journal of Orthopaedics. 2013;47(5):437–42.
32. McGuire RA, Chen Z, Donahoe K. Dual fibular allograft dowel technique for sacroiliac joint arthrodesis. Evid Based Spine Care J. 2012;3(3):21–8.

David W. Polly, Jr.

Introduction

This chapter discusses the inherent implications involving the sacroiliac joint (SIJ) when a long lumbosacral fusion is performed. It will discuss direct effects on the SIJ due to adjacent stress from the more modern methods being used to attain a solid lumbosacral fusion. Current instrumentation techniques to fixate the SIJ while performing a long lumbosacral fusion will be discussed as well as the hazards of over zealous bone graft harvesting and positive sagittal balance.

Adjacent Segment Disease

Long fusions are being done more frequently today than in the past. Technology has enabled spine surgeons to fix problems that previously could not be fixed. The advantage of this technological advance is that more patients can be treated but the disadvantage is that this places much greater stress on the SIJ and the pelvis. We are now recognizing the SIJ and the pelvis as adjacent segments that can undergo degeneration just like other spinal segments. For the lumbar

D.W. Polly, Jr., M.D. (✉)
Department of Orthopaedic Surgery,
University of Minnesota, 2450 Riverside Avenue
South, Suite R 200, Minneapolis, MN 55454, USA
e-mail: pollydw@umn.edu

spine the rate of adjacent segment degeneration can be as much as 16 % at 5 years and 31 % at 10 years [1]. A recent study by Ha et al. [2] reports that 75 % of patients who were fused to the pelvis demonstrated radiographic degenerative changes within the SIJ. In patients who had a floating fusion, this only occurred 38 % of the time.

Implications of Long Fusions to the Sacrum

Long fusions to the sacrum/pelvis have a higher incidence of pseudarthrosis. The success rate with noninstrumented fusions was low. The next incremental advance involved the Galveston technique which involved placing rods into the pelvis, especially in neuromuscular scoliosis [3]. This improved the deformity correction and the fusion rate. However, it was not perfect, and in many patients halo formation developed about the intra-iliac portion of the rods. Presumptively this is due to the persistent motion across the SIJ, which is unfused with this technique. The clinical revision rate for this technique is on the order of 36 % [4].

The next step forward was the development of a modular screw, which could be connected to a rod [5–7]. This made this technique easier to technically accomplish and has been the predominant technique for perhaps 20 years. The revision rate for this technique is 14 %, but when combined with bicortical S1 screws, it drops to 8.5 % [4]. The disadvantage of this technique is

B.E. Dall et al. (eds.), *Surgery for the Painful, Dysfunctional Sacroiliac Joint*,
DOI 10.1007/978-3-319-10726-4_13, © Springer International Publishing Switzerland 2015

that the implants are much more prominent than the Galveston technique. This necessitates removal in a significant number of patients. The connector mechanisms can be technically demanding exercises adding time to the surgery. In addition to prominence as a source of pain, it is also possible that the SIJ itself can be a source of pain in these patients who are symptomatic. In my own experience, at least 35 % of these patients have significant symptoms at the posterior superior iliac spine requiring intervention.

The recognition of the role of anterior column support has been well recognized. Anterior column fusion improves the healing rate. Structural interbody support decreases the strain on posterior spinal instrumentation [8, 9]. There has been debate about the relative value of anterior interbody fusion compared to posterior interbody techniques [10–12].

The relative comparative stiffness of lumbosacral fixation has now been well studied. Iliac fixation provides the most benefit [13–15]. So we can now do a much better job matching the biomechanical demands to the capabilities of the fixation technique in terms of achieving fusion of the spine but still with the potential for adjacent segment degeneration [16].

Sacroiliac Joint Fixation with Long Lumbosacral Fusions

Recently a new technique of fixation, the S2 alar iliac screw, has been popularized and studied [17–19]. This technique places a screw directly through the SIJ and into the ilium. This technique has greater insertional torque as it crosses multiple cortices (dorsal sacrum, sacral outer table, ilium inner table) and then engages bone in the suprasciatic notch. This technique lowers the profile of the implants compared to conventional iliac screws by having the rod directly landing into the screw, avoiding the need for a connector [20]. It is also more deeply seated below the ilium than a typical iliac screw. There is not clear data to look at relative amount of halo formation, but individual series anecdotal experience (Polly, unpublished data) seems to indicate a lower rate of halo formation and a lower rate of need for

subsequent implant removal. Similar anecdotal experience shows a lower rate of symptomatic SIJs with the S2AI screws. Perhaps this provides adequate stabilization for the joint due to the rigid fixation of the screw across the joint.

The advent of transiliac sacral fixation (in the path used by iliosacral screws) poses a new challenge to long segment fusion to the pelvis. These devices (rods, cages, etc.) occupy a large cross-sectional volume of the SIJ. This may make it impossible to place conventional iliac screws or S2AI screws. The inability to place this fixation will make it more challenging to achieve successful fusion. This can even be the case when image-guided navigation is utilized.

Effects of Associated Iliac Bone Graft Harvesting

Iliac crest bone graft harvesting for long fusions probably adds to the stress upon the SI joint. With long fusions surgeons are more likely to be aggressive in harvesting the ilium. This harvesting takes bone substance away from this area of high stress leading to greater force per unit area of bone. In addition there is some rate of inadvertent SIJ violation with iliac crest bone graft harvesting [21, 22]. Finally if the ilium has been harvested and the SIJ becomes sufficiently symptomatic to require stabilization, this stabilization will be more difficult due to decreased ilium available for purchase.

Positive Sagittal Balance, Especially in Elderly Patients

Today the surgeon faces the dilemma of both the spine and the SIJ especially in the middle-aged to elderly patient. If the patient has positive sagittal balance, then they are profoundly incapacitated [23]. This alignment will also place significant additional stress on the long dorsal ligaments of the posterior SIJ. Physical exam and diagnostic injections can in fact confirm the SIJ as a pain generator. Fixing the SIJ will relieve the local pain but will not resolve the positive sagittal balance issues. If implants are used to traverse the SIJ, then that will make it difficult or impossible to place subsequent iliac fixation for the spinal realignment. Conversely iliac fixation may make it impossible to place implants across the SIJ. This is a dilemma that the surgeon must consider in choosing what order to do things. An alternative strategy is to fix the spinal alignment first using S2AI screws, transfixing the SIJ to see if this solves both problems.

Case Study

A patient presented with bilateral SIJ pain confirmed by physical exam provocation maneuvers and image-guided diagnostic injections. The patient was only interested in having his SIJs addressed and not his spine (Figs. 13.1, 13.2, and 13.3).

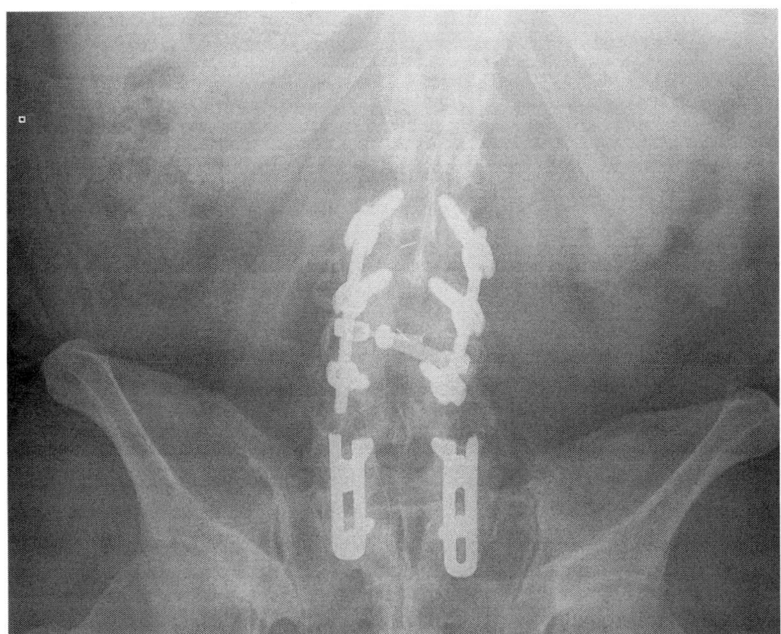

Fig. 13.1 AP X-ray of previous lumbosacral instrumented fusions

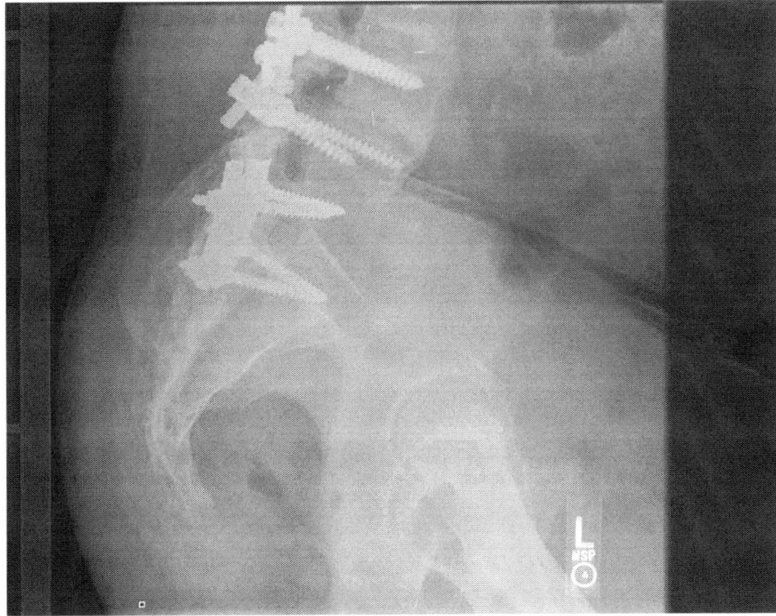

Fig. 13.2 Lateral X-ray of previous instrumented lumbosacral fusions

The patient noted significant pain relief after his SI joint fusions; however, he had persisting symptoms consistent with flat back syndrome, also known as positive sagittal imbalance (Figs. 13.4, 13.5, and 13.6).

The patient then underwent spinal reconstruction with a lumbar pedicle subtraction osteotomy. Distal fixation was challenging with the SI joint implants in place. The patient is quite satisfied with his clinical improvement (Figs. 13.7, 13.8, 13.9, and 13.10).

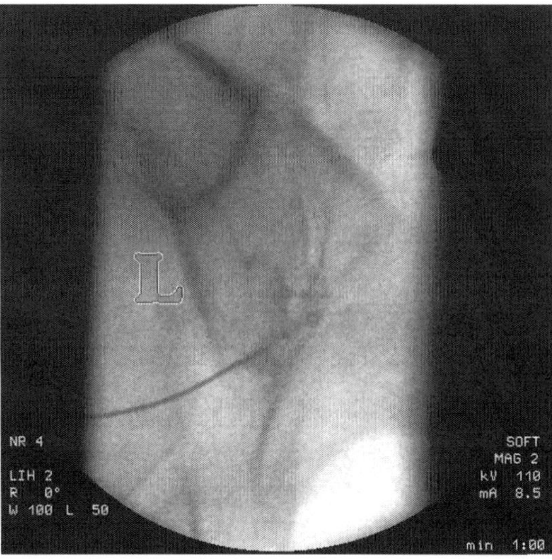

Fig. 13.3 Image guided diagnostic injection verified diagnosis

Conclusion

It is now recognized that adjacent segment degenerative disease does affect the SIJ when a long lumbosacral fusion is performed. If the SIJ is fixated when performing a long lumbosacral fusion, certain pitfalls such as over abundant iliac bone graft harvesting, with its associated potential effects on the SIJ and the ramifications of positive sagittal balance, especially in the elderly, must be considered by the spine surgeon proactively to avoid potential long-term complications. When both positive sagittal balance and the SIJs are symptomatic and require surgery, the spine surgeon must be cognizant of the best methods to use and in what sequence to use them in order to achieve the best overall result for the patient.

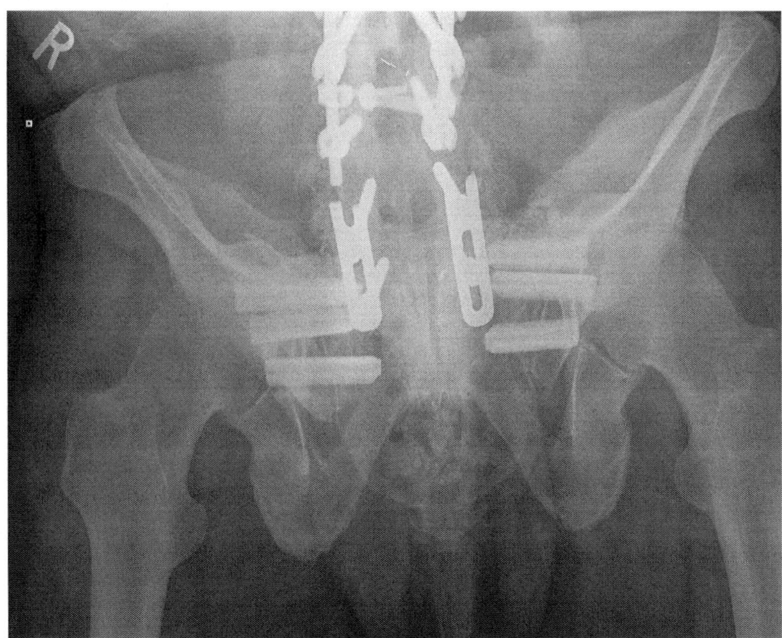

Fig. 13.4 Postoperative AP X-ray showing bilateral SIJ instrumentation

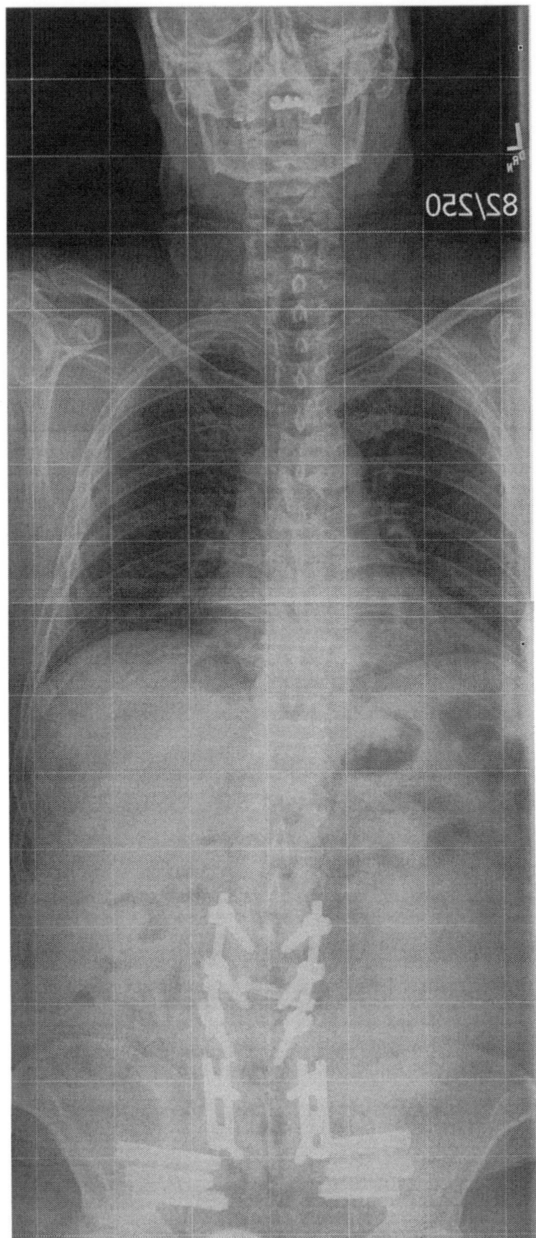

Fig. 13.5 PA scoliosis film

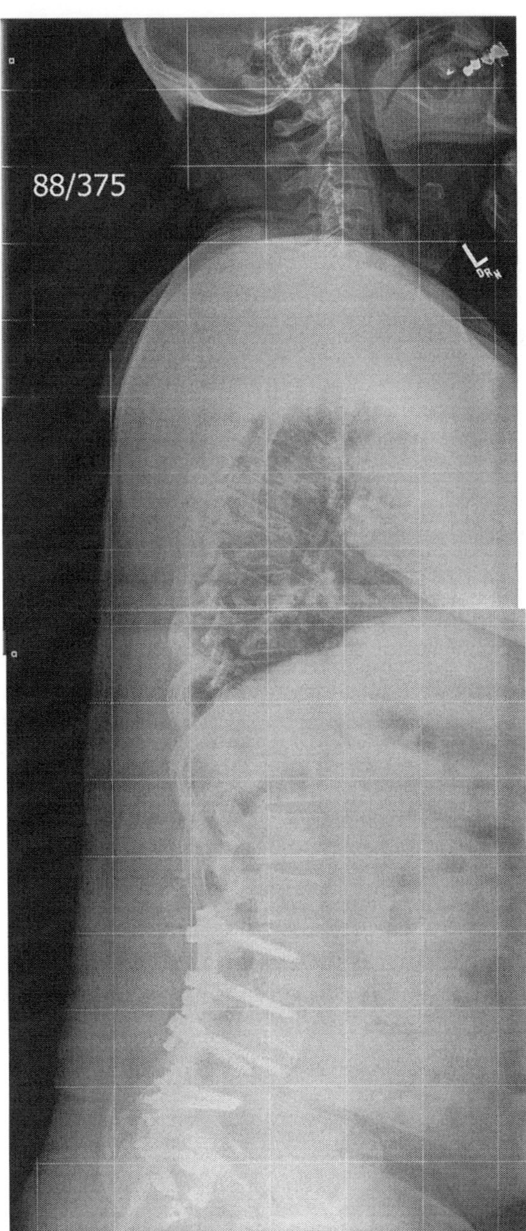

Fig. 13.6 Lateral scoliosis film showing "flat back" syndrome

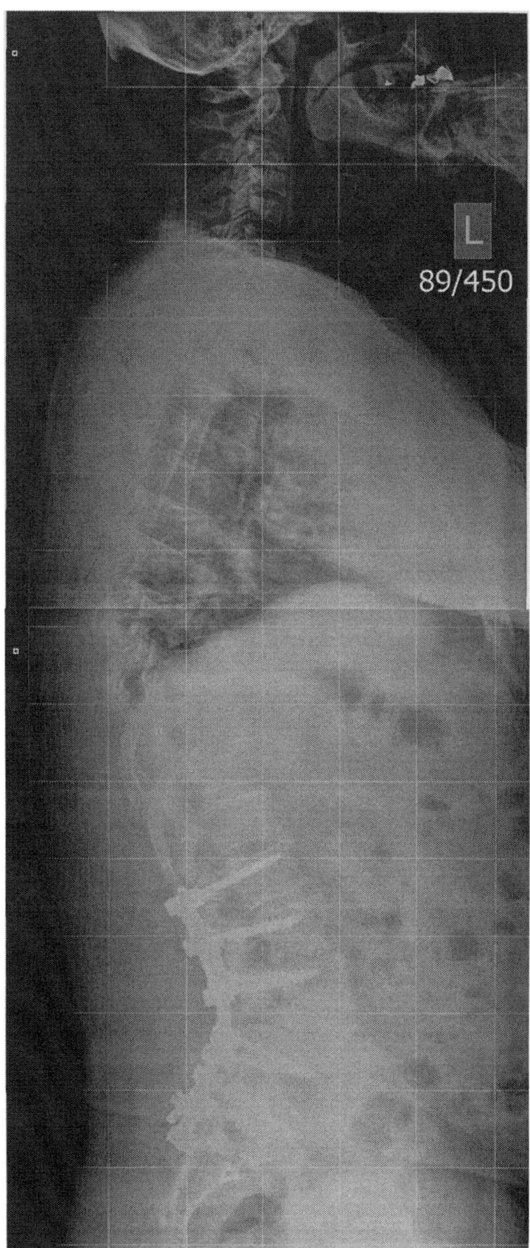

Fig. 13.7 Postoperative lateral scoliosis film after subtraction osteotomy

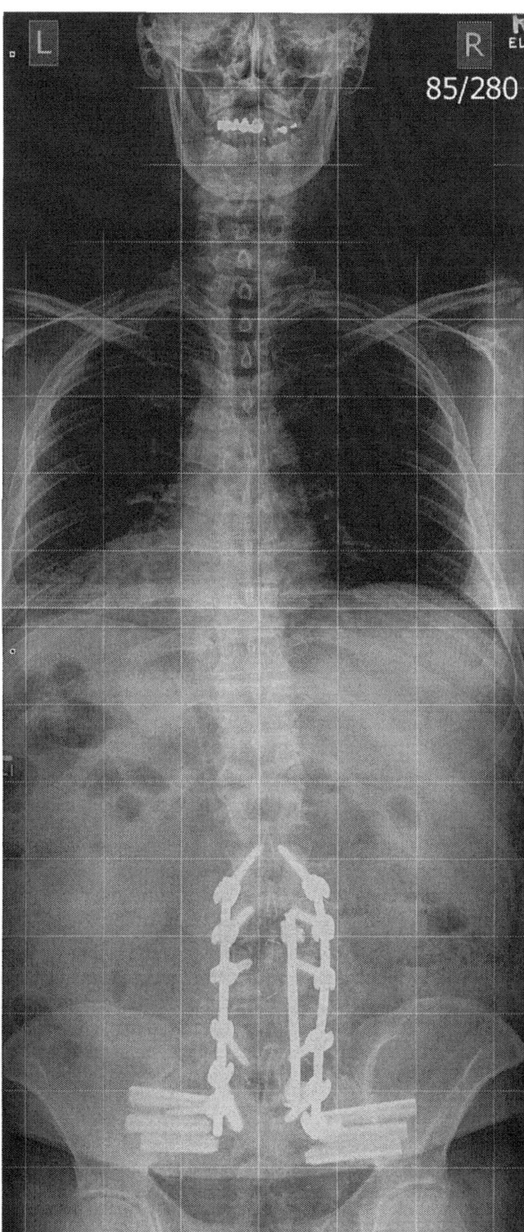

Fig. 13.8 Postoperative PA scoliosis film after subtraction osteotomy

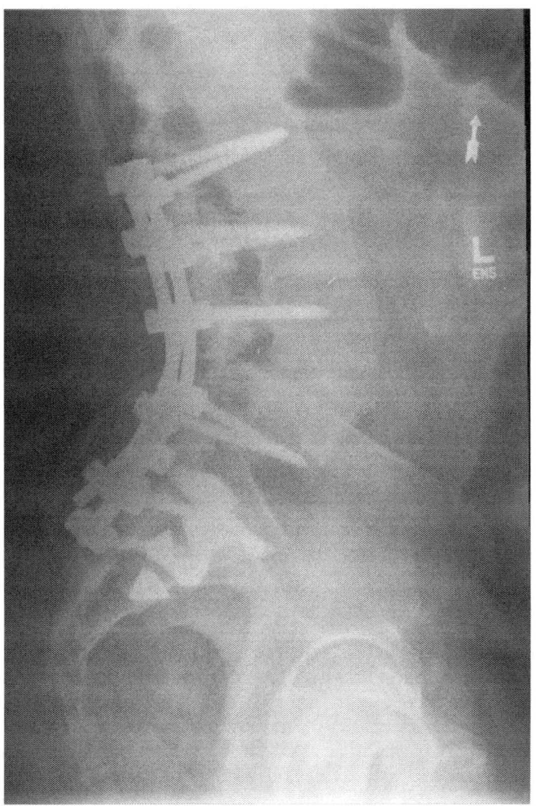

Fig. 13.9 AP X-ray after subtraction osteotomy

Fig. 13.10 Lateral X-ray after subtraction osteotomy

References

1. Ghiselli G, Wang JC, Bhatia NN, et al. Adjacent segment degeneration in the lumbar spine. J Bone Joint Surg Am. 2004;86-A(7):1497–503.
2. Ha KY, Lee JS, Kim KW. Degeneration of sacroiliac joint after instrumented lumbar or lumbosacral fusion: a prospective cohort study over five-year follow-up. Spine. 2008;33(11):1192–8.
3. Allen Jr BL, Ferguson RL. The Galveston technique for l rod instrumentation of the scoliotic spine. Spine (Phila Pa 1976). 1982;7(3):276–84.
4. Emami A, Deviren V, Berven S, et al. Outcome and complications of long fusions to the sacrum in adult spine deformity: Luque-Galveston, combined iliac and sacral screws, and sacral fixation. Spine (Phila Pa 1976). 2002;27(7):776–86.
5. Peelle MW, Lenke LG, Bridwell KH, et al. Comparison of pelvic fixation techniques in neuromuscular spinal deformity correction: Galveston rod versus iliac and lumbosacral screws. Spine (Phila Pa 1976). 2006;31(20):2392–8. discussion 2399.
6. Tis JE, Helgeson M, Lehman RA, et al. A biomechanical comparison of different types of lumbopelvic fixation. Spine (Phila Pa 1976). 2009;34(24):E866–72.
7. Yu BS, Zhuang XM, Zheng ZM, et al. Biomechanical advantages of dual over single iliac screws in lumbo-iliac fixation construct. Eur Spine J. 2010;19(7):1121–8.
8. Cunningham BW, Polly Jr DW. The use of interbody cage devices for spinal deformity: a biomechanical perspective. Clin Orthop Relat Res. 2002;394:73–83.
9. Polly Jr DW, Klemme WR, Cunningham BW, et al. The biomechanical significance of anterior column support in a simulated single-level spinal fusion. J Spinal Disord. 2000;13(1):58–62.
10. Crandall DG, Revella J. Transforaminal lumbar interbody fusion versus anterior lumbar interbody fusion as an adjunct to posterior instrumented correction of degenerative lumbar scoliosis: three year clinical and radiographic outcomes. Spine (Phila Pa 1976). 2009; 34(20):2126–33.
11. Dorward IG, Lenke LG, Bridwell KH, et al. Transforaminal versus anterior lumbar interbody fusion in long deformity constructs: a matched cohort analysis. Spine (Phila Pa 1976). 2013;38(12):755–62
12. Jiang SD, Chen JW, Jiang LS. Which procedure is better for lumbar interbody fusion: anterior lumbar interbody fusion or transforaminal lumbar interbody fusion? Arch Orthop Trauma Surg. 2012;132(9):1259–66.
13. Cunningham BW, Lewis SJ, Long J, et al. Biomechanical evaluation of lumbosacral reconstruction techniques for spondylolisthesis: an in vitro porcine model. Spine (Phila Pa 1976). 2002;27(21):2321–7.
14. Cunningham BW, Sefter JC, Hu N, et al. Biomechanical comparison of iliac screws versus interbody femoral ring allograft on lumbosacral kinematics and sacral screw strain. Spine (Phila Pa 1976). 2010;35(6):E198–205.
15. Lebwohl NH, Cunningham BW, Dmitriev A, et al. Biomechanical comparison of lumbosacral fixation techniques in a calf spine model. Spine (Phila Pa 1976). 2002;27(21):2312–20.

16. Santos ER, Sembrano JN, Mueller B, et al. Optimizing iliac screw fixation: a biomechanical study on screw length, trajectory, and diameter. J Neurosurg Spine. 2011;14(2):219–25.
17. Bederman SS, Hahn P, Colin V, et al. Robotic guidance for s2-alar-iliac screws in spinal deformity correction. J Spinal Disord Tech. 2013. doi:10.1097/BSD.Ob013e3182a3572b
18. O'Brien JR, Yu W, Kaufman BE, et al. Biomechanical evaluation of s2 alar-iliac screws: effect of length and quad-cortical purchase as compared with iliac fixation. Spine (Phila Pa 1976). 2013;38(20):E1250–5.
19. Zhu F, Bao HD, Yuan S, et al. Posterior second sacral alar iliac screw insertion: anatomic study in a Chinese population. Eur Spine J. 2013;22(7):1683–9.
20. Chang TL, Sponseller PD, Kebaish KM, et al. Low profile pelvic fixation: anatomic parameters for sacral alar-iliac fixation versus traditional iliac fixation. Spine (Phila Pa 1976). 2009;34(5):436–40.
21. Bojescul JA, Polly Jr DW, Kuklo TR, et al. Backfill for iliac-crest donor sites: a prospective, randomized study of coralline hydroxyapatite. Am J Orthop (Belle Mead NJ). 2005;34(8):377–82.
22. Dhawan A, Kuklo TR, Polly Jr DW. Analysis of iliac crest bone grafting process measures. Am J Orthop (Belle Mead NJ). 2006;35(7):322–6.
23. Glassman SD, Bridwell K, Dimar JR, et al. The impact of positive sagittal balance in adult spinal deformity. Spine (Phila Pa 1976). 2005;30(18):2024–9.

Postsurgical Rehabilitation

14

Michael D. Rahl

Introduction

Surgical interventions to treat sacroiliac joint (SIJ) dysfunction have changed over time with advancements in medicine and surgery. In the early twentieth century, surgery to treat the SIJ often required invasive procedures resulting in significant tissue disruption and severe scarring. Long periods of immobilization were required and time frames until complete recovery were uncertain. Today, surgical options include minimally invasive procedures and instrumentation leading to SIJ fusion. These approaches and techniques minimize tissue disruption, immobilization, and recovery time. Little agreement exists, considering the uniqueness of each patient and presentation, as to which approach, surgical technique, and instrumentation placement are optimal.

Guidelines for Rehabilitation

A thorough understanding of the surgical procedure used to fuse the SIJ is important for safe rehabilitation. Different approaches to the SIJ may lead to more stable fusions but can disrupt different tissues to varying degrees (Fig. 14.1).

M.D. Rahl, PT, DPT, OCS, CSCS (✉)
Full Potential Physical Therapy, 286 Hoover
Boulevard, Holland, MI 49423, USA
e-mail: michael@fullpotentialpt.com

Knowing which tissues were interrupted, and in some approaches reapproximated, is essential to avoid unnecessary complications. The instrumentation used to fixate the SIJ and adjacent structures involved will affect the rehabilitation protocol. The graft material placed within the joint and any intra-articular hardware used to fuse it might also require different precautions.

Most postsurgical SIJ fusion patients will fall into one of three categories. The first category involves patients that have minimal restrictions at their initial 1–6-week post-op physical therapy visit (Table 14.1). Often, these patients have undergone a posterior midline or posterior lateral approach with minimal tissue disruption. Weight bearing is full and restrictions are minimal. The second category involves patients that have the same restrictions as the first category plus weight-bearing limitations. These patients have often undergone a direct lateral approach. Weight bearing is limited to toe touch only. The toe is allowed to touch the ground in order to unload the SIJ and surrounding soft tissue, but minimal force is transferred through the limb. The third group involves patients who have undergone a concurrent lumbosacral fusion. In these instances, the postsurgical lumbosacral fusion protocol is defaulted to.

Many surgeons performing SIJ fusions have specific rehabilitation protocols, while others do not. Contacting the referring surgeon to assure proper adherence to all precautions is important throughout the rehabilitation process.

B.E. Dall et al. (eds.), *Surgery for the Painful, Dysfunctional Sacroiliac Joint*,
DOI 10.1007/978-3-319-10726-4_14, © Springer International Publishing Switzerland 2015

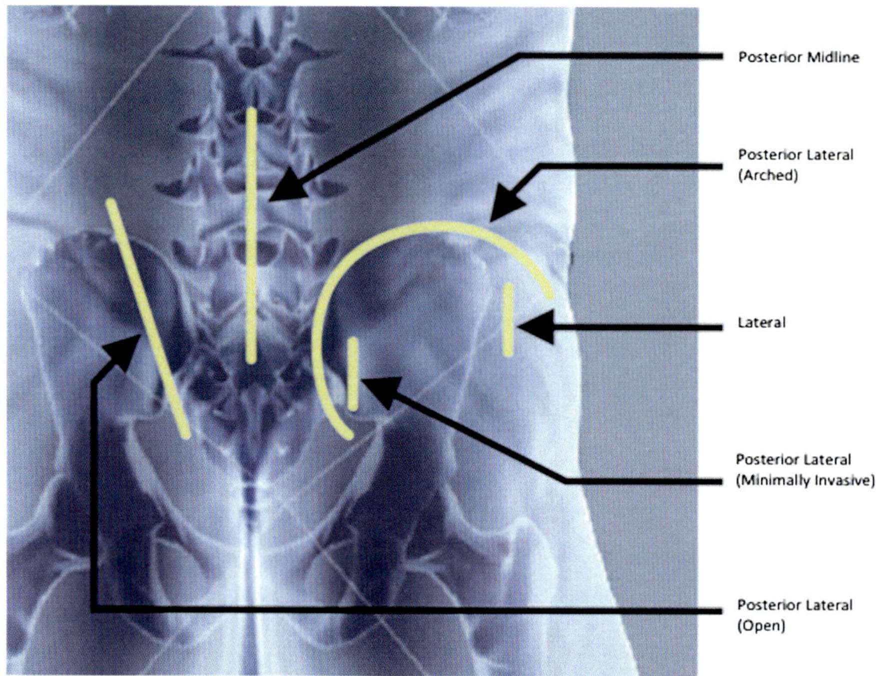

Fig. 14.1 Incision sites for various surgical approaches to the sacroiliac joint (used with permission from Borgess Health)

Table 14.1 Surgical approaches to the sacroiliac joint and associated precautions[a]

Approach	Restrictions	Brace/assistive device	Initiate PT
Posterior midline	No bending, lifting (>10 lbs), twisting for 12 weeks Full WB	Pelvic belt for 6–12 weeks Walker/no pelvic belt (obese pts)	6 Weeks post-op
Lateral (minimally invasive)	No bending, lifting (>10 lbs), twisting for 12 weeks Toe-touch WB for 3–6 weeks	Pelvic belt for 6–12 weeks Crutches/walker for 3–6 weeks	6 Weeks post-op
Posterior lateral (minimally invasive)	No bending, lifting (>10 lbs), twisting for 12 weeks Full WB	Pelvic belt for 6–12 weeks Walker/no pelvic belt (obese pts)	1–2 Weeks post-op
Posterior lateral (open)	Toe-touch WB for 6–8 weeks	Crutches for 6–8 weeks	6–8 Weeks post-op
Posterior inferior	WB as tolerated	Crutches/walker for 3–6 weeks	6 Weeks post-op
Concurrent lumbosacral fusion	No bending, lifting (>10 lbs), twisting for 12 weeks	TLSO (pantaloon attachment)	6–10 Weeks post-op

WB weight bearing, *TLSO* thoracolumbosacral orthosis, *Pts* patients
[a]Guidelines obtained from surgeons performing specific approach frequently

Failure to do so may result in negative consequences and poor outcomes.

While the SIJ and lumbar spine are close in proximity, rehabilitation following surgical fusion is different for each. The lumbar spine has many direct muscle attachments and can be stabilized via interventions aimed at these muscles. The sacrum has less direct muscular attachments and joint support, which requires interventions directed at adjacent structures both cephalad and caudal to the SIJ. Structural and force symmetry are also more of an issue with unilateral SIJ fusions compared to fusions of the lumbar spine.

The following rehabilitation guidelines (Table 14.2) are meant to be used in conjunction with sound clinical judgment. Some patients may

Table 14.2 Rehabilitation guidelines for postsurgical sacroiliac joint fusions

Phase	Time frame post-op	PT goals	Sample interventions
1	Weeks 1–5	Patient education Pain control Bracing/assistive device training Proper body mechanics with ADLs Gait training	Cryotherapy Pelvic belt instruction Walker/crutches instruction (WB restrictions) Transfers, sleeping/sitting position instruction Stair training Aquatic therapy
2	Weeks 6–11	Patient education Pain control Promote tissue remodeling Correct tissue dysfunction Initiate stabilization exercises Gait training Improve mobility/activity level HEP	Cryotherapy, TENS Scar mobilization Soft tissue techniques Hip ERs, HS, hip flexor stretches Eliminate compensatory patterns of muscles Gentle hip, facet mobilizations Draw-in maneuver, table-top exercises Kegel exercises Postural training Light cardiovascular exercise (walking) Gait mechanics correction Aquatic therapy
3	Weeks 12–19	Patient education Promote tissue remodeling Correct tissue dysfunction Progress stabilization exercises Initiate resistance exercises Increase activity level HEP Return to work	Stretches to maintain flexibility Gluteal, hip ERs, HS strengthening Dynamic stabilization (Swiss ball, unstable surfaces) Single-leg stance exercises (bird dip, balance reach) Compound exercises (multi-planar) Cardiovascular exercise (recumbent bike) Workstation ergonomic evaluation
4	Weeks 20+	Prior level of function Sport-specific training HEP	Dynamic stabilization Return to gym Running Agility exercises

HEP home exercise program, *WB* weight bearing, *TENS* transcutaneous electrical nerve stimulation, *ERs* external rotators, *HS* hamstrings

be progressed faster or slower at the discretion of the referring surgeon. Specific exercises, volumes, and intensities will not be presented in detail. All patients are unique. Patient-specific interventions and education based on patient goals, current evidence, and clinician experience are the essential components to successfully rehabilitate a postsurgical SIJ fusion.

Phase 1, Weeks 1–5

Following SIJ surgery, the patient may remain in the hospital for up to several days. If iliac bone was harvested, a drain may be placed but will usually be removed within 24 h. The goals of physical therapy are pain control, to monitor the surgical site looking for signs and symptoms of possible infection, and patient education on activities of daily living (ADL), mobility, and precautions. Modalities, such as cryotherapy, may be used to control pain at the surgical site and surrounding tissues. Redness, swelling, increased pain in the buttock, and fever may indicate an underlying infection. If these symptoms are observed, contact the surgeon immediately.

Education should consist of verbal descriptions, visual demonstrations, and written instructions. Each patient's preferred learning style should be taken into consideration when educating the patient and his or her family. The patient should be instructed to avoid any bending, lifting (>10 lbs), or twisting at the waist for 12 weeks. Sleeping may be uncomfortable depending on the patient's preferred sleeping position. If the patient prefers to sleep in side lying, a pillow can

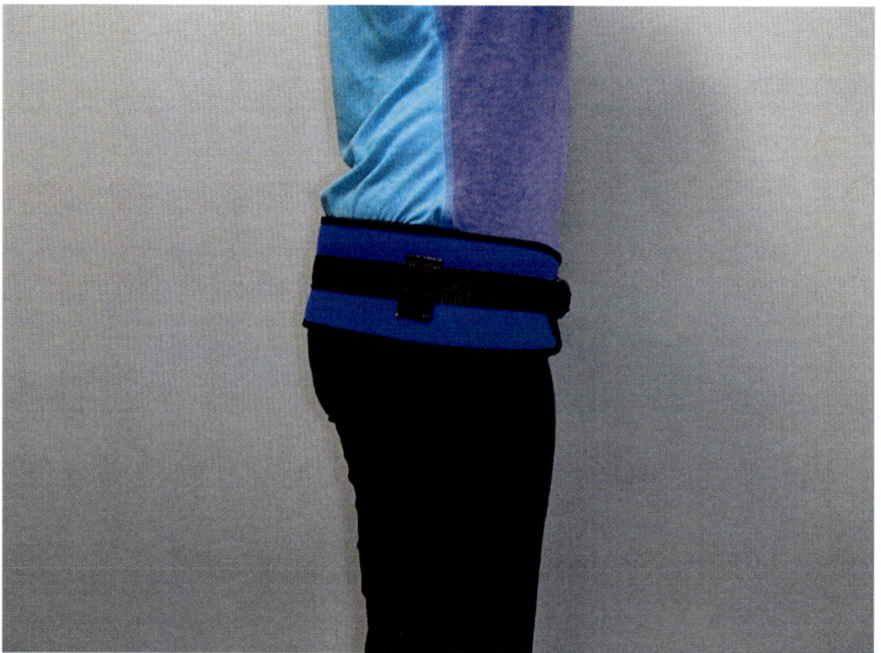

Fig. 14.2 A sacroiliac belt and proper placement just proximal to the greater trochanters

be used between the knees and thighs to minimize hip adduction and stress on the fusion site. Be sure the patient is able to recall all postsurgical precautions prior to discharge.

Some patients may be required to wear a brace or use an assistive device. Education on how to get in and out of the brace as well as when it needs to be worn is important. Improper adherence to bracing can be detrimental to the fusion process. A pelvic belt can help support the SIJ by compressing the pelvis and increasing force closure at the SIJs (Fig. 14.2).

As the belt tightens, the alae of the ilium are approximated and the ventral part of the SIJ is compressed. The dorsal ligaments and fascia tighten as the posterior superior iliac spines (PSISs) try to separate and approximate the dorsal aspect of the joint (Fig. 14.3).

It is recommended that the belt be worn just proximal to the greater trochanter with a tension force of 50 N or about 11.0 lbs [1, 2]. The pelvic belt should be worn when the patient is upright for 6–12 weeks until referral to physical therapy and the initiation of core stabilization can begin. A pelvic belt will be ineffective in obese patients secondary to excessive adipose tissue around the

midsection, so these patients are encouraged to use a walker for all ambulation for up to 12 weeks.

Assistive devices may also be required secondary to weight-bearing restrictions or due to the acute side effects of medication used during and/or after surgery. After SIJ fusions using a direct lateral approach, toe-touch weight bearing is required and the patient will use crutches or a walker for 3–6 weeks. Using proper technique with all assistive devices is imperative for safety, surgical site protection, and energy conservation.

Ascending and descending stairs may also be difficult. Proper adherence to weight-bearing restrictions is challenging on stairs with the safety of the patient being the primary goal. Ascending stairs using the uninvolved limb first and descending stairs with the involved limb first while also using a rail or rails to unload the limb further is the best way to start. As the patient gets further out from surgery and strength and stability improve, the step-to-step pattern will transition to a step-over-step pattern. In cases of bilateral fusions, clinician discretion and patient comfort will guide treatment.

Patients with and without weight-bearing restrictions are good candidates for aquatic

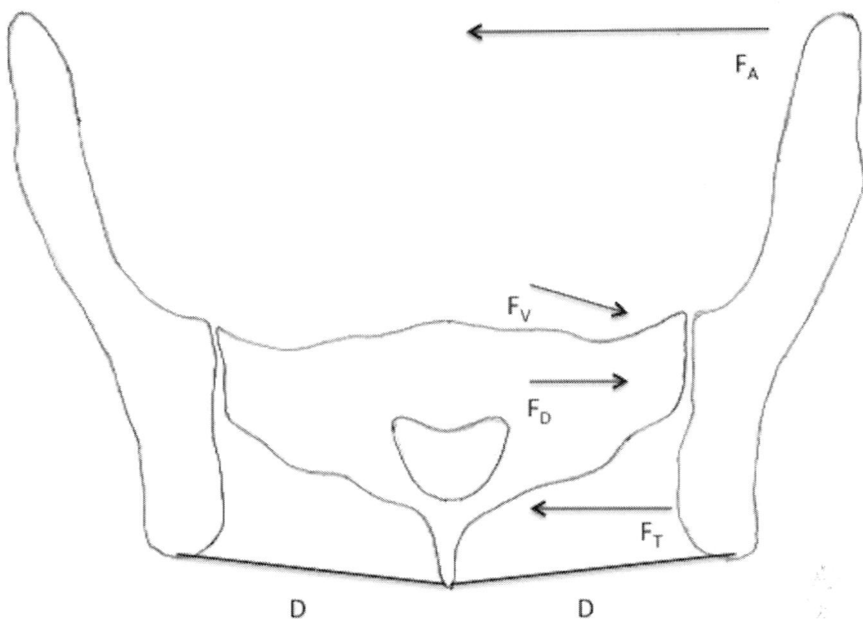

Fig. 14.3 Force closure of the sacroiliac joint. The deep abdominals contract and pull the ilia medially, which compresses the ventral aspect of the sacroiliac joint. This tensions the dorsal ligaments, which compresses the dorsal aspect of the sacroiliac joint. D=dorsal sacroiliac ligaments, F_A=force of the contracting deep abdominals (or pelvic belt), F_D=force compressing the dorsal joint, F_T=force of the tensioned dorsal ligaments, F_V=force compressing the ventral joint

therapy. While immersed in the water up to his or her xiphisternum (about 70 % immersed), the patient will experience 25–50 % and 50–75 % weight bearing through his or her lower extremities during static stance/slow-speed walking and fast-speed walking, respectively [3] (Fig. 14.4).

Standing or floating in deeper water will unload the lower extremities further still. Being in the water can allow for the initiation and progression of exercises that may not be possible on land at that time. Aquatic therapy should focus on stretching, stabilization, balance, and strengthening.

Most patients will be discharged from the hospital and referred to physical therapy after 6 weeks. Healing and bone callus formation usually occurs within 6–8 weeks but may take longer in more complex cases. The timing of referral to physical therapy depends on the approach used during the surgery, which structures were operated on, and progression of the patient. The operating surgeon will decide if physical therapy is needed or not.

Phase 2, Weeks 6–11

During this phase of rehabilitation, physical therapy will focus on pain control, the promotion of tissue remodeling, correcting tissue dysfunction, initiation of stabilization exercises, and mobility. Postsurgical precautions and adherence to the postsurgical rehabilitation protocol provided by the surgeon are still important. Continued patient education is also necessary for the patient to have realistic goals, an understanding of time frames, and proper exercise compliance. A home exercise program (HEP) is started and progressed throughout Phase 2. The HEP progression will be based on patient progress and goals and will continue on for several months to years.

Evaluation

A thorough subjective and objective examination and evaluation should be completed before performing any interventions. Knowledge of whether the fusion was unilateral, bilateral, and/or involved the lumbar spine will help direct the

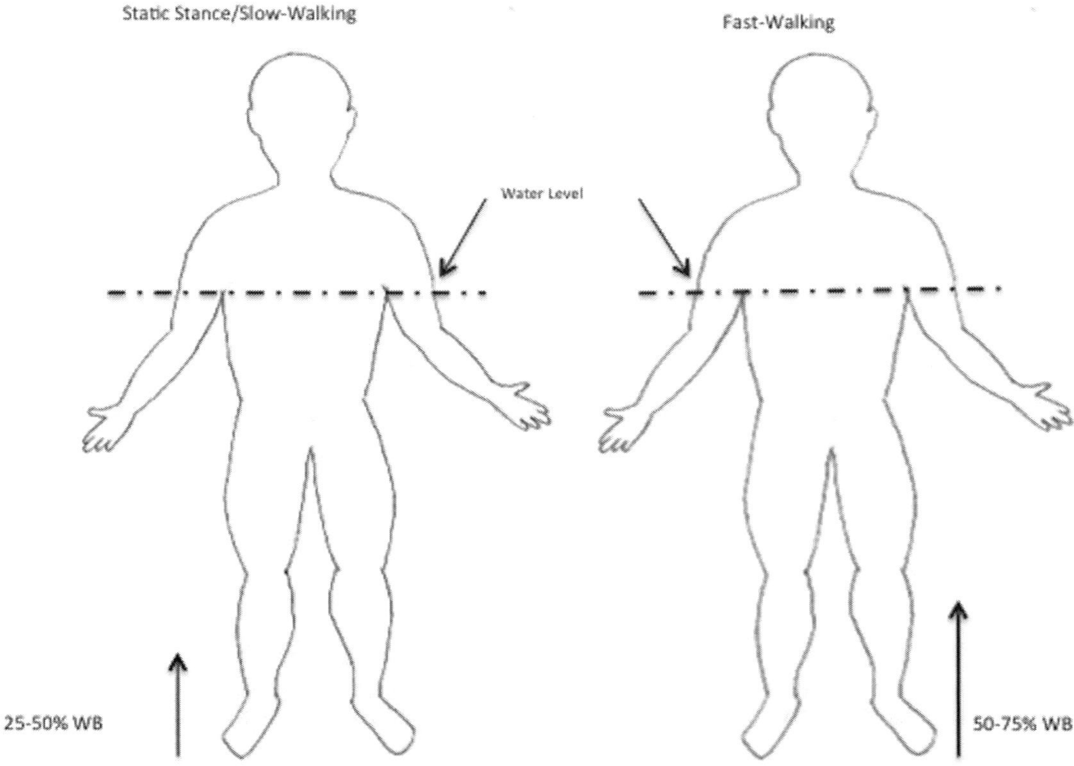

Fig. 14.4 Percent weight bearing through the lower extremity when submerged to the level of the xiphisternum. Note that increased walking speed increases the force up through the lower extremity

evaluation. An examination of the surgical site or sites and any pain in the area should be clearly documented. Discomfort in the region of the surgery is normal and intermittent increases are not uncommon with the start of physical therapy. Severe or constant pain in the area of the surgery or down into the lower extremity requires discussion with the referring surgeon or possible referral back to his or her office.

An evaluation of the patient's mobility can be performed directly or indirectly by observing specific tasks instructed to the patient or observing how he or she moves from one task to the next. Specific tasks and transfers should be evaluated under direct supervision and instruction. A gait assessment and proper use of any assistive devices must also be conducted. Noting any structural or biomechanical asymmetries, such as a leg-length discrepancy, is important and needs to be addressed immediately.

Gross strength and range of motion (ROM) should be documented. The extremes of hip ROM should be avoided secondary to the accompanying stress placed on the SIJs. Soft tissue lengthening during ROM testing must also be performed with caution to avoid disruption of any surgical reapproximation or disruption of the fusion site. Lumbar spine ROM should not be tested until at least 12 weeks postsurgery. Manual muscle testing of any muscle with direct attachment to the sacrum or ligamentous structures supporting the SIJs should be done with caution or avoided. Muscles to take caution with are the hip extensors, hip lateral rotators, and low back extensors. Hip flexion strength should not be assessed in patients with concurrent lumbar fusions.

A complete neurological examination should also be conducted. Reflexes and sensation should be tested and documented. Decreasing sensation in the buttock or lower extremity is not to be expected and needs careful evaluation for possible referral back to the surgeon.

Pain Control and Tissue Remodeling

Pain is a natural consequence of surgery. Pain control is important and can be achieved in a variety of ways. Medication prescribed by the surgeon can be helpful, but side effects such as lethargy and impaired balance can interfere with the goals of physical therapy. Ice can be used on the site of pain for periods of 20 min. At least 20 min should pass before reapplying the ice to protect the skin. Other modalities such as transcutaneous electrical nerve stimulation (TENS) can also be used in cases of moderate to severe pain. Ultrasound should not be used over any surgical implants or fusion sites.

Scar mobilizations are helpful to break up any adhesions that may form during the scarring process. Surgical scars resulting from various approaches can range from one or several small scars, found in minimally invasive procedures, to large scars, found in open procedures. Tissue tightens when scarred and manual mobilizations can help to soften it and promote proper collagen realignment.

Correcting Tissue and Joint Dysfunction

Patients may present with structural dysfunction that has developed over many months or years prior to surgery. A patient who had been dealing with chronic pain for several years is not uncommon. Addressing this dysfunction, such as weakness, tightness, hypermobility, and/or hypomobility, is important.

Stretching and strengthening soft tissue in the surrounding areas can help optimize the biomechanics in the area of the SIJ. Some of the larger, more superficial muscles such as the gluteus maximus, biceps femoris, and erector spinae attach in the area of the SIJs and have a direct or indirect effect on SIJ motion via their attachments to bone and ligamentous structures [4]. The lateral rotators of the hip and hamstrings should be gently stretched avoiding unnecessary strain on the SIJs and/or surgical site and minimizing any neural irritation (Fig. 14.5).

The hip flexors may also be tight or under spasm and require stretching; however, this should be avoided initially in patients with concurrent lumbar fusions. The quadratus lumborum may also be under spasm and can be corrected with different manual techniques and biomechanical modifications.

Strengthening of the low back, buttock, hip, posterior thigh, and abdominal musculature is important. Resistance exercises should be avoided in Phase 2 and gradually integrated in Phase 3. Good coordination and contribution of the surrounding musculature is important to minimize compensation and overactivation of neighboring muscles. Single-leg stance exercises should be avoided at this time.

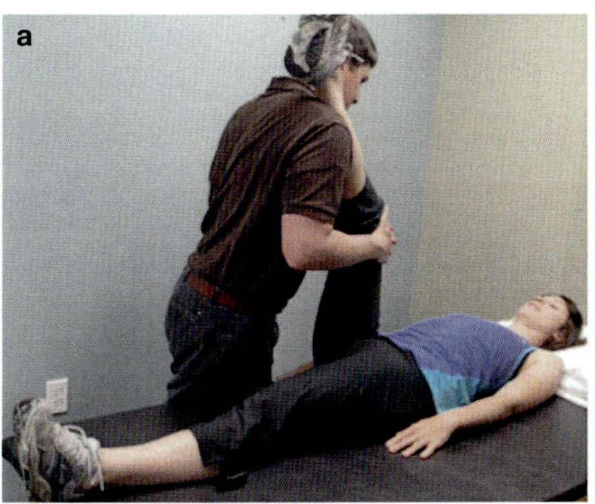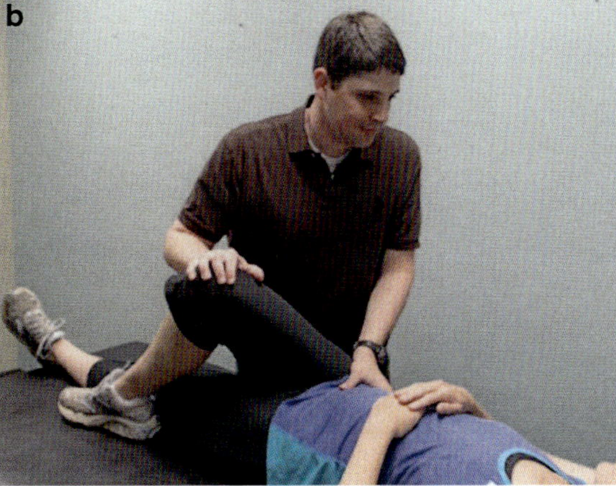

Fig. 14.5 (**a**) Stretch for the hamstrings. (**b**) Stretch for the lateral rotators of the hip

Joint mobility of the hips and thoracolumbar spine should be addressed. If stiffness is present in one or both hips, gentle mobilizations should begin. It is important to avoid end-range hip motion since this will place excessive stress on the fusion site and surrounding tissues. Mobility through the thoracic and lumbar spine is also important to allow for minimal stress on the fusion site and to prepare these areas for slight increases in mobility demands due to the decreased motion at the SIJ following the fusion. Mobilization techniques used through the thoracic and lumbar spine should also be gentle. Vigorous mobilizations can lead to increased symptoms and delayed progress. If symptoms experienced by the patient increase, the mobilizations targeting that area should be discontinued.

Stabilization

Reeducation of the core musculature must begin immediately. Improving on when, how much, and for how long muscles around the SIJ are activated will help optimize the biomechanics of the area surrounding the fused SIJ. Abnormal activation patterns of the gluteus maximus, biceps femoris, deep abdominals, and epaxial muscles are common in patients with SIJ dysfunction prior to surgery [5]. The deep abdominals and multifidi help to improve the stability of the SIJ by increasing force closure via their attachment to the ilium, lumbosacral spine, and thoracolumbar fascia [6] (Fig. 14.3). When motion is decreased at one joint, there tends to be compensation for that loss at adjacent joints. In the case of a unilateral SIJ fusion, the fused joint will no longer move but will likely put extra, and asymmetrical, stress on the contralateral SIJ and lumbar spine. If not controlled, this motion can possibly lead to pathology at these tissues. The draw-in maneuver, to activate the deep abdominals and multifidi, should be instructed and proper technique should be ensured (Fig. 14.6).

Progression of core stabilization exercises is made on an individual basis with the physical therapist using his or her discretion. The patient must demonstrate proper technique and body awareness before any stabilization exercise can be progressed.

Pelvic floor muscle reeducation is also important. These muscles form a sling through the pelvis to support the pelvic viscera and are active during respiration. They activate prior to movement and

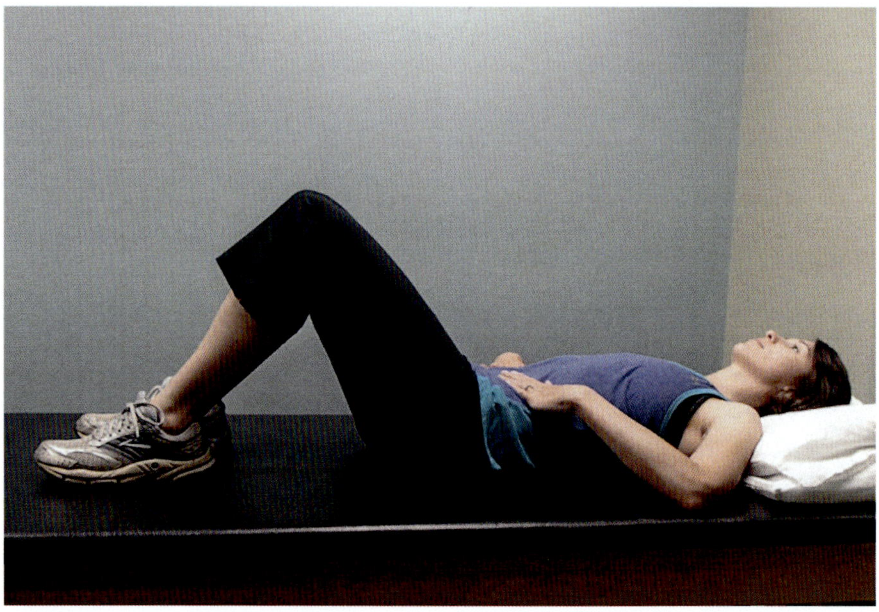

Fig. 14.6 Abdominal draw-in maneuver: engaging the deep abdominals to stabilize the lumbar spine and pelvis while continuing to breathe

increases in intra-abdominal pressure [7, 8] and often demonstrate abnormal activation patterns in patients with SIJ dysfunction [9]. The pelvic floor muscles also help to increase the stiffness of the SIJs via their attachments to the coccyx and sacrum and ability to oppose lateral motion of the coxal bones [10, 11]. Kegel exercises to help retrain this muscle group should be initiated early on in Phase 2.

Mobility

Activity should be less than moderate intensity and consist of ADLs, walking, and/or other light cardiovascular activities. Prolonged positions should be avoided, especially sitting. Patients should be instructed to sit for no more than 20 min with forces distributed evenly over their buttocks, using a firm cushion, while keeping their lumbar spine in a neutral position (natural lordotic curve). A lumbar roll can be used to help assist the patient in keeping their lumbar spine in the neutral position. Long or bumpy car rides should be avoided. Stabilization and postural exercises performed during this phase of rehabilitation will improve the patient's body awareness and core support to help optimize lumbar spine position.

Position transfers must be performed with caution and with proper technique. Increased stress is placed on the SIJs with changes in position, especially going from supine to standing [12–14]. While supine, the sacrum is at near end-range counternutation or sacral extension. As the patient sits up and finally stands, the sacrum is now at near end-range nutation or sacral flexion. Educating the patient how to logroll from supine to sitting and then with the spine held in neutral transition to standing is very important to minimize stress across the fusion site.

Single-leg stance should be avoided until complete bony fusion of the SIJ has occurred. Shear force through the SIJ is increased while standing on one leg [12, 15]. The ridges and depressions found throughout the auricular surface of the SIJ help to increase the coefficient of friction and reduce shear [16]. However, motion still occurs and could be harmful to the fusion site if not careful.

Similar to single-leg stance, a leg-length discrepancy can also cause asymmetrical forces through the SIJs. A leg-length discrepancy of 1.0 cm can increase the force up through the SIJ on the side of the longer limb 6-fold, while a 3.0 cm discrepancy can increase it 20-fold [17]. Correction of the discrepancy with a heel lift or other modifiable means may be helpful during the healing phase. However, caution with long-term use is recommended secondary to altered biomechanics at other body parts.

Gait training will start immediately. Improving gait symmetry and normalizing the biomechanics associated with gait is the long-term goal. Early on, patients may need to be instructed to decrease their step length. This will decrease pelvic rotation and minimize single-leg stance time. Also, a decreased step length can lessen the stress on the biceps femoris at the end of swing phase and beginning of stance phase. The biceps femoris often has attachment to the sacrotuberous ligament and can impart an extension force on the sacrum when stressed [18]. Upper body rotation is important and is reciprocal to lower body rotation. This coupled motion is due to the relationship of the latissimus dorsi and contralateral gluteus maximus [19]. Stiff and guarded motion will promote more stiffness and tissue dysfunction. Immediate verbal cueing and feedback can help break abnormal gait patterns quickly.

Phase 3, Weeks 12–19

At 3 months postsurgery, activity level should be of moderate intensity and most patients will return to work with or without modifications in time and duties. Patients with sedentary jobs will need to be educated on continued avoidance of prolonged positions, especially prolonged sitting. A workstation ergonomic evaluation may be necessary and frequent standing breaks every 20 min will be required. Some people may even find it beneficial to temporarily raise their workstations to elbow height and stand for the majority of the day, taking seated breaks as necessary.

Single-leg stance exercises may begin during this phase. Single-leg stance exercises can be

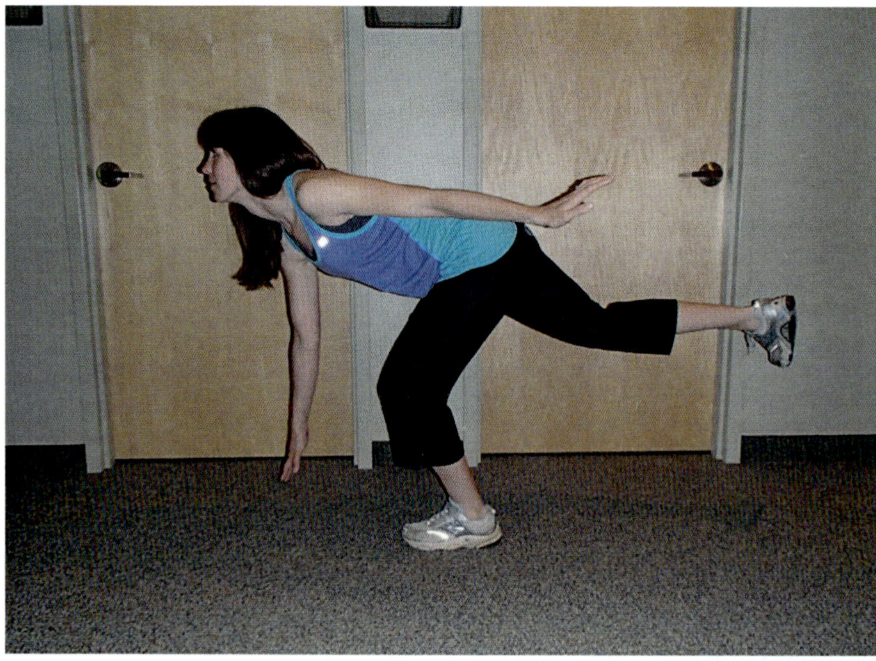

Fig. 14.7 Single-leg bird dip: the lumbar spine and pelvis are held in a neutral position, while flexion occurs at the hip

used to challenge hip and core stability and to improve balance (Fig. 14.7). High impact exercises like bounding and skipping should be avoided.

The HEP continues to progress with the addition of more challenging exercises and increased repetitions. Resistance exercises targeting muscles around the SIJ may be initiated. Compound exercises using the sagittal, coronal, and axial planes simultaneously are incorporated and progressed. The patient must be reminded that compliance with the HEP is still very important and needs to be completed 4–5 times per week.

Phase 4, Weeks 20 and Up

Most patients will have no restrictions with everyday activities at this time. The exception is contact sports. Football, volleyball, and/or any other sport or activity that may potentially lead to excessive forces on the body that can cause injury must be avoided. Patients are encouraged to continue with the HEP and to stay active to promote proper tissue remodeling. Tissue remodeling can

continue for up to 2 years postsurgery. Patients should now have the tools they need in regard to knowledge and exercises to manage flare-ups and to keep steady progress.

Sport-specific exercises and/or higher impact exercises can be initiated. Proper exercise technique is important, and the patient should be instructed to make good decisions and to listen to his or her body. If symptoms begin to increase, he or she must cease the provocative activity immediately. Clearance from the referring surgeon must be obtained before any return to sport. The body should now have a stable foundation with optimized biomechanics and will be able to tolerate these higher-level activities without further injury.

Summary

Postsurgical rehabilitation for a SIJ fusion can be complex. Knowledge of which surgical approach was used and whether the fusion was unilateral, bilateral, and/or involved the lumbar spine is very important. Tissues heal at different speeds, and being aware of what tissues are stressed and how long it has been since surgery is important. The rehabilitation process should be individualized to each patient and close communication with the referring surgeon is essential. Progress is rarely linear and often varies day to day. However, weekly progress should be seen. Building symmetry in muscle strength, stability, flexibility, and force transfer is essential for progress, patient satisfaction, and prevention of future injury.

References

1. Mens JM, Damen L, Snijders CJ, Stam HJ. The mechanical effect of a pelvic belt in patients with pregnancy-related pelvic pain. Clin Biomech (Bristol, Avon). 2006;21:122–7.
2. Vleeming A, Buyruk HM, Stoeckart R, et al. An integrated therapy for peripartum pelvic instability: a study of the biomechanical effects of pelvic belts. Am J Obstet Gynecol. 1992;166:1243–7.
3. Harrison RA, Hillman M, Bulstrode S. Loading of the lower limb when walking partially immersed: implications for clinical practice. Physiotherapy. 1992;78(3):64–167.
4. van Wingerden JP, Vleeming A, Buyruk HM, et al. Stabilization of the sacroiliac joint in vivo: verification of muscular contribution to force closure of the pelvis. Eur Spine J. 2004;13:199–205.
5. Hungerford B, Gilleard W, Hodges P. Evidence of altered lumbopelvic muscle recruitment in the presence of sacroiliac joint pain. Spine. 2003;28(14):1593–600.
6. Richardson CA, Snijders CJ, Hides JA, et al. The relation between the transversus abdominis muscles, sacroiliac joint mechanics, and low back pain. Spine (Phila Pa 1976). 2002;27:399–405.
7. Hodges PW, Sapsford R, Pengel LH. Postural and respiratory functions of the pelvic floor muscles. Neurourol Urodyn. 2007;26:362–71.
8. Sapsford RR, Hodges PW. Contraction of the pelvic floor muscles during abdominal manoeuvres. Arch Phys Med Rehabil. 2001;82:1081–8.
9. O'Sullivan PB, Beales DJ, Beetham JA, et al. Altered motor control strategies in subjects with sacroiliac joint pain during the active straight-leg-raise test. Spine (Phila Pa 1976). 2002;27:E1–8.
10. Pel JJ, Spoor CW, Pool-Goudzwaard AL, et al. Biomechanical analysis of reducing sacroiliac joint shear load by optimization of pelvic muscle and ligament forces. Ann Biomed Eng. 2008;36:415–24.
11. Pool-Goudzwaard AL, Hoek van Dijke GA, van Gurp M, Mulder P, Snijders CJ, Stoeckart R. Contribution of pelvic floor muscles to stiffness of the pelvic ring. Clin Biomech. 2004;19:564–71.
12. Egund N, Olsson TH, Schmid H, Selvik G. Movements in the sacroiliac joints demonstrated with roentgen stereophotogrammetry. Acta Radiol Diagn. 1978;19:833–46.
13. Sturesson B, Uden A, Vleeming A. A radiostereometric analysis of movements of the sacroiliac joints during the standing hip flexion test. Spine. 2000;25(3):364–8.
14. Weisl H. The movements of the sacro-iliac joint. Acta Anat. 1955;23:80–91.
15. Kissling RO, Jacob HA. The mobility of the sacroiliac joint in healthy subjects. Bull Hosp Jt Dis. 1996;54(3):158–64.
16. Vleeming A, Stoeckart R, Volkers AC, et al. Relation between form and function in the sacroiliac joint. Part I: clinical anatomical aspects. Spine (Phila Pa 1976). 1990;15:130–2.
17. Kiapour A, Abdelgawad AA, Goel VK, et al. Relationship between limb length discrepancy and load distribution across the sacroiliac joint – a finite element study. J Orthop Res. 2012;30:1577–80.
18. Vleeming A, van Wingerden JP, Snijders CJ, et al. Load application to the sacrotuberous ligament; influences of sacroiliac joint mechanics. Clin Biomech. 1989;4(4):204–9.
19. Mooney V, Pozos R, Vleeming A, et al. Exercise treatment for sacroiliac pain. Orthopedics. 2001;24:29–32.

Arnold Graham Smith

Introduction

This chapter will discuss the generalities of common types of complications as they pertain to any general orthopedic surgical procedure and some suggestions as to how to avoid certain pitfalls that may lead to such complications. The discussion will then focus on specific complications for sacroiliac joint (SIJ) fusion as they pertain to the approach used to obtain that fusion. Considerations for salvage are then discussed.

Generalities

All operative treatment may be accompanied by complications due to infection or venous thrombosis due to the natural increase in platelet adhesiveness that comes with surgery. As preventative, antibiotics are given before and during surgery, and many patients are fitted with elastic hose, which they are required to wear for 14 days, at which time platelet adhesiveness returns to normal. Cardiovascular problems and pulmonary problems may also occur, for which general medical clearance is advisable before the operation.

It is well documented that smokers are less likely to heal bony fusion (Patel et al. [1]; Al-Hidathy et al. [2]), so discussing this with the patient and offering nicotine skin patches or Wellbutrin tablets to enable the patient to stop smoking before the surgery may improve outcome. Similarly, smokers and an increasing number of older patients are known to have a risk of osteopenia and osteoporosis [3], which are most frequently seen on X-rays or CT scans. DEXA scans with bone density measurements may be indicated before the operation. In cases of severe decrease in bone density, treatment by an endocrinologist or a rheumatologist may be needed before surgery, as with any procedure that attempts to utilize instrumentation to stabilize and fuse bones together, SIJ Fusions are subject to malposition, loosening, breakage, and failure to achieve the fusion as well.

Complications Specific to SIJ Fusion

The Original "Postero Lateral Long Arc" Incisional Approach

Specific complications for this approach include:
- Cluneal nerve injury.
- Injury to the superior gluteal artery.
- Injury to the sciatic nerve.
- Gluteal muscle injury resulting in abductor weakness.
- Fracture of the iliac wing.
- Failure of fusion.

A.G. Smith, M.D., P.A. (✉)
Orthopaedic surgery, Baptist Medical Center – South,
9191 R.G. Skinner Pkwy #103, Jacksonville,
FL 32256, USA
e-mail: backchap2@aol.com

B.E. Dall et al. (eds.), *Surgery for the Painful, Dysfunctional Sacroiliac Joint,*
DOI 10.1007/978-3-319-10726-4_15, © Springer International Publishing Switzerland 2015

Smith-Petersen and Rogers first described this approach [4].

In this posterior procedure, extensive stripping of the gluteus maximus muscle was required, leading to the possibilities of developing a hematoma or injuring the gluteal artery and nerve and also to postoperative muscle scarring. The ilium is cut through to enable a direct approach to the SIJ. This is the bone from which bone marrow is harvested, so significant blood loss may be encountered. In their account of 26 cases, these complications are not mentioned. No internal fixation is described so the nerves that travel through the sacrum are not at risk. However, the cluneal nerves are at risk in the cephalad portion of the incision.

The Anterior Approach

Specific complications for this approach include:
- Injury to the lateral cutaneous nerve during initial exposure.
- Injury to the deep nerves and vessels.
- Special consideration for the L4, L5, and S1 nerve roots overlying the anterior joint surface.
- Injury to gastrointestinal and genitourinary structures.
- Hematoma formation.
- Osteoporosis of the sacrum causing poor screw fixation.
- Failure of fusion.

Orthopedic trauma surgeons, who are very familiar with pelvic anatomy, may more often use the anterior approach. A long (20 cm) incision is made along the anterior iliac crest. The lateral cutaneous nerve of the thigh is vulnerable, especially if the leg is extended, so it is important to keep the hip flexed. Access to the front of the joint is by subperiosteal dissection deep to the iliacus muscle, on which lie the great vessels, and, at the caudal portion of the joint, the sciatic nerve. Retraction may lead to thrombosis or nerve damage, and the deepest part of the joint, which is caudal, cannot easily be reached by an anterior approach. Removal of cartilage, grafting,

and plating have to be done lateral to the L5 and S1 nerves, in the superior, shallow part of the joint. Bone is harvested from the inner table of the pelvis, giving rise to the potential for hematoma formation.

The Posterior Approach

Specific complications for this approach include:
- Cluneal nerve injury.
- Deep vessel or nerve injury if the anterior sacrum is penetrated.
- Potential chronic pain from prominent posterior hardware.
- Hematoma formation.
- Failure of fusion.
- Incisional problems if closure is not complete and tight.
- Bony prominence at fusion site if proper deep fascial closure is not performed correctly.

The safest approach is directly dorsal to the joint. Initially using a 10 cm incision, which lies medial to the cluneal nerves and has now been reduced to 3 cm, as described by Dr. Donner (personal communication, 2013), the cartilage from both sides of the joint can be curetted, followed by decortication and grafting. Using the longer incision, internal fixation is easy and safe. A pedicle screw [5] may be placed in the S1 pedicle, and a second screw may be placed between the tables of the ilium, using care because the ilium is sloping outward at an angle of about 50°. Often, the prominence of the posterior superior iliac spine has been harvested for bone graft, making placement of the second screw easier. A short rod between the two screws will help to hold the SIJ securely while fusion occurs. The patient is encouraged to be non-weight bearing until all pain has gone. In the account by Belanger and Dall [5], they suggested that a midline incision with a fascial splitting approach can be used to achieve the same outcome with minimal risk to the cluneal nerves. Also the approach allows for deep fascia to fascia closure over the instrumentation and bone grafting, and full weight bearing is allowed postoperatively.

The Direct Lateral Approach

Specific complications for this approach include:
- Superior gluteal artery injury.
- Sciatic nerve injury.
- Nerve root injury in the S1 or S2 foramina.
- Deep vessel or nerve injury if anterior sacrum penetrated.
- Bowel injury if anterior sacrum is penetrated.
- Iliac wing fracture.
- Failure of fusion.

It is the lateral approach to the joint that carries most hazards. The L5 nerve leaves its foramen and travels on the anterior surface of the sacrum to join the S1 nerve on the piriformis muscle, on the anterior surface of the SIJ. The S1 nerve, having passed over the L5-S1 disc, enters its own tunnel to emerge half way down the SIJ, moving obliquely and laterally. Both of these nerves are vulnerable to fixation devices inserted from lateral to medial. Cannulated screws [6], or the more recently described minimally invasive surgery (MIS) systems [7–9], cannot be accurately located by fluoroscopy alone and require CT studies, either intraoperatively or postoperatively, to assure the surgeon that they are safely placed. EMG intra-operative testing has been found to be deficient, for it only records abnormality if the nerve is in direct contact with an implant.

CT Scanning Considerations

Much has been written recently about the radiation hazards of CT scans [10]. Consequently, they are to be used strategically, and not repeated unnecessarily. A preoperative CT scan is most helpful in planning the operation, for anatomical variation in the shape of the sacrum can be seen no other way [11]. The author finds that the coronal reconstruction is often surprisingly informative. A CT scan during the operation, or in the first 24 h after surgery, ensures that the patient is able to leave the hospital secure in the knowledge that emergency readmission for neurological reasons will not occur. Subsequent scans may not be needed if symptom improvement is achieved and maintained.

When Pain Returns

Unexpected symptoms may still arise postoperatively. One patient who was greatly relieved of pain following an MIS approach had recurrent symptoms after a motor vehicle accident and had to be bone grafted later in the year in order to get better. Another patient experienced increased back pain once the buttock pain had been relieved, and additional testing was required for the lumbar spine to determine the origin of the pain. This was not a complication, but the recognition of an ongoing symptom after the buttock pain had been relieved.

Salvage

SIJ surgical salvage is difficult to do successfully, and it is important for the patient to understand that this may be their last chance to reduce disabling buttock symptoms. No time lines can be accepted for healing a salvage operation.

If the symptoms of the patient persist, it is necessary to check that they are coming from the SIJ. Diagnostic injection into the SIJ, followed by a CT scan, will indicate whether the joint is still painful, and the CT scan will show if the bone graft has healed and if there is a problem with instrumentation. If it has healed, and the injection does not help, an alternative source of pain must be sought. This may implicate a facet joint, or a disc, or even an irritated nerve. It must always be remembered that, as Bernard and Kirkaldy-Willis wrote in 1987 [12], patients may have multiple pathology, of which the SIJ is only one part.

Nonunion of bone graft sometimes responds well to re-fixation. The author has a small number of cases in which pedicle screws have worked loose, and improved stabilization, using SI-Bone rods, has been rewarding. There are also cases in which stabilization alone has not provided adequate pain relief. This author believes it is very difficult to remove SI-Bone rods that have been in place for many weeks. In some cases, the addition of bone graft to the instrumentation, which the author refers to as the "hybrid operation," has led to significant improvement. Adequate length of incision is needed for this last operation, and cosmesis may need to be sacrificed in order to end disability.

Conclusion

This chapter has briefly touched on some of the general and specific complications that can be associated with procedures that fuse the SIJ. Also discussed were some items that might be utilized to prevent or lessen the possibility of a complication occurring. A few considerations on salvaging an unsuccessful SIJ fusion were discussed.

References

1. Patel RA, Wilson RF, Patel PA, Palmer RM. The effect of smoking on bone healing: a systematic review. Bone Joint Res. 2013;2(6):102–11.
2. Al-Hadithy N, Sewell MD, Bhavikatti M, Gkas PD. The effects of smoking on fracture healing and on various orthopaedic procedures. Acta Orthopaedica Belgica. 2012;78(3):285–90.
3. Dempster DW. Osteoporosis and the burden of osteoporosis-related fractures. Am J Manag Care. 2011;17:S164–9.
4. Smith-Petersen MN, Rogers WA. End-result study of arthrodesis of the sacro-iliac joint for arthritis – traumatic and non-traumatic. J Bone Joint Surg. 1926;8(1):118–36.
5. Belanger TA, Dall BE. Sacroiliac arthrodesis using a posterior midline fascial splitting approach and pedicle screw instrumentation: a new technique. J Spinal Disord. 2001;14(2):118–24.
6. Lippitt AB. Recurrent subluxation of the sacroiliac joint: diagnosis and treatment. Bull Hosp Joint Dis. 1995;54(2):94–102.
7. Al-khayer A, Hegarty J, Hahn D, Grevitt MP. Percutaneous sacroiliac joint arthrodesis: a novel technique. J Spinal Disord Tech. 2008;21(5):359–63.
8. Khurana A, Guha AR, Mohanty K, Ahuja S. Percutaneous fusion of the sacroiliac joint with hollow modular anchorage screws: clinical and radiological outcome. J Bone Joint Surg (Br). 2009;91-B:627–31.
9. Rudolf L. Sacroiliac joint arthrodesis-MIS technique with titanium implants: report of the first 50 patients and outcomes. Open Orthop J. 2012;6:495–502.
10. Brenner DJ, Hall EJ. Cancer risks from CT scans: now we have data, what next? Radiology. 2012;265(2):330–1.
11. Prassopoulos PK, Faflia CP, Voloudaki AE, Argyro E, Gourtsoyiannis NC. Sacroiliac joints: anatomical variants on CT. J Comput Assist Tomo. 1999;23(2):323–7.
12. Bernard TN, Kirkaldy-Willis WH. Recognizing specific characteristics of nonspecific low back pain. Clin Orthop Relat Res. 1987;217:266–80.

E. Jeffrey Donner

Moderator: Bruce E. Dall
Attendees: E. Jeffrey Donner, Michael Moore,
Sonia Eden, Arnold Graham Smith,
Michael Rahl

Question #1:
- What formal training have you had for diagnosing and treating both conservatively and surgically the dysfunctional sacroiliac joint (SIJ)?

BD: Jeff, would you start out with that?

EJD: Sure. Over 25 years ago I was trained in orthopedics and subsequently completed a spinal surgery fellowship in Philadelphia. I can confidently say, at that time, there was no discussion about sacroiliac dysfunction, pain, or treatment in either of those training programs other than if the patient had some type of pelvic trauma. Even within that group of patients with residual sacroiliac pain, the prognosis was "your pain will go away in time," and there was no direction beyond this.

BD: OK, Michael Rahl. You are our only physical therapist in the author group, and we would certainly be interested to hear what a physical therapist was taught about the dysfunctional SIJ.

MR: Well, sure. When I was in school, I think we spent one laboratory session, so about 2 h worth, talking about the biomechanics of the SIJ and learning different special tests to try to help identify SIJ dysfunction. We discussed how the reliability and sensitivity of the special tests were lacking and how cluster testing could be useful to help identify the SIJ or surrounding areas as the pain generator. We also discussed how special tests used to identify abnormal motion of the SIJ were not useful. In regard to treating dysfunction of the SIJ, there was really no discussion on treatment, what would be effective, or what would be the best approach to improving these patients. I think the instructors, like many PTs out there, were not well versed in the SIJ. I think, unfortunately, we as students left the class with the same lack of understanding. Since that point, I have tried to improve my knowledge of the SIJ through continuing education courses, reading the current literature, and talking with others involved with treating the SIJ.

E.J. Donner, M.D. (✉)
Colorado Spine Institute, 5285 McWhinney
Boulevard, Suite 145, Loveland, CO 80538, USA

University of Colorado Health, Medical Center
of the Rockies, 2500 Rocky Mountain Avenue,
Loveland, CO 80538, USA
e-mail: ejdonner@gmail.com

B.E. Dall et al. (eds.), *Surgery for the Painful, Dysfunctional Sacroiliac Joint*,
DOI 10.1007/978-3-319-10726-4_16, © Springer International Publishing Switzerland 2015

BD: Thank you very much. OK, the floor is open. Who else would like to comment on this?

BD: OK, I would have to say after lecturing to groups of orthopedic surgeons and groups of physical therapists, I was really amazed at the lack of understanding or knowledge base either of these groups had. I actually put on a symposium in our region in 2001 associated with Michigan State University on the diagnosis and treatment of the dysfunctional SIJ. The reason I did that was because I knew very little about it. I invited people from multiple disciplines to come in and lecture on it for a day. It was an extremely eye-opening experience for all of us, which probably is culminating in me wanting to put this book together 10 or 15 years later.

MM: Could I respond, Bruce?

BD: Yes.

MM: I had the good fortune of actually having some training during residency at the University of California at San Diego by one of the members of our faculty, David Gershuni, who is primarily a trauma surgeon. He would take care of most of the major pelvic trauma that came into our Level I trauma unit. In the course of following up some of these patients and other patients who did not have major pelvic trauma, we had a small number of patients who seemed to have pain arising from the SIJ. David is now deceased, but he basically taught me as a senior resident that some people do have pain arising from the SIJ. The way you diagnose it is by doing a CT-guided injection of local anesthetic into the synovial portion of the joint. If that relieves their pain transiently, they will respond positively to a sacroiliac fusion. We had about five patients on whom we operated and he showed me a modified Smith-Peterson technique of performing that surgery. What I recalled at the end of residency is that those patients had all done well. That was the extent of my formal training. I started looking for the problem as a fellow during my spine surgery fellowship and also early in practice. It was really quite by happenstance and by having this experience with that particular attending that I did receive some small portion of formal training, which ended up being a very positive experience in terms of developing an interest in this.

BD: Thank you very much. Let's go on to the second question.

Question #2:

–   How do most of your patients end up coming to your office?

BD: Who would like to answer that question?

BD: I would answer that question by saying we have actually studied this at our institution. The people who do not send SIJ patients to a surgeon like me for potential SIJ fusion are chiropractors and pain doctors; at least that has been my experience. Many of the patients I have ultimately operated on had been in years of continuous chiropractic treatment as well as getting injections one after another in situations where a firm diagnosis of SIJ dysfunction had long been made by the injecting clinician. In our study we found over half of the patients referred to our office, who ultimately went on to have an SIJ fusion, were referred by either their primary care physician or by their physical therapist. The rest of them literally found our office through the Internet after being told by their injection pain doctor "you need a SIJ fusion," but not being able to tell their patients where to go to get that done.

BD: Someone else?

EJD: One of the main referrers to my practice is me. I initially incorporated fluoroscopic injections into my practice a year after I went into clinical practice. I did not learn this in training, but I was very frustrated with the fact there were a lot of people I would see and could not give them the answer as to why they were having the variety of pains in their back, buttock, and leg. I also became very involved in the International Spinal Injection Society, which is now called International Spinal Interventional Society (ISIS). I learned these injection techniques and found I was eventually able to diagnose sacroiliac pain under fluoroscopy by blocking the SIJ if I could not reproduce pain with discography or eliminate it with facet injections. I believe a lot of these patients I see come to me because no one else could identify the source of their problem, especially 25 years ago when very few people were doing this. This experience led to my early adoption of sacroiliac dysfunction as a legitimate diagnosis and eventually, especially with Dr. Moore's help, I identified ways to treat this surgically.

BD: Very good. Thank you Jeff.

AGS: Bruce, can I answer the last question?

BD: Yes, please go ahead.

AGS: I would say the same that the Internet has been a steady source of referrals. Having taught in the community and in the state of Florida, I have found the people in the community and elsewhere in Florida who did not want to get involved in sacroiliitis would send the patients to me. So, I have had in-state referrals from local teaching and out-of-state referrals from the Internet.

BD: OK, thank you, Arnold.

Question #3:

 – As a surgeon, do you feel you can treat all cases of dysfunctional SIJs with one type of surgery, or do you feel you should have alternate procedures to fuse the SIJ under certain circumstances?

BD: Anyone want to tackle that?

MM: If I could respond to that, I believe at this point my first choice in treating someone with SIJ dysfunction would be one of the minimally invasive types of interventions of which there are several available now. I think there are some patients for whom that is not a practical consideration. For example, someone who has had a very extensive bone graft harvest from the ilium on the affected side may not have sufficient bone stock for one of the minimally invasive techniques to be successful. Again, this is just a personal bias based on dealing with these patients and is not really based on the data because such data does not exist. I think there are some patients for whom an open procedure is necessary because of unfavorable anatomy or because of prior surgery. If you need to perform extensive bone grafting in order to achieve an arthrodesis or stabilization, I think an open procedure may be preferable to one of the minimally invasive procedures. So, I do think there are some circumstances in which you have to modify your preferred procedure in order to accommodate the patient's pathology.

BD: Thank you, Mike.

SE: This is Sonia Eden. I just wanted to add that I agree with that. In addition, in certain patient populations, when we are addressing both spine and SIJ pathology on them simultaneously, there are some options for fusions of the SIJ in those patients that we can do at the same time we are doing the spine surgery. These may not necessarily have to be the lateral approach but perhaps could be the posterior approach that we do at Borgess.

BD: Thank you. Anyone else?

BD: OK, let's go onto the fourth question.

Question #4:

 – Should the SIJ be realigned before performing an SIJ fusion?

AGS: My response is to say if the patient is asleep, then the position in which the joint finds itself is perfectly good for me to fuse and I do not need to manipulate it while they are asleep.

BD: OK, anyone else?

EJD: There are a lot of patients who feel like their joint is not aligned. There are also a lot of providers in the chiropractic and physical therapy domains that are convinced the patient's symptoms are not only pain but also malalignment. As we know, the joint is a very complex structure with matching undulating surfaces. It does not take much of what we call malalignment, or displacement, of those normal surfaces to markedly increase the joint contact forces, which make the patient feel like there is significant malalignment. We have seen malalignment and subtle instability in shoulders as well as other joints in orthopedics. I think the SIJ is a unique joint, which can be very painful if there is minimal malalignment, but I don't recall seeing one that had been grossly malaligned after doing hundreds of these with an open approach. I do believe that if a patient and some medical provider feel like malalignment is an issue, the technique I presently use can potentially resolve that issue either by identifying it as not malaligned or attempting to realign the joint by operative techniques under direct visualization. I have not, however, seen a major shift, like 1 cm, you will often see in some of the medical reports by these providers.

BD: All right, thank you.

BD: In this textbook I suggested they do not need to be realigned and I gave the illustration of coming to this opinion by doing open posterior midline approaches to the SIJ on a few hundred patients. During that approach, I actually exposed the whole dorsal joint, removing the posterior superior iliac spine, removing all the posterior ligaments, and actually creating a space down into the joint itself which I then packed with bone before I put in all of the instrumentation. Part of the instrumentation was to put a fixation screw in the ilium and in the S1 pedicle. With those two screws in and grabbing them with large instruments (this is with the patient asleep and paralyzed and with all of the ligaments removed), I could barely move that joint. Most of the time I could not see the joint move. I recreated that situation in a cadaver study, which is also in this textbook as a chapter. The results were exactly the same, very little movement. So, I have trouble thinking that

anything dramatic is happening with realignment. We do know, when chiropractors "realign" the painful SIJ, that the patient frequently walks away less painful. So something positive happens with this process. I think we need more science to figure out what being realigned really means and what it is actually accomplishing on a biological level. It is good to talk about this subject.

BD: Anyone else? OK, question five.

Question #5:
 – Should bilateral SIJs be performed? If so, under what circumstances?

AGS: Well, it is just very difficult for the patient to be non-weight bearing if both SIJs are operated on at the same time. If they have a wheelchair and someone to push the wheelchair, fair enough. But it is asking an awful lot to be non-weight bearing while the graft heals. It is very difficult to be non-weight bearing if neither foot is allowed to touch the ground. That's all.

BD: OK, anyone else?

EJD: In my experience, bilateral SIJ fusion outcomes tend to be less favorable than unilateral SIJ surgeries. I believe it is for the same reasons Arnold suggested. Usually, I try to stage them, but the patients seem to say, "No, I really want to get this over with at one time; I will not weight bear and I will follow instructions." But that is really hard to do as Arnold suggested. I am really reluctant to do bilateral fusions at this time until we improve our technology.

BD: Thank you Jeff.

BD: I have performed several hundred SIJ fusions and I have done all of them from a posterior approach, which was either a posterior midline approach or a minimally invasive posterolateral approach. I have never had any patient partially weight bearing after any of these surgeries. I have allowed immediate weight bearing as tolerated every time. I have published papers on the surgeries I do on the SIJ with the most recent one in 2008, where we did a minimally invasive posterolateral approach with cages. Actually, over one-third of the patients in that study were bilateral, and there was no correlation between unilateral or bilateral in outcomes, and the outcomes were about 80 % successful (Fig. 7.12). I have continued to find that out. I am currently working on a paper to counter the paper written by Shutz [1] relating his terrible results from bilateral SIJ fusions. Our study has 15 patients followed for greater than two years with overall satisfaction of 87 % and a statistically valid drop in pain scores on the VAS. I frequently have fused SIJs bilaterally after which I use a sacral belt for immobilization unless a lumbar or lumbosacral fusion has simultaneously been performed and a TLSO with a pantaloon is used. So, it is sounding like my experience is quite different from others in this group.

EJD: Bruce, can I ask you a question?

BD: Yes.

EJD: Did you use INFUSE (Medtronic, Inc.) on these patients?

BD: Yes, I pretty much used INFUSE, off-label, my whole career, well once it was available. For example, INFUSE was used in all of the cages in the study that I published in 2008 on minimally invasive SIJ fusions. I can honestly say I never had a problem with INFUSE used for SIJ fusions. I do have more to say on that subject in reference to its use and the specific approach used by other surgeons, but I feel that is a subject for another day.

Question #6:
  – Is there a learning curve for performing SIJ fusions?

BD: The reason I put that question in here is because there are a lot of surgeons out there who obviously have not been trained in the SIJ fusion. They are interested in it, want to get involved in it, but they want to know what the learning curve is. I think all of us have been working on our learning curve for so many years that I guess the question becomes do you think there is a learning curve in the modern era with better knowledge, better teaching, and better equipment?

MM: I will respond to that. I think there is definitely a learning curve and I think the most important part of the learning curve is patient selection, because it is ultimately picking the right patient that has the biggest impact on clinical success, I believe. Having said that, I think there is a learning curve for performing the surgery. I think some of the new techniques are available with very good didactic and laboratory teaching programs that allow that curve to be much more abbreviated than it was compared to those of us who sort of had to feel our way along with doing the surgery. I think the most important part of the learning curve is patient selection, and I think it is easier for surgeons now if they have become comfortable with that to obtain specific training for procedures to fuse the SIJ.

BD: Mike, would you have an opinion as to whether the average SIJ fusion patient is a pretty straightforward patient or possibly a very complex patient with a lot of history behind them? Do you have an opinion on that?

MM: I think it is highly variable depending upon the subgroup you are discussing. I think someone who has had a multiply operated back and has either SIJ dysfunction as a consequence of prior lumbar surgery that involves the sacrum or perhaps has had coexistent pathology that has been treated and their SIJ dysfunction has not been identified until recently as a problem certainly is a more difficult patient to deal with. The subgroup of patients who have isolated SIJ pathology certainly have the best clinical success in my experience. Unfortunately, I would not say these are rare, but they are not the most common presentation. I would say it is more common that patients present with either coexistent or derivative pathology, and it is much more difficult to sort those out. However, if a practitioner is looking for and is conscious of the possibility of SIJ dysfunction being part of the differential diagnosis of low back pain, patients will present who are in that less complicated group and very good results can be expected.

BD: Thank you, Mike.

BD: Let's move on to question seven.

Question #7:

– Is morbid obesity a rate-limiting factor in performing SIJ fusions? If so, why?

SE: I do think morbid obesity may be a rate-limiting factor if you are using a minimally invasive approach because you rely a lot on x-ray imaging. If you cannot get adequate imaging on a patient because of their body habitus, then it makes it difficult to perform the fusion by that approach.

BD: OK, anyone else?

AGS: I would agree, but I would agree for a different reason. I think the minimally invasive procedure in very heavy patients is asking an awful lot for the minimally invasive support system to work. So, I think very heavy patients either need a lot more minimally invasive placed instrumentation, that is to say instead of three rods, they need four rods, five rods, or six rods; or they need an open procedure. I do not think the typical minimally invasive procedure is going to work very well in a very obese patient.

BD: In review of our institutional data on SIJ surgeries in the morbidly obese patient, we have found that having a BMI of >35 portended a more unsatisfactory result. Since 2008 we have operated on more than thirty morbidly obese patients, many bilateral, using both the posterior midline approach and the posterior lateral minimally invasive approach without hardware failure at long-term follow-up. I believe we need studies showing the stress to failure rates in cadavers using all these various approaches with the various different instrumentation types to see if there are significant differences between

them. If so, such data could help in deciding what type of approach and fixation device might offer the best benefit for a given patient.

Question #8

– Have you performed revision surgery for previous SIJ fusions? If so, what were the challenges you faced?

EJD: I would like to start off with my first experience resulting in a poor outcome over 20 years ago when I attempted to obtain a fusion expecting a good result using the Smith-Petersen approach even after being instructed by Dr. Moore who was very experienced. I found that this was a very challenging operation where I was passing a chisel in an area that seemed very unusual for me to operate on let alone all of the anatomy that could get you in trouble, so I am sure my poor result had something to do with that fear factor and inexperience. That being said, I had to revise the patient anteriorly after she failed to improve with that technique and a spica cast, which was a nightmare. The anterior approach led to a significant bleeding problem, which gave me gray hairs early on in my career. I am surprised I continued on this endeavor despite this experience, but I was convinced these patients really did have an SIJ problem and there had to be a better way to obtain reliable results with fewer complications. So, I decided to do more of a traditional orthopedic approach and remove the anatomy in my way, i.e., the PSIS, in order to get down to the articular cartilage, which I believed was the source of the pain in most of these patients and in most other painful joints, and then pack that joint with bone. Next, I ran a couple of screws across the joint under fluoroscopy. With that technique and then some modifications like you described using the pedicle screws in S1 and the iliac bone, I was able to increase the stability and fusion rates. My go-to operation would have been that open posterior approach, but I did find there was quite a bit of recovery from that approach and the eventual need to remove the hardware in the S1 area where the rod crosses the ilium. Consequently, what I did was try to eliminate all of those potential sources of pain and perform an approach that minimally interferes with all of the potential structures, which can cause post-op problems, like the cluneal nerve, gluteal neurovascular bundle, and the PSIS, and work in the zone above the sciatic notch and below the PSIS. I remove the cartilage and pack the joint with bone and some spacers, which help stabilize it. I think this is also a very valuable technique in patients who have failed to improve with screws or rods, which are still in place because you can still work below these devices and remove the cartilage leaving a wide surface area to perform a fusion, which is what you need. This is the technique I now prefer.

BD: OK, thank you. Anyone else?

AGS: I think we are all going to be involved in doing revision surgery. I have had a number of patients who have gone on the Internet and decided which procedure they want, and then they come to see me because I am listed as a surgeon who is familiar with the procedure. As a result, some of my patients demand an MIS procedure, and if it does not work, a revision is going to be required. Sometimes this is less than 1 year out and sometimes it may be 2 or 3 years. The laterally placed implants are often difficult to remove, so I have had to add bone graft dorsally, achieving a bone-to-bone fusion, leaving the implants in place. I have done this operation, which I refer to as a "hybrid" procedure, on five occasions and all have been pleased with the end result. There are more awaiting revision. The problem is that patient selection is being made more difficult as patients believe everything they read on the Internet.

BD: I have revised both failed lateral and posterior attempts at fusing the SIJ. Some of the most challenging cases are when instrumentation is inside the joint, such as cages or bone dowels, or the retained hardware is in a plane 90° from the plane being used for the insertion of new hardware or bone graft. We have used the Stryker Virtual Navigation system to maneuver around existing hardware in an effort to obtain fusions in challenging cases. The figure (Fig. 9.17) illustrates a complex case of a middle-aged female with a failed posterior midline fusion. After her index procedure she had the posterior hardware removed which did not relieve her pain. With the assistance of my Neurosurgical Spine partner, Dr. Mark Krinock, who was well versed in use of the Stryker Navigation System, she was revised and ultimately successfully fused.

BD: Anyone else? Well, let's get into a little of the theory.

Question #9:
 – Do you feel there are types of lumbosacral pathology that can mimic SIJ pain clinically even in the presence of a positive valid SIJ injection?

AGS: Bruce, please define what you mean by a positive valid SIJ injection.

BD: It was an intra-articular injection using an anesthetic agent, a steroid, and some dye. The dye verified that it was an intra-articular injection. The patient had much greater than 2 h of complete pain relief at least until the anesthetic wore off, which I think is the gold standard for saying that pain is coming from the SIJ. Does anyone feel when someone has something like that; there could actually be associated or causative pathology in the lumbar spine that could eliminate that pain if treated?

BD: The reason I threw this question in is because I have been confused by this situation more than once. The situation was the patient did have a valid injection as I have defined it and did get pain relief. Under normal circumstances, the patient would have had an SIJ fusion. But they also had significant lateral foraminal stenosis at the L4–L5 foramen. Because that was so apparent, that was injected also at a different setting, like two weeks later, and their pain went away again. So, the foramen was opened as their only procedure, and they quit having any symptoms at all. I have run into that scenario 2–3 times now and it makes me wonder if anyone else has come across such a combination of symptoms in such a patient. This is one of the reasons that the algorithm (Chap. 6) states to treat all the verified lumbar pathology first before proceeding to the SIJ.

BD: OK, well we will let that one go. Perhaps someone reading this discussion will be able to identify with this scenario. It does make me realize that with all the overlap in pain radiating musculoskeletal pathology in this region of the body, more work is needed to understand it all and nothing about the diagnosis of SIJ dysfunction seems to be straightforward.

Question #10:
 – How do you think the dysfunctional mostly stable SIJ generates pain? For example, do you feel it is all about micromotion and micro-instability? Is it about joint contact points or overstressing a pelvic ring causing one or most of the above? Or something else?

EJD: I believe this is like most things in orthopedics with multiple causes, and a lot of times they are overlapped. I look at this as I do other orthopedic joints, although it is unique as we have already described. No doubt, for the reasons we discussed earlier about the joint undulations, how minimally that joint has to be malaligned, and how minor trauma can sublux the joint enough to substantially increase the joint contact forces and cause degenera-

tion and pain over time, I have yet to see a grossly unstable or malaligned joint like we have discussed, but I think this concept of a keystone type compression joint with marked surface forces, the obesity problem, and the lumbosacral spine fusions are all compounding the problem.

BD: It is a complicated question and my feeling is likewise that it is multifactorial. We did a study at Globus Medical, Inc. (Audubon, PA) using cadavers. They were stripped of all muscle. What we did was to sequentially transect the posterior iliosacral ligament and then all of the posterior ligaments, each time testing the motion. It so happens, in the intact specimen, the joint under eight Newton meters of torque showed 1° or less of motion. When you cut these ligaments, it showed about 1.5° of motion, not a lot of motion. So, with our surgeries, we are literally stopping 1°, 1.5°, or 2° of motion and the pain stops. This is very interesting to me and makes me consider that motion does play a role of some kind in the pain production, but other variables are certainly at work.

BD: Let's go onto the last question.

Question #11:
 – Where do you see the surgical treatment for the dysfunctional SIJ going in the future? Do you think we will have total joints? Do you think we will have some sort of a moveable spacer?

EJD: Bruce, I feel very strongly that the majority of this pain is articular. Based on that and being an orthopedic surgeon who treats other articular problems, this surgical treatment either involves removing those surfaces and fusing them together or providing some type of surface replacement. We have been developing that latter technology. Although, as you can imagine especially in the United States and with the FDA, that is going to be a major challenge. The idea certainly has fit with other orthopedic principles and technologies, but I think extending that to the SIJ will be challenging.

BD: I do too. Right now there are a significant number of lateral devices for SIJ fusion. One of the reasons for that is because it is easy to get a device cleared by the FDA using the 510(k) application if you can prove whatever it is you are coming up with is somewhat similar to what was being marketed before May 28, 1976. The problem going into the future is that anything that goes directly into the joint from a posterior minimally invasive or a posterior open approach will be looked at by the FDA as new uncharted ground, and that gets to be very expensive for corporations to start going in that direction. I think the FDA is really going to be one of the rate-limiting factors for progress in SIJ surgery as we move ahead.

EJD: Well, Bruce, just a brief comment on that concept. I have found that in pre-submission meetings the FDA has been open to these concepts based on appropriate analogies, supporting science and biomechanical data. With that information, we are proceeding with developing technology specifically down the joint.

BD: This concludes the round-table discussion. It certainly has provided thought-provoking ideas and opinions. I want to thank all the authors who participated and look forward to more discussions like this one.

Reference

1. Schutz U, Grob D. Poor outcome following bilateral sacroiliac joint fusion for degenerative sacroiliac joint syndrome. Acta Orthopaedica Belg. 2006;72: 296–308.

Appendix A
LITERATURE SEARCH: Sacroiliac Joint Fusion Surgery—Outcomes/Complications

Prepared for Sonia Eden MD by Jennifer Barlow MILS, Borgess Library

April 11, 2013

Searches conducted in PubMed, EMBASE, CINAHL, Web of Science

Search 1: sacroiliac concept + surgery concept + fusion concept

Search 2: sacroiliac concept + surgery concept + fusion concept + outcomes concept

Search 3: sacroiliac concept + surgery concept + fusion concept + complications concept

Limits: Human subjects, English language

B.E. Dall et al. (eds.), *Surgery for the Painful, Dysfunctional Sacroiliac Joint,*
DOI 10.1007/978-3-319-10726-4, © Springer International Publishing Switzerland 2015

PubMed Search

Search	Query	Items found
#25	Search (#14 AND #24) Filters: Humans; English Sort by: PublicationDate	60
#26	Select 60 document(s) (SEARCH 3 RESULTS)	60
#24	Search (#21 OR #22 OR #23) Filters: Humans; English	1446753
#23	Search adverse effects[MeSH Subheading] Filters: Humans; English	1049685
#22	Search postoperative complications[MeSH Terms] Filters: Humans; English	260667
#21	Search complication*[Title/Abstract] Filters: Humans; English	382360
#19	Search (#14 AND #18) Filters: Humans; English Sort by: PublicationDate	45
#20	Select 45 document(s) (SEARCH 2 RESULTS)	45
#18	Search (#16 OR #17) Filters: Humans; English	981307
#17	Search treatment outcome[MeSH Terms] Filters: Humans; English	497352
#16	Search outcome*[Title/Abstract] Filters: Humans; English	653844
#14	Search (#3 AND #7 AND #10) Filters: Humans; English Sort by: PublicationDate	93
#15	Select 93 document(s) (SEARCH 1 RESULTS)	93
#13	Search (#3 AND #7 AND #10) Filters: English	100
#12	Select 120 document(s)	120
#11	Search (#3 AND #7 AND #10) Sort by: PublicationDate	120
#10	Search (#8 OR #9)	137510
#9	Search spinal fusion[MeSH Terms]	15534
#8	Search fusion[Title/Abstract]	131404
#7	Search (#4 OR #5 OR #6)	2811909
#6	Search surgical procedures, operative[MeSH Terms]	2246906
#5	Search surgical[Title/Abstract]	626989
#4	Search surgery[Title/Abstract]	715707
#3	Search (#1 OR #2)	4432
#2	Search sacroiliac joint[MeSH Terms]	3000
#1	Search sacroiliac[Title/Abstract]	2961

EMBASE Search

No.	Query	Results
#28	sacroiliac:ti AND [humans]/lim AND [english]/lim OR (sacroiliac:ab AND [humans]/lim AND [english]/lim) OR ('sacroiliac joint'/exp AND [humans]/lim AND [english]/lim) AND (surgery:ti AND [humans]/lim AND [english]/lim OR (surgery:ab AND [humans]/lim AND [english]/lim) OR (surgery:lnk AND [humans]/lim AND [english]/lim) OR (surgical:ti AND [humans]/lim AND [english]/lim) OR (surgical:ab AND [humans]/lim AND [english]/lim) OR ('surgery'/exp AND [humans]/lim AND [english]/lim)) AND (fusion:ti AND [humans]/lim AND [english]/lim OR (fusion:ab AND [humans]/lim AND [english]/lim) OR ('spine fusion'/exp AND [humans]/lim AND [english]/lim)) AND (complication*:ti AND [humans]/lim AND [english]/lim OR (complication*:ab AND [humans]/lim AND [english]/lim) OR ('postoperative complication'/exp AND [humans]/lim AND [english]/lim) OR ('adverse effects' AND [humans]/lim AND [english]/lim) OR ('adverse effect'/exp AND [humans]/lim AND [english]/lim)) (SEARCH 3 RESULTS)	42
#27	complication*:ti AND [humans]/lim AND [english]/lim OR (complication*:ab AND [humans]/lim AND [english]/lim) OR ('postoperative complication'/exp AND [humans]/lim AND [english]/lim) OR ('adverse effects' AND [humans]/lim AND [english]/lim) OR ('adverse effect'/exp AND [humans]/lim AND [english]/lim)	909491
#26	'adverse effect'/exp AND [humans]/lim AND [english]/lim	215598
#25	'adverse effects' AND [humans]/lim AND [english]/lim	66945
#24	'postoperative complication'/exp AND [humans]/lim AND [english]/lim	298599
#23	complication*:ab AND [humans]/lim AND [english]/lim	444084
#22	complication*:ti AND [humans]/lim AND [english]/lim	60450
#21	sacroiliac:ti AND [humans]/lim AND [english]/lim OR (sacroiliac:ab AND [humans]/lim AND [english]/lim) OR ('sacroiliac joint'/exp AND [humans]/lim AND [english]/lim) AND (surgery:ti AND [humans]/lim AND [english]/lim OR (surgery:ab AND [humans]/lim AND [english]/lim) OR (surgery:lnk AND [humans]/lim AND [english]/lim) OR (surgical:ti AND [humans]/lim AND [english]/lim) OR (surgical:ab AND [humans]/lim AND [english]/lim) OR ('surgery'/exp AND [humans]/lim AND [english]/lim)) AND (fusion:ti AND [humans]/lim AND [english]/lim OR (fusion:ab AND [humans]/lim AND [english]/lim) OR ('spine fusion'/exp AND [humans]/lim AND [english]/lim)) AND (outcome*:ti AND [humans]/lim AND [english]/lim OR (outcome*:ab AND [humans]/lim AND [english]/lim) OR ('treatment outcome'/exp AND [humans]/lim AND [english]/lim)) (SEARCH 2 RESULTS)	49
#20	outcome*:ti AND [humans]/lim AND [english]/lim OR (outcome*:ab AND [humans]/lim AND [english]/lim) OR ('treatment outcome'/exp AND [humans]/lim AND [english]/lim)	1260038
#19	'treatment outcome'/exp AND [humans]/lim AND [english]/lim	728764
#18	outcome*:ab AND [humans]/lim AND [english]/lim	781175
#17	outcome*:ti AND [humans]/lim AND [english]/lim	166270
#16	sacroiliac:ti AND [humans]/lim AND [english]/lim OR (sacroiliac:ab AND [humans]/lim AND [english]/lim) OR ('sacroiliac joint'/exp AND [humans]/lim AND [english]/lim) AND (surgery:ti AND [humans]/lim AND [english]/lim OR (surgery:ab AND [humans]/lim AND [english]/lim) OR (surgery:lnk AND [humans]/lim AND [english]/lim) OR (surgical:ti AND [humans]/lim AND [english]/lim) OR (surgical:ab AND [humans]/lim AND [english]/lim) OR ('surgery'/exp AND [humans]/lim AND [english]/lim)) AND (fusion:ti AND [humans]/lim AND [english]/lim OR (fusion:ab AND [humans]/lim AND [english]/lim) OR ('spine fusion'/exp AND [humans]/lim AND [english]/lim)) (SEARCH 1 RESULTS)	124
#15	fusion:ti AND [humans]/lim AND [english]/lim OR (fusion:ab AND [humans]/lim AND [english]/lim) OR ('spine fusion'/exp AND [humans]/lim AND [english]/lim)	65348
#14	'spine fusion'/exp AND [humans]/lim AND [english]/lim	12313
#13	fusion:ab AND [humans]/lim AND [english]/lim	58356
#12	fusion:ti AND [humans]/lim AND [english]/lim	15182
#11	surgery:ti AND [humans]/lim AND [english]/lim OR (surgery:ab AND [humans]/lim AND [english]/lim) OR (surgery:lnk AND [humans]/lim AND [english]/lim) OR (surgical:ti AND [humans]/lim AND [english]/lim) OR (surgical:ab AND [humans]/lim AND [english]/lim) OR ('surgery'/exp AND [humans]/lim AND [english]/lim)	2241657

(continued)

No.	Query	Results
#10	'surgery'/exp AND [humans]/lim AND [english]/lim	1879248
#9	surgical:ab AND [humans]/lim AND [english]/lim	418000
#8	surgical:ti AND [humans]/lim AND [english]/lim	90096
#7	surgery:lnk AND [humans]/lim AND [english]/lim	1066667
#6	surgery:ab AND [humans]/lim AND [english]/lim	517864
#5	surgery:ti AND [humans]/lim AND [english]/lim	153798
#4	sacroiliac:ti AND [humans]/lim AND [english]/lim OR (sacroiliac:ab AND [humans]/lim AND [english]/lim) OR ('sacroiliac joint'/exp AND [humans]/lim AND [english]/lim)	3386
#3	'sacroiliac joint'/exp AND [humans]/lim AND [english]/lim	2458
#2	sacroiliac:ab AND [humans]/lim AND [english]/lim	2330
#1	sacroiliac:ti AND [humans]/lim AND [english]/lim	872

CINAHL Search

#	Query	Limiters/Expanders	Results	Action
S15	S4 AND S10 AND S14	Expanders—Apply related words; Also search within the full text of the articles Search modes—Find all my search terms (SEARCH 1 RESULTS)	7	
S14	S11 OR S12 OR S13	Expanders—Apply related words; Also search within the full text of the articles Search modes—Find all my search terms	2,377	
S13	MH spinal fusion	Limiters—English Language; Human Expanders—Apply related words; Also search within the full text of the articles Search modes—Find all my search terms	1,336	
S12	AB fusion	Limiters—English Language; Human Expanders—Apply related words; Also search within the full text of the articles Search modes—Find all my search terms	1,968	
S11	TI fusion	Limiters—English Language; Human Expanders—Apply related words; Also search within the full text of the articles Search modes—Find all my search terms	784	
S10	(S5 OR S6 OR S7 OR S8 OR S9)	Expanders—Apply related words; Also search within the full text of the articles Search modes—Find all my search terms	43,235	
S9	AB surgica	Limiters—English Language; Human Expanders—Apply related words; Also search within the full text of the articles Search modes—Find all my search terms	19,412	
S8	TI surgical	Limiters—English Language; Human Expanders—Apply related words; Also search within the full text of the articles Search modes—Find all my search terms	5,333	
S7	MH surgery, operative	Limiters—English Language; Human Expanders—Apply related words; Also search within the full text of the articles Search modes—Find all my search terms	2,214	
S6	AB surgery	Limiters—English Language; Human Expanders—Apply related words; Also search within the full text of the articles Search modes—Find all my search terms	25,038	

#	Query	Limiters/Expanders	Results	Action
S5	TI surgery	Limiters—English Language; Human Expanders—Apply related words; Also search within the full text of the articles Search modes—Find all my search terms	10,165	
S4	(S1 OR S2 OR S3)	Expanders—Apply related words; Also search within the full text of the articles Search modes—Find all my search terms	349	
S3	AB sacroiliac	Limiters—English Language; Human Expanders—Apply related words; Also search within the full text of the articles Search modes—Find all my search terms	250	
S2	TI sacroiliac	Limiters—English Language; Human Expanders—Apply related words; Also search within the full text of the articles Search modes—Find all my search terms	151	
S1	MH sacroiliac joint	Limiters—English Language; Human Expanders—Apply related words; Also search within the full text of the articles Search modes—Find all my search terms	223	

Web of Science Search

Topic = (sacroiliac) AND Topic = (surgery) AND Topic = (fusion)
Refined by: Languages = (ENGLISH)
Timespan = All Years. Databases = SCI-EXPANDED, SSCI, A&HCI, BKCI-S, BKCI-SSH.

Results = 35 (SEARCH 1 RESULTS)
Topic = (sacroiliac) AND Topic = (fusion) AND Topic = ((outcome* OR complication*))
Refined by: Languages = (ENGLISH)
Timespan = All Years. Databases = SCI-EXPANDED, SSCI, A&HCI, BKCI-S, BKCI-SSH.

B.E. Dall et al. (eds.), *Surgery for the Painful, Dysfunctional Sacroiliac Joint*,
DOI 10.1007/978-3-319-10726-4, © Springer International Publishing Switzerland 2015

ROM (degrees) left	Flexion-extension	Intact	Posterior sacrotuberous ligament cut	Plus the dorsal sacroiliac ligaments and the interosseous ligament	Plus L5-S1 pedicle screws and rod	Normalized ROM (% intact)	Flexion extension	Intact	Ilio sacro ligament cut (l-ISL cut)	Posterior ligaments cut (L-PL complex cut)	L5-S1 rods
	Spine 1	0.38	0.41	0.59	0.89		Spine 1	100	109	156	236
	Spine 2	0.13	0.25	0.39	0.52		Spine 2	100	190	302	400
	Spine 3	1.45	1.54	1.61	1.64		Spine 3	100	106	111	113
	Spine 4	2.39	2.58	3.43	3.49		Spine 4	100	108	144	146
	Spine 5	1.01	0.97	1.16	1.45		Spine 5	100	96	114	143
	Spine 6	0.47	0.48	0.58	0.82		Spine 6	100	102	124	176
	Spine 7	0.46	0.55	0.67	0.69		Spine 7	100	121	147	151
	Mean	0.90	0.97	1.21	1.36		Mean	100	119	157	195
	Stdev	0.79	0.83	1.07	1.03		Stdev	0	32	66	98
Test direction			Increase	Increase	Increase		95 % CI		24	49	73
Paired t statistic	0	0	-2.424871131	-2.27476237	-3.303140472		95 % CI Upper Bound		143	206	268
p-Value	0	0	0.025760279	0.031626404	0.008171891		95 % CI Lower Bound		95	108	122
Sig. at .05 level			*	*	*						

Lateral bending	Intact	Ilio sacro ligament cut (l-ISL cut)	Posterior ligaments cut (L-PL complex cut)	L5-S1 rods
Spine 1	0.09	0.10	0.09	0.08
Spine 2	0.09	0.07	0.10	0.10
Spine 3	0.37	0.36	0.37	0.36
Spine 4	0.51	0.51	0.62	0.64
Spine 5	0.19	0.19	0.19	0.19
Spine 6	0.10	0.10	0.11	0.09
Spine 7	0.17	0.18	0.25	0.25
Mean	0.22	0.22	0.25	0.24
Stdev	0.16	0.16	0.19	0.20
		Increase	Increase	Increase
		0.353553391	−1.917276549	0.603022689
		0.63211757	0.051828407	0.715714372

Lateral bending	Intact	Ilio sacro ligament cut (l-ISL cut)	Posterior ligaments cut (L-PL complex cut)	L5-S1 rods
Spine 1	25	25	23	20
Spine 2	66	57	77	80
Spine 3	25	25	25	25
Spine 4	21	21	26	27
Spine 5	19	19	19	18
Spine 6	21	22	23	20
Spine 7	37	40	54	55
Mean	31	30	35	35
Stdev	17	14	22	24
95 % CI		10	16	17
95 % CI upper bound		40	52	53
95 % CI lower bound		20	19	18

Axial rotation	Intact	Ilio sacro ligament cut (l-ISL cut)	Posterior ligaments cut (L-PL complex cut)	L5-S1 rods
Spine 1	0.25	0.25	0.31	0.33
Spine 2	0.30	0.27	0.32	0.31
Spine 3	0.99	1.03	1.03	1.37
Spine 4	1.25	1.22	1.45	1.42
Spine 5	0.48	0.49	0.52	0.56
Spine 6	0.28	0.26	0.29	0.32
Spine 7	0.37	0.39	0.46	0.41
Mean	0.56	0.56	0.62	0.68
Stdev	0.40	0.40	0.45	0.50
		Increase	Increase	Increase
		0.141421356	−2.354911186	−0.969189495
		0.553917039	0.028338378	0.184940177

Axial rotation	Intact	Ilio sacro ligament cut (I-ISL cut)	Posterior ligament cut (L-PL complex cut)	L5-S1 rods
Spine 1	67	66	81	86
Spine 2	233	211	249	242
Spine 3	69	71	71	95
Spine 4	53	51	61	60
Spine 5	47	49	51	56
Spine 6	61	56	61	69
Spine 7	81	84	101	90
Mean	87	84	96	100
Stdev	65	57	69	65
95 % CI		43	51	48
95 % CI upper bound		127	148	148
95 % CI lower bound		42	45	52

ROM (degrees) right	Flexion-extension	Intact	Lateral bending	Intact	Axial rotation	Intact
	Spine 1	0.34	Spine 1	0.07	Spine 1	0.23
	Spine 2	0.11	Spine 2	0.08	Spine 2	0.32
	Spine 3	1.54	Spine 3	0.39	Spine 3	1.04
	Spine 4	2.46	Spine 4	0.58	Spine 4	1.30
	Spine 5	0.94	Spine 5	0.19	Spine 5	0.45
	Spine 6	0.49	Spine 6	0.09	Spine 6	0.26
	Spine 7	0.44	Spine 7	0.17	Spine 7	0.36
	Mean	0.90	Mean	0.22	Mean	0.57
	Stdev	0.83	Stdev	0.19	Stdev	0.42

Index

B.E. Dall et al. (eds.), *Surgery for the Painful, Dysfunctional Sacroiliac Joint*,
DOI 10.1007/978-3-319-10726-4, © Springer International Publishing Switzerland 2015